Blood Feuds

BLOOD FEUDS

AIDS, BLOOD, AND THE POLITICS OF MEDICAL DISASTER

Edited by

ERIC A. FELDMAN, J.D., Ph.D
Institute for Law and Society
New York University

RONALD BAYER, Ph.D
Joseph L. Mailman School of Public Health
Columbia University

New York   Oxford
OXFORD UNIVERSITY PRESS
1999

Oxford University Press

Oxford   New York
Athens Auckland Bangkok Bogotá Buenos Aires Calcutta
Cape Town Chennai Dar es Salaam Delhi Florence Hong Kong Istanbul
Karachi Kuala Lumpur Madrid Melbourne Mexico City Mumbai
Nairobi Paris São Paulo Singapore Taipei Tokyo Toronto Warsaw

and associated companies in
Berlin   Ibadan

Library of Congress Cataloging-in-Publication Data
Blood feuds : AIDS, blood, and the politics of medical disaster /
edited by Eric A. Feldman and Ronald Bayer.
p. cm. Includes bibliographical references and index.
ISBN 0-19-512929-6 (cloth)—ISBN 0-19-513160-6 (paper)
1. AIDS (Disease)—Social aspects. 2. AIDS (Disease)—Political aspects.
3. AIDS (Disease)—Transmission. 4. Blood—Collection and preservation—Government policy.
5. Blood banks—Government policy. 6. Blood—Transfusion—Safety measures.
I. Feldman, Eric A. II. Bayer, Ronald.
RA644.A25B583 1999   362.1'969792—dc21   98-47064

9 8 7 6 5 4 3 2 1

Printed in the United States of America
on acid-free paper

To Stephanie and Jane,
to whom we are tied by choice,
and to all who, bound by blood,
have suffered in the bitter blood feuds,
we dedicate this book.

Acknowledgments

This book evolved from our discussions several years ago about the contours and content of AIDS policy disputes in a number of industrialized nations. A planning grant from the Social Science Research Council's Joint Committee on Japanese Studies permitted us to develop our ideas fully and to pursue funding for a full-scale project. That support ultimately and generously came from the Toyota Foundation and the Japan Foundation's Center for Global Partnership. Without their backing, this volume would not have been written. At the Toyota Foundation, we want to give special thanks to Chimaki Kurokawa, Director, and Kyoichi Tanaka. At the Center for Global Partnership, we are especially indebted to Junichi Chano, Kohki Kanno, Kim Gould Ashizawa, and Norio Furushima. Additionally, our work was facilitated by support from the Merieux Foundation, which hosted our second meeting in Annecy, France, and the Rockefeller Foundation, which hosted our final meeting at its Conference Center in Bellagio, Italy.

Eric Feldman's work on this project was supported in part by the Robert Wood Johnson Foundation's Scholars in Health Policy Research Program, and by Yale University's Center for Interdisciplinary Research on AIDS (funded by the National Institute of Mental Health [NIMH] and the National Institute on Drug Abuse, Grant No. PO1 MH/DA56826-01A1). Ronald Bayer's work was partially supported by an NIMH Senior Research Scientist Award (Grant No. KO5 MH01376).

A number of our collaborators are not represented in this volume, although they contributed immeasurably to our work: Dr. Robert Beal, International Society of Blood Transfusions; Dr. Zarin Bharucha, Tata Memorial Hospital, Bombay, India; Dr. Jean C. Emmanuel, Blood Safety Unit, World Health Organization; John Gagnon, Department of Sociology, State University of New York at Stonybrook; Dr. Atsuaki Gunji, Faculty of Medicine, University of Tokyo; Jerry Mashow, Yale Law School; Ugo Mattei, Hastings College of Law and the University of Trento, Italy; David Mvere, National Blood Transfusion Service, Zimbabwe; Dr. Alvin Novick, Yale University; Dr. Chaivej Nuchprayoon, National Blood Center, Thai Red Cross; Harvey Sapolsky, Massachusetts Institute of Technology; Shinichi Sugiyama, Harago & Partners Law Offices, Tokyo; Rosemary Taylor, Community Health Program, Tufts University; Dr. Peter Tomasulo, Haemonetics SA, Geneva; Bert deVroom, Faculty of Public Administration and Public Policy, University of Twente, The Netherlands;

David Wolff, The Wilson Center, Washington, DC; Takao Yamada, Faculty of Law, Yokohama National University, Japan; and Shohei Yonemoto, Division of Social and Life Sciences, Mitsubishi-Kasei Institute of Life Sciences, Japan.

Along the way, our work was facilitated by remarkable research assistance provided by Alexandra Kowalski-Hodges, Beck Young, Kaori Yamada, and Catherine Stayton. Stephen Scher prepared the index with uncommon attention to detail. Sergej Zoubok provided administrative support, computer wizardry, and editorial contributions at a multitude of critical moments, and James Melo helped with crises large and small. Lela Cooper, with intelligence and forbearance, helped to organize meetings, coordinate travel plans, typed, retyped, and retyped again the many revisions of the chapters in this volume.

New York City   E. F.
June 1, 1998   R. B.

Contents

Part II
Comparative Perspectives on the Politics of Medical Disaster

Contributors

ERIK ALBÆK is Associate Professor of Public Administration at the University of Aarhus, Denmark. His research has focused on agenda setting, evaluation, and the utilization of social science knowledge in public policy making.

JOHN BALLARD is a political scientist at the Australian National University. He has advised and written extensively on AIDS issues in Australia and in developing countries.

RONALD BAYER is Professor at the Joseph L. Mailman School of Public Health, Columbia University. For the past 15 years his research has focused on ethical, legal, and policy issues raised by the AIDS epidemic. He is author of *Homosexuality and American Psychiatry* (1981); *Private Acts, Social Consequences: AIDS and the Politics of Public Health* (1989); with David Kirp, co-editor of *AIDS in the Industrialized Democracies: Passions, Politics and Policies* (1992); and, with Gerald Oppenheimer, co-editor of *Confronting Drug Policy* (1993).

PATRICIA A. DILLON is Assistant Majority Leader and chair of the Appropriations Subcommittee on Health and Hospitals of Connecticut's General Assembly. Her extensive work on health policy in Connecticut includes her leading role in shaping the state's legislative response to HIV. An architect of Connecticut's needle exchange and AIDS pharmacy programs, she has also authored key legislation concerning the disabled, maternal and child health, mental health, and addiction.

STEPHAN DRESSLER is a physician and philosopher and a former employee of the Federal AIDS Center, FR Germany. His research has focused on philosophical anthropology, ethical aspects of AIDS, and philosophy and children. He was cofounder of the European AIDS Treatment Group (EATG) and is currently working as editor of *AIDS Treatment Update*, published by Deutsche AIDS-Hilfe.

ERIC FELDMAN is Associate Director of New York University's Institute for Law and Society. He has been a Robert Wood Johnson Health Policy Research Scholar at Yale University's Institution for Social and Policy Studies, and a Fulbright Fellow at the University of Tokyo's International Center for Comparative Law and Politics. His articles on law and society, Japanese health policy, and HIV/AIDS have appeared in edited volumes and publications, including the *Los Angeles Times, American Journal of Comparative Law, Social and Legal Studies, Hastings Center Report,* and *The Lancet.* He has recently completed a book on rights assertion and social policy in Japan.

NORBERT GILMORE is Professor of Medicine at the McGill Centre for Medicine, Ethics and Law, and Associate Director of the McGill AIDS Centre. He is also a Senior Physician in the Division of Clinical Immunology and the Immunodeficiency Unit of the Royal Victoria Hospital. Dr. Gilmore was a chair of the National Advisory Committee on AIDS (NAC-AIDS) from its inception in 1983 until his resignation in 1989. His research has involved analysis of ethical, legal, and policy issues relating to AIDS, public health, drug use, prisons, and immigration.

SHERRY GLIED is Associate Professor and head of the Division of Health Policy and Management at the Joseph L. Mailman School of Public Health, Columbia University. Her research has focused on the role of economic institutions in the outcome of the HIV- infected blood problem. She is the author of *Chronic Condition.*

UMBERTO IZZO is an attorney and a Ph.D. candidate in comparative law at the University of Trento, Italy. The author of several articles on AIDS law and medical tort law in Italy, his research is focused on issues surrounding the relationship of law and medicine. He is currently completing a comparative analysis on the status of complementary medicine in the world's legal systems.

DAVID KIRP is Professor of Public Policy at the Goldman School of Public Policy, University of California at Berkeley. His research spans the gamut of social policy concerns, including education, race, and housing, as well as AIDS. His most recent books are *Learning by Heart: AIDS and Schoolchildren in America's Communities, Our Town: Race, Housing and the Soul of Suburbia,* and (co-edited with Ronald Bayer) *AIDS in the Industrialized Democracies: Passions, Politics and Policies.*

THEODORE R. MARMOR is Professor of Public Policy and Management at the Yale School of Management, where he specializes in the modern welfare state with an emphasis on medical care and health issues. A consultant to government agencies and foundations since the mid-1960s, Professor Marmor frequently testifies before Congress about medical care reform, Social Security, and welfare issues. He has written for a wide range of scholarly journals, leading newspapers, and magazines; his most recent of eight books is *Understanding Health Care Reform* (Yale Press, 1994). He is currently working on a third edition of his book *The Politics of Medicare* (Aldine de Gruyter, 1973).

DOROTHY NELKIN is University Professor at New York University in the Department of Sociology and School of Law. Her research is in the area of science, technology, and society. She is a member of the National Academy of Sciences' Institute of Medicine and a fellow and former director of the American Association for the Advancement of Science. Her books include *Controversy: Politics of Technical Decisions*; *Selling Science: How the Press Covers Science and Technology*; *Dangerous Diagnostics: The Social Power of Biological Information* (with L. Tancredi); and *The DNA Mystique* (with S. Lindee).

STEPHEN SCHER is a philosopher who works as an academic editor and writer in Cambridge, Massachusetts. He has taught at Harvard Medical School, Yale School of Management, and Harvard Business School. He writes on ethics, law, politics, and public policy, and is completing a book on bioethics for Yale University Press.

MARGARET A. SOMERVILLE is Gale Professor in the Faculty of Law, and Professor in the Faculty of Medicine at McGill University, and Founding Director of the McGill Centre for Medicine, Ethics and Law. Her research areas include the ethical, legal, social, and economic impact of HIV infection and AIDS on individuals and society. Through frequent media appearances she engages in public debate on these issues and consults government and international agencies regarding the formation of public policy concerning them.

MONIKA STEFFEN is researcher at the *Centre National de la Recherche Scientifique* and is affiliated with the CERAT, University of Grenoble, France. Her work focuses on health policies and international comparisons in Europe. She edited with B. Jobert *Les Politiques de Sante en France et en Allemagne* (Espace Social European, Observatoire des Politiques Sociales Europenes, Paris, 1994). She is author of *The Fight Against AIDS: A Public Policy Comparison: France, Great Britain, Germany, Italy* (Presses Universitaires de Grenoble, Grenoble, France, 1996).

Introduction

Understanding the Blood Feuds

Ronald Bayer and Eric Feldman

Blood—its color, its flow, its scientific properties, its social significance—has long captured the imagination. With magical associations that exceed its biological functions, blood encompasses a spectrum of meanings that are complex, controversial, and often contradictory. Blood has been viewed as the apogee of purity and the nadir of filth; cited as both the basis for unity and the justification for war; analyzed as a gift that brings life and a source of death; and sold as a commodity that has been called priceless.

Only in the twentieth century did it become possible to use blood therapeutically: initially for battlefield transfusions, later in response to accidents and in surgery, and finally as pharmaceutical products made from technologically transformed blood components. Blood thus became a lifesaving medical intervention. The healing uses of blood inevitably would have unintended side effects; along with the new curative powers flowed dangerous pathogens that made blood and its components a medium for disease transmission. The infection of soldiers with hepatitis in the 1940s was among the first occasions for the expression of concern about blood-borne disease. Half a century later, anxiety about whether mad cow disease might be transmitted by blood provides the most recent instance of controversy. The transmission of HIV through blood, and the bitter and protracted controversies it engendered, however, is by far the most serious crisis to have confronted the blood system. International in scope, it presents a poignant opportunity to examine the reactions and interactions of blood systems, health care institutions, policy-makers, physicians, and injured parties as they faced a deadly threat.

The development of clotting agents for hemophiliacs, all made from blood plasma, set the stage for an iatrogenic (medically induced) tragedy. Factor VIII blood concentrate transformed the lives of hemophiliacs by reducing debilitating, often crippling, bleeding. A few short years later, tainted products wreaked havoc. In 1982 the U.S. Centers for Disease Control and Prevention (CDC) identified blood as a medium that could transmit the as-yet-unknown etiologic agent responsible for the newly identified lethal disease, AIDS. From that moment, the collection, fractionation, distribution and consumption of blood became the subjects of bitter legal and political disagreements.

Even before the first cases of AIDS were identified in the United States, HIV had entered the world's bloodstream. Starting in the late 1970s, until the blood supply was made safer by testing for viral antibody and by heat treatment, those dependent on blood or blood products were at risk for HIV infection. In that period of less than a decade, tens of thousands of people, primarily in the developed world, received blood or blood products infected with a lethal virus. Blood—with its spectrum of social and medical meanings—had become the vector for an international iatrogenic catastrophe.

The risk of being infected with HIV-tainted blood or blood products, like all other risks in technologically advanced societies, was not evenly distributed. Patients requiring transfusions of whole blood typically received supplies donated by several persons, depending on how much blood was needed. Their overall risk depended on the prevalence of HIV infection in the local blood-donating population, and it was limited by the small chance that any given donor was infected. In the industrialized nations, where millions of people annually receive blood transfusions, the proportion of those infected with HIV was but a fraction of one percent.

Hemophiliacs, on the other hand, do not receive whole blood from small numbers of donors. Instead, as a result of therapeutic advances, blood clotting elements known as factors VIII and IX are extracted from the pooled blood of hundreds, thousands, even tens of thousands of donors. A single infected source of plasma can contaminate an entire lot of factor concentrate. Consequently, in the late 1970s and early 1980s, hemophiliacs had a high risk of receiving contaminated blood products even when the overall prevalence of HIV infection in a given society was relatively low. The political economy of blood further compounded the risk to which hemophiliacs were exposed. Sixty percent of the world's plasma supply was purchased from plasma sellers in the United States, where it was then made into factor concentrate. The fact that the background prevalence of HIV infection in the United States was higher than in any other industrialized nation had fatal consequences.

As a result of these epidemiological, technological, and economic factors, hemophiliacs were compelled to bear an extraordinary burden. Half of the hemophiliacs in many countries were infected with HIV. Entire families have succumbed to AIDS as infected men with hemophilia—fathers, brothers, and sons—transmitted HIV infection to their wives, who in turn infected their children.

A single viral infection thus endangered the universe of blood therapeutics. Unlike the refusal of viruses to honor national boundaries, however, the practice of medicine and the shaping of policy is profoundly affected by the specificities of culture and politics. Beyond the intrinsic importance of understanding widespread medical disasters with terrible human costs, the study of conflicts over HIV-tainted blood is significant because it provides an unusual opportunity for a comparative understanding of power, politics, policy, and markets in the context of an epidemic disease. Because the unfolding of conflicts over contaminated blood occurred almost simultaneously in different nations, blood became the vantage point from which to analyze the way in which countries with distinctive historical legacies managed a common crisis. The national case studies included in this volume focus on HIV and blood, and the plethora of concerns related to them. These studies also serve as an empirical base on which to ground analyses of fundamental institutions of industrialized democratic societies. Public health systems, the processes of dispute resolution, identity politics and interest group formation, and forms of economic association are all brought into comparative focus by studying conflicts over tainted blood.

Another striking fact makes studying the tragic nexus of blood and AIDS intriguing; unlike many of the battles that characterized the early years of the AIDS epidemic, which had ebbed by the late 1980s, the controversy surrounding blood persisted. Indeed, the intensity of the controversy over blood and AIDS underwent a process of amplification in the early 1990s. The explosive issues of who bore responsibility for the infection of those dependent on blood and blood products, and what if anything was owed to the infected, were being confronted simultaneously in many nations. Here, too, comparative analysis could be revealing.

In the course of conflicts over blood, long-established convictions about the moral and political status of the institutions responsible for the blood supply were shattered. Symbols of altruism and national solidarity, such as Red Cross societies, became the targets of escalating criticism. The reputations of many who had cared for hemophiliacs, some of whom contributed to therapeutic advances that ushered in the era of hemophilia normalization, were destroyed. Abject apologies were forced from corporate officials and government administrators. In some dramatic instances, those held responsible for the catastrophe were jailed. Hemophiliacs, once docile patients, transformed themselves into activists demanding justice and recompense from those they held responsible for their plight. As a result, nation after nation came to the determination that those infected through blood deserved special compensation. In some instances, the sums involved dwarfed other funds for AIDS-related activities.

The nations discussed in this volume—the United States, Japan, Australia, Canada, Denmark, France, Germany, and Italy—have all experienced deep and sustained conflict as a result of the contamination of blood with HIV. In some the conflict escalated to the level of high scandal. In all eight nations, the awareness that AIDS could be transmitted through blood, the discovery that heat treatment could kill HIV, and the development of an antibody test that would detect the viral cause of AIDS were well-known scientific achievements. Dispute centered on when emerging scientific and epidemiological evidence was sufficient to provide a basis for public action. In the heat of controversy, no nation escaped the tendency to treat blood as a metaphor for the connection between the individual and society, thereby making domestic blood a symbol of virtue and foreign blood one of impurity. This volume seeks to provide an understanding of both the commonalities of the conflicts evoked by blood and AIDS and an appreciation of the importance of differences in epidemiological burdens, institutional histories, political traditions, and legal conventions for the response to a common challenge.

A series of questions informed our efforts[1]:

How did the epidemiology of AIDS, and the structure of the system of blood collection, distribution and fractionation, ultimately affect the pattern of HIV infection among those who were dependent on whole blood transfusions and factor concentrate for the treatment of hemophilia?

To what extent did the national capacity for self-sufficiency in blood products affect the fate of hemophiliacs?

How, when, and under what circumstances did officials first become aware that those dependent on blood and blood products were at increased risk for *contracting* AIDS?

When were proposals to exclude from the donor pool those who might be at increased risk for *transmitting* AIDS first made, and what political reaction did these proposals evoke from those to be excluded?

What accounted for the timing of the introduction of antibody testing for HIV, once it became technologically feasible, and the heat treatment of factor concentrate, once evidence suggested that it might kill HIV?

To what extent and with what degree of success did those infected turn to the courts for redress?

How did prior experiences with mass torts, and the legal regime surrounding blood, set the stage for such litigation?

How and when did hemophiliacs begin to confront their own hemophilia societies as agents of betrayal, and to demand compensation for their injury?

What response did calls for compensation elicit from those who had been infected sexually and those with other medically induced injuries?

Was compensation ultimately provided to those who were infected—and their families—and how was such compensation justified?

How did the experience of the AIDS tragedy affect thinking about the steps necessary to safeguard the blood supply?

Some of these questions emerged from the unique confluence of factors associated with AIDS. Others, particularly those concerning the relationship between the structure of the blood system, the extent to which blood was donated or sold, and blood safety, were first asked by Richard Titmuss in his 1971 classic, *The Gift Relationship,* and have remained contentious ever since.

Five core issues have animated conflicts over contaminated blood, to varying degrees, in all industrialized democracies. They provide a framework for both a retrospective understanding of controversy over HIV-tainted blood and an attempt to identify the central policy questions that must be answered if the threat of blood-borne pathogens is to be minimized in the future, and the social burden they create is to be managed equitably.

Managing Threats to Blood Safety

The first indication that blood could transmit AIDS came in mid-1982 in the United States. The CDC's *Morbidity and Mortality Weekly Report* reported three hemophiliacs with symptoms virtually identical to those found in some homosexual men and

Haitians, suggesting the possibility that members of all three groups were victims of a common, new, and poorly understood syndrome. In retrospect it is clear that those first cases were warnings of a potential catastrophe. To those examining the evidence available at the time, however, the picture was rife with uncertainty. Beyond the contested baseline question of whether the blood supply was contaminated, the appropriate course of action was the subject of controversy because of disagreement about which (if any) interventions would enhance blood safety. How should such ambiguous and inconclusive evidence have been judged? Which institutional forces shaped and constrained decision making? What scientific and clinical factors informed the behavior of those in positions of responsibility?

In the face of uncertainty, both action and inaction had potential costs. An immediate change in blood collection, processing, and distribution could make authorities vulnerable to charges of overzealousness if their action proved unnecessary or ineffective. It could increase costs and decrease supplies of whole blood and blood products. It could require hemophiliacs to return to burdensome therapeutic interventions. Inaction, on the other hand, could lead to disastrous clinical consequences. In the end, the concept of "acceptable risk," in this instance as well as others, inevitably produces the question, "acceptable to whom?"

Confronted with uncertainty about the danger of blood and blood products as vectors for AIDS transmission, decision makers retreated to a well-established paradigm of blood safety developed in response to hepatitis B. From the 1970s, patients, physicians, and blood safety experts were united in accepting that the lifestyle benefits hemophiliacs enjoyed from blood products outweighed the substantial risk of contracting hepatitis B from those products. By 1980, progress in developing a test for hepatitis B reinforced the view that the burden of hepatitis B would be time-limited as well as worth bearing. Those who produced, distributed, prescribed, and consumed blood products were therefore accustomed to stressing the significant benefits of the products and minimizing their risks.

Once it became clear that a viral blood-borne agent was responsible for AIDS, decision makers confronted a range of policy options. They included the introduction of antibody testing, the mandating of heat treatment, and the withdrawal of blood and blood products on the shelves before safety-enhancing measures were introduced. The speed with which those responsible for blood and blood products introduced safety measures, and their willingness to bear the costs of withdrawing potentially unsafe products, varied from country to country, despite reference to shared epidemiological data. Sometimes the differences could be measured in months, but the impact of even small differences would become epidemiologically and politically significant.

In retrospect, it is known that some cases of HIV infection in those dependent on blood occurred before the first blood-associated cases of AIDS were identified. Other persons were infected in the period between the identification of the first cases and the technical availability of safety-enhancing measures; still others between the time when such measures were available and when they were introduced. In each of these periods, the issues of risk assessment and management were different. So, too, are the lessons to be drawn.

The disaster of HIV contamination, and the outrage it has spawned, has profoundly affected how those responsible for public health now view questions of blood safety. It has shaped their understanding of how new and uncertain risks to the blood supply should be managed, especially risks that are small but costly to eliminate. In the United States, for example, p24 antigen testing was introduced to reduce the risk of HIV transmission, but did so only marginally at a cost of millions of dollars per averted case. In Australia as well as Denmark, a decision was made to screen for the viruses HTLV I/II. Danish estimates indicated that such efforts would prevent only one case of cancer in the next 30 to 60 years. In many nations, there has been a shift in presumptions governing decision making under conditions of uncertainty, one that emphasizes risk aversion at any cost.

As a result, the need to balance high levels of safety with reasonable costs has been subsumed by an impulse to maximize safety, irrespective of the price. Despite the obvious social benefits of blood safety, there are some degrees of safety that require vast expenditure and bring small benefit. Sometimes, possibilities to improve safety marginally must be forgone. Such determinations should be made under conditions that maximize public accountability, without regard to commercial or other narrow interests. They must take into consideration individual needs and broad social welfare concerns. In most cases, there will be a tendency to mask decisions that accept "imperfect" safety; such decisions have high political costs. Such tendencies must be resisted. Those who may be placed at risk by the decision to forgo costly safety-enhancing measures have a right to know about the situation they confront as they make medical decisions. Consent to undergo treatment in such circumstances should not be confused with a willing acceptance of risk. Therefore, those who may suffer injury may have a legitimate claim to some form of compensation.

In a world where absolute safety is unattainable, decision makers are compelled to make policy choices based on ambiguous, incomplete, and conflicting information. Such decisions implicate ethical concerns about the distribution of the burdens and benefits of treatment with blood and blood products. In short, the question of managing risk must confront the question of justice.

Voluntarism, Markets, and the Supply of Blood

Since Richard Titmuss posited a direct relationship between blood safety and voluntary, unremunerated donation, the idea that all blood should be freely given has achieved the status of an international orthodoxy. What made his proposition all the more attractive was the claim that the goals of social solidarity and safety were, in the case of blood, linked through the altruistic donor. Here, at any rate, markets and market-inspired behavior seemed not to provide a model for the organization of a critical domain of social life. Despite sustained criticism of Titmuss' views by those who claimed that carefully selected "paid donors" could provide a source of blood that was both safe and reliable, voluntarism has survived the increasingly hegemonic status of market perspectives in recent decades.

The aura that has come to surround volunteer blood donors and altruistic blood donation has exacted a price that only became apparent in the context of the AIDS epidemic. Because donors were viewed as selfless, and because the process of donation was viewed as an expression of solidarity, it was politically and ethically difficult to develop policies that distinguished among potential donors. Blood authorities could not simply exclude those who might pose a risk because of their behavior or because they came from nations or groups thought to present increased risk to the blood supply. Indeed, some of the most contentious encounters in nations as diverse as the United States, Australia, and Denmark (in terms of the status of gay men) centered on the potential benefits from and consequences of efforts to exclude gay blood donors, who viewed such actions as a manifestation of homophobia and a threat to the goal of social equality. Gay men were not the only ones affected in this way. In France, prison officials were reluctant to exclude inmates, many of whom were drug users, from the donor pool because giving blood was viewed as a step toward social integration.

In the aftermath of the AIDS epidemic, the mythic equivalence of the voluntary donor and the safe donor has been shattered. What will be the consequences for the future of blood policy and practice? Now that tensions have emerged between the ends of solidarity and safety—twinned by Titmuss—how will they be resolved? In nations where donor organizations have been influential, what role will they play when matters of safety are under consideration? Will they be viewed as representing a narrow sectional concern or the overarching interests of those dependent on blood and blood products?

As blood plasma is increasingly subject to transformation by pharmaceutical firms, it is difficult to sustain the symbolic attachments evoked by whole blood. So too is it difficult to preserve the centrality of the whole blood donor when plasma donation requires a kind of "professional" commitment in both time and effort that is hardly compatible with the amateur voluntarism so praised by Titmuss. It remains a striking feature of the world supply of plasma that much of it is still purchased from blood sellers in the United States at for-profit plasmapheresis centers.

As scientific advances continue to open the way to new therapeutic developments, the blood system is increasingly shaped by concerns about safety and the avoidance of liability. How the commercial world of sellers and fractionators confronts that of donors and blood banks is a central component of the evolving transformation of the blood industry.

Safety and the Ideology of Self-Sufficiency

In an era of globalization, in which national borders increasingly give way to regional and international economic forces, both international and national health authorities continue to regard self-sufficiency as the fundamental principle of blood policy. From Australia to Japan, from the United States to France, the idea that nations should be self-sufficient in blood is the holy grail of public health policy.

HIV infection caused by the distribution of contaminated blood offers an opportunity to disentangle the meanings of and justifications for self-sufficiency, and to question the faith placed in it as both a moral and medical aspiration. Because HIV was spread through whole blood transfusions and treatment with blood products, it has made possible a discussion of the relevance of self-sufficiency for both whole blood and the pharmaceutically transformed products derived from blood and its components.

There are a number of concerns about the sale and/or donation of blood across borders that make autarky in blood and its components appealing. Among the most pragmatic is that whole blood and its components have storage requirements that make it difficult to ship them over long distances. If they are not stored properly, and used rapidly, they become useless. Furthermore, international dependence rather than national self-sufficiency might diminish the sense of belonging to a community in which blood freely circulates as a common currency; it might diminish the willingness to donate; it could result in shortages not remediable through local action; the effectiveness of local regulatory control could be reduced; and injuries or accidents caused by "foreign" blood could lead to accusation and recrimination infused with racism and xenophobia.

There is considerable justification for whole blood and component self-sufficiency, particularly when compared to the possibility of dependence on distant nations. Still, the justification for self-reliance of blood components is least compelling in bordering or geographically close nations with similar economic, social, and regulatory configurations. The primary public health concern ought to be that of obtaining an adequate supply of safe blood from donors among whom there is likely to be a low prevalence of blood-borne infectious agents. That goal is not necessarily advanced by an ideology of self-sufficiency that values the citizenship of the blood donor over the medical needs of recipients.

In the case of clotting factors, it is more difficult to justify the importance of national self-sufficiency. Unlike blood components, which do not require an expensive or technologically sophisticated infrastructure, blood products pose difficulties for both collection and manufacture. Donating whole blood components is neither invasive, time-consuming, nor costly; providing plasma for blood products takes time and incurs the cost of plasmapheresis. For these reasons, much of the world's plasma supply is purchased, not donated, regardless of whether or not a nation is self-sufficient.

There are, however, nations that derive much of their plasma supply from whole blood donations rather than from plasmapheresis.

The practical impediments to international trade in whole blood do not arise with blood products and derivatives, and their manufacture into pharmaceutical agents differentiates them from whole blood, with its powerful cultural associations. Nevertheless, in nations where hemophiliacs became infected as a consequence of the use of clotting factor made from American plasma, import dependency became the target of outrage. Had local "pure" plasma been used, it is claimed, catastrophe could have been prevented. The claim is well received by the media, the public, those interested in the blood system and, most importantly, by victims seeking to pinpoint blame. The lesson commonly drawn from the spread of HIV through blood products is that never again must nations import products made from blood drawn in other nations. Self-sufficiency is therefore promoted as a principle by which injury from future blood-borne pathogens can be avoided.

The evidence at hand does not substantiate the popular perception of a link between import dependence and heightened risk. The United States, which produced its own supply of concentrate from American plasma, had one of the highest rates of HIV infection among hemophiliacs. In Australia as well as in France, domestic factor VIII also produced high rates of infection among hemophiliacs. On the other hand, hemophiliacs in nations such as Japan, which depended on American imports, had similarly high infection rates. These data indicate that self-sufficiency itself does not answer the question of how best to ensure the safety of blood products, because the risk of contamination by blood products is determined, in part, by the underlying serological risks of the population from whom plasma is collected.

Since it is impossible to know where the next blood-borne pathogen will arise, it is equally impossible to determine the safest source of blood products. Carefully regulating plasma collection and fractionation centers to ensure that they meet the highest possible international safety standards is more likely than national self-sufficiency to limit the distribution of tainted products. The ideology of self-sufficiency that gives pride of place to the nationality of blood donors masks the most basic concern of those in need of blood: relative safety. The importance of minimizing the possibility that blood will be a vector for the transmission of infectious disease, not the need for self-sufficiency, ought to serve as the fundamental lesson of the AIDS years.

Justice and Compensation for the Victims of Blood-Borne Pathogens

In every country we have studied, persons infected with HIV through whole blood or blood products have demanded compensation. They have done so in part by turning to the courts as individuals or classes of the aggrieved. More dramatically, they have pressed governments to make payment either through the public treasury or by coordinating payments from public and private sector sources. Both implicitly and explicitly, those who have sought compensation have distinguished themselves from persons infected through sexual activity and injection drug use. Unlike those who acted in ways that placed themselves at risk, the claim goes, blood transfusion recipients and those who took factor concentrate prescribed to them by their physicians did not make a "choice." By highlighting their medical vulnerability and their dependence on heath care providers, "victims" of blood-borne HIV infection have asserted a special claim on society's resources.

To a remarkable degree, these claims have been successful. In Japan, each person infected with HIV through the blood supply receives compensation payments of close to $500,000. In France, claimants receive between $150,000 and $400,000; in Denmark, $120,000. Even the United States finally adopted a compensation act in late 1998, with the promise of a payment of about $100,000 for each claimant. In no country do those with HIV infection caused by sexual or needle-sharing behavior, the primary modes of transmission, receive compensation payments. A deep moral and financial wedge has consequently been driven between those infected with HIV through blood and others with HIV infection.

The financial contours of national compensation schemes and the legal and political maneuvering that led to their creation are detailed in the following chapters. Everywhere, the timing of compensation, the generosity of the payments, and the designation of those eligible were political determinations. Those most able to organize, lobby, sue, and marshal the influence of the media were most likely to succeed. Even the language of justice and compensation has been contested. From Canada to Japan, from Australia to Denmark, debate has raged over whether the money paid to those infected by HIV-contaminated blood should be called compensation, relief, or extraordinary assistance. The choice of terminology depends on one's view of whether those responsible for blood safety failed to exercise due care, whether such failure constituted negligence, and whether such negligence rose to the level of criminal culpability.

The pitched battles over HIV and blood experienced in every nation, the recognition that there had been a medical tragedy and the knowledge that many would die as a result, made it difficult to think carefully and fairly about whether particular individuals and groups infected with HIV had a special claim to financial compensation. The time is now ripe for the kind of analytical—perhaps skeptical—consideration that was so difficult in the face of human misery. That process might start with the following questions:

> To what extent is justice served by providing state compensation to people infected with HIV through the blood supply when others who suffer iatrogenic injury are not similarly compensated?

Should all who were infected through blood and blood products be treated equally regardless of the extent to which their infections were preventable?

Should a no-fault system of compensation be created to manage future blood-related claims?

Should national legislatures, administrative agencies, or courts be responsible for developing and managing compensatory schemes?

Nations guarantee different levels of medical care and social security to those who are ill and disabled. Individuals infected with HIV in one country may receive care that is life-long and free, along with publicly funded social support for themselves and their families. Those in another may have no claim to affordable or adequate care and will have to call on their own resources. Given such differences, it is difficult to arrive at a cross-national standard for what constitutes just compensation. If outrage at the failure of the United States to provide public compensation is rooted, at least in part, in concern about how those infected will pay for their medical care, how might compensation be justified in western European nations that provide not only medical care but robust social insurance?

Compensation payments are generally viewed as a way of making injured parties whole. They are not always linked to judgments about fault. In almost every legal system, there are instances in which injuries occur and compensation payments are made, but blame is not assigned. Such schemes reflect a certain rationality. Tragedies do not require travesties. Technological achievements inevitably bring with them the possibility of unintended harms. No-fault compensation schemes are appealing under such circumstances because of their efficiency, their low transaction costs, the relative ease with which injured parties can be compensated, and the extent to which economic burdens of injury are borne by those most able to pay.

However, such schemes fail to "make whole" when they do not recognize the psychological needs of individuals or the social needs of communities to hold to account those deemed responsible for actions that caused injury. In France and Japan, where demands for compensation were met with cash payments, many injured parties rejected the proffered funds as insufficient. They did not simply desire a financial payment; they insisted on the identification of responsible actors and the apportionment of blame. No-fault compensation fails in such cases because it emphasizes money and denies the need to censure guilty individuals and institutions.

Nations must develop efficient and compassionate schemes to meet the economic needs of those who will in the future be victims of unavoidable iatrogenic injuries. Such efforts will not substitute, in the case of negligence-related harms, for effective mechanisms that hold to account those in whom the public has invested its trust.

Blood, Bureaucracy, and Organizational Reform

In the effort to understand why they were infected, those who contracted HIV through blood and blood products sought to identify individuals who had failed to protect the safety of the blood supply. In the United States, hemophilia activists denounced a well-known hemophilia expert as "The Mengele of the Hemophilia Holocaust." Denmark's Minister of the Interior was castigated as "Blood Britta." French and Japanese officials were subject to criminal prosecution.

In addition to the search for guilty individuals, there was an attempt to determine what went wrong with the very institutions responsible for blood safety. Investigative commissions in nation after nation concluded that in the late 1970s and throughout the 1980s, governmental structures and other organizations responsible for the blood supply were ill-equipped to understand, evaluate, or respond effectively to the challenge of HIV-contaminated blood. Blood experts, whatever their individual beliefs or policy desires, had been constrained by institutional loyalties and concerns that made bold action anathema. The blood bureaucracy had failed.

Common denunciation of past bureaucratic arrangements has linked the perspective of independent commissions of inquiry charged in many nations with the task of uncovering the roots of policy failure. Virtually everywhere it was asserted that the long history of collaboration between regulators and the regulated poorly served the goals of blood safety. The lack of accountability to consumers of blood and blood products was almost everywhere viewed as a guarantee that narrow commercial and institutional interests would prevail on the blood policy agenda. Despite these elements of commonality, striking variation exists in the attempt to pinpoint the cause of systemic failure. The fault in one nation may be viewed as a willingness to accept the burden of hepatitis B as the price of progress; in another, the failure to appreciate the data on AIDS is underscored. In some nations the dead weight of bureaucratic control is highlighted; in others it is the failure to impose careful and stringent bureaucratic regulations. Some have argued that market forces corrupted the goals of public health; others claim that market-driven behavior was more salutary than the behavior of those in organizations that are formally not-for-profit.

Hope that comparing different national experiences with HIV and blood would result in clear and simple lessons for the future has not been realized. Indeed, the lessons to be learned are more easily read as cautionary tales about the many possible bureaucratic arrangements. Despite systems that varied significantly in terms of degree of centralization, links between state actors and the private sector, responsiveness to public input, the power of the medical lobby, and the overall power of bureaucracy, the initial response to the possibility that HIV could contaminate the blood supply was remarkably similar. Confronted with uncertainty and lacking transparency in policy-making, the various blood bureaucracies did too little (in some cases, far too little), at least initially, about the threat of HIV.

In the aftermath of infection, often in response to the calls of national commissions for bureaucratic reform, some features of national blood systems have begun to converge. In the broadest sense, one reaction to conflict, blame, and litigation over HIV-tainted blood has been a move toward greater centralization. The virtues of pyramid-like governmental structures have been extolled, while the well-known costs of such arrangements have been minimized. Ironically, centralizing governmental control of blood has proceeded despite a political climate in many nations that has led to calls for "less regulation" in many other sectors. Even where greater degrees of centralization have not been achieved, the recognition that certain agencies (like Japan's former Pharmaceutical Affairs Bureau, and the Canadian Red Cross) were themselves tainted by the conflict over blood has generated wide-scale institutional reorganization.

Stung by accusations of inaction and apathy, regulators in all of the countries we have studied have come to realize the high costs of political paralysis. They now accept that it is their responsibility to investigate publicly and skillfully potential risks to the blood supply. While action may not be required, active decision making is imperative. In addition, the relationship between regulatory agencies and the entities they are charged with overseeing has come under attack. Concern that the agencies were "captured" by interested parties, in part as a result of their near-monopoly on technical expertise, has led many nations to restructure the formal ties permitted between the blood sector and the state. Industry involvement in the U.S. FDA's Blood Products Advisory Committee, a hallmark of the earlier era, has been denounced as a recipe for disaster. A new regime that seeks to limit industry's influence has been embraced. At the same time, consumer participation on such committees, and in other aspects of blood regulation, has increased.

What remains unclear is whether changes in the bureaucratic agencies that manage blood will result in effective responses to future blood-borne pathogens. Despite the long conflict over HIV and blood, we still cannot clearly specify the most desirable institutional arrangements for limiting the potential for a future iatrogenic tragedy caused by blood.

This volume is concerned with a medical disaster that was largely confined to advanced industrial nations. Although the HIV pandemic has had a profound impact on Third World nations, many of those nations have been spared the tragedy related to transfusion- and blood product–associated AIDS. The most impoverished nations have avoided conflicts over HIV and blood because, unlike the sexual transmission of AIDS, blood-related transmission requires the existence of a medical and technical infrastructure, and the economic capacity to pay for pharmaceuticals such as factor concentrate. Here the data are stark. Approximately 80% of the world's blood collection and usage occurs in 20% of the world's nations. In poorer nations, blood transfusions, where they are available, rarely involve more than 2 units of blood, because there is not enough blood to meet demand. Most boys with severe hemophilia die of their disease before reaching adulthood and they rarely, if ever, receive clotting factor concentrate.

While limited, however, transfusions are not unknown in many Third World countries, especially in large cities. With the background level of HIV infection rising, the epidemiological picture is changing. A report from Vietnam in late 1997, for example, revealed that at least 100 people had contracted HIV infection from blood transfusions. Although Vietnamese blood is screened for HIV antibody, such testing can fail to detect the presence of infection during the first months after a donor contracts HIV. Where the incidence of new infections is high, this can pose a serious threat to blood safety. Moreover, because the majority of blood is collected from professional blood sellers in urban areas, where rates of HIV are higher than in the countryside, blood shipped from the city is introducing HIV into areas that previously had low rates of infection. A similar pattern has emerged in China, making the blood supply a major source for the spread of AIDS.

While the threat of blood-borne HIV infection may be emerging in the Third World, it has clearly receded in the advanced industrial nations; there the bitter feuds that erupted in the wake of the iatrogenic disaster spawned in the early 1980s have all but been brought to an end. The lessons of the past 15 years are many. They emerge from the experiences of the nations whose encounters with HIV are detailed in this volume. As one considers these accounts, it is crucial not to lose sight of an overriding theme: The saga of AIDS and blood involved both a tragedy that could not have been averted and a disaster that was the consequence of individual malfeasance and institutionally structured misjudgments. Both aspects of the story must be borne in mind as we think about the demands that securing a safer blood supply should impose on us and about the limits of public policy in securing that safety.

The challenges of the next years will center on the capacity of sophisticated medical systems to detect and respond to the first signs of contamination in a way that limits the potential for disaster. They will also center on the importance of developing social policies to meet the needs of those who, despite the best of efforts, will be exposed to pathogenic injuries during the course of their treatment. Already, the recognition of a widespread hepatitis C epidemic has caused an international conflict over risk and responsibility for medically induced disease. Disagreement between public health authorities, blood bankers, and patients about whether those who might have been exposed to hepatitis C should be notified and offered testing was the first sign that the era of blood scandal had not come to an end. In Canada and Australia, political turmoil over who was at fault and who should bear the financial costs of compensating those infected through blood transfusions has been acute; the other industrialized democracies discussed in this volume are destined to experience similar controversy. The questions raised by hepatitis C make clear that blood feuds did not end with conflicts over HIV, but have been indelibly marked by the experience of the AIDS years.

It is the uniqueness of blood that is the focus of analysis in this volume. Yet the controversies that have surrounded blood in the age of AIDS share common features with others endemic in advanced industrial societies. Technological achievements are Janus-faced: along with their promise of progress almost always come unintended social burdens. How to manage those threats without impeding the innovative impulse and how to assure that the benefits and burdens of progress are equitably borne remain fundamental challenges of governance in societies ever more dependent on scientific developments.

NOTE

1. The conceptualization of these core issues, and indeed this volume, emerged from an international collaborative project that involved three meetings over the course of one year. The first, held in July 1996, brought together 25 project participants—authors of national case studies, as well as those who were to write comparative analyses focused on politics, policy, culture, and economics. Country experts circulated drafts of their papers, each of which was discussed at the three-day meeting. The meeting provided an opportunity for authors to refine their work, probed by colleagues who had examined the same issues in other nations, and by those who came to the project primarily interested in cross-national concerns. Authors invited to write comparative papers used the occasion to secure from country experts the data they needed to begin writing their analytical chapters.

Comparative essays were the focus of the second project meeting. The comparativists profited from the in-depth understanding of those who prepared country studies, just as those who prepared country studies benefited from the insights of those writing comparative analyses. At the final project meeting held in June 1997, we sought to synthesize the emerging understanding of the decade-long controversy involving AIDS and blood with an eye toward anticipating the challenges posed by future pathogenic threats to the blood supply.

I

NATIONAL ENCOUNTERS WITH BLOOD AND AIDS

1

Blood and AIDS in America

Science, Politics, and the Making of an Iatrogenic Catastrophe

Ronald Bayer

On July 16, 1982, three cases of *Pneumocystis carinii* pneumonia were reported among hemophiliacs in the Centers for Disease Control's *Morbidity and Mortality Weekly Report*.[1] Two had died; one remained critically ill. All three were heterosexual. None had a history of intravenous drug use. In commenting on these cases, the CDC stated, "Although the course of the severe immune dysfunction is unknown, the occurrence among the three hemophiliac cases suggests the possible transmission of an agent through blood products." These were the sentinel cases of an iatrogenic catastrophe that would affect the lives of thousands of blood transfusion recipients and hemophiliacs dependent on factor VIII concentrate for the treatment of their disorder. And although the numbers affected would be relatively small compared to the hundreds of thousands who would become infected through sexual contact and intravenous drug use, the plight of those infected through blood would, because of its implications for the vulnerability of all Americans, take on special significance.

In *The Gift Relationship*, Richard Titmuss has given us a metaphor for blood collection and distribution that underscores the bitter ironies that have emerged over the past 15 years as the tragedy of blood and AIDS has unfolded in the United States. The gift of life had been transformed into its opposite, something deadly. If blood and its exchange were symbolic of the bonds of community, the saga of AIDS and the blood supply would test the durability of those ties. How would those charged with the responsibility of securing "the gift" respond to an emerging threat of unknown dimensions? How would efforts to protect the blood supply affect the boundaries of community? And in the end, how would the political community meet the needs of those who had fallen victim to the "poisoned gift"?[2]

Titmuss's 1972 study of blood policy in the United States and Great Britain was more than a sermon on sharing. It was a scathing attack on American practices. Reliance on paid donors (what an oxymoron) in the United States, as contrasted with Britain's all-volunteer donor pool, was bad for public health as well as for public values. By paying donors, those most at risk for hepatitis were drawn into the donor pool. Hence, the critical problem of transfusion-associated hepatitis could only be addressed if America were to radically transform its approach to blood banking. It mattered little that Titmuss's analysis was based on factually problematical assumptions about the extent to which whole blood was derived from paid donors. His critique was broadly accepted[3] and led to a fundamental reexamination of the American blood system.

In the wake of the publication of *The Gift Relationship*, a special task force of the U.S. Department of Health, Education and Welfare undertook a thorough study of the American blood system and concluded that there were indeed major systemic flaws. Blood was of uneven quality, and commercial blood contributed to the unacceptably high rate of posttransfusion hepatitis; inefficiencies resulted in wastage of blood products, while shortages sometimes resulted in a blood supply that was inadequate to meet patient need; and the cost of therapy involving blood and blood products represented an economic burden to many.[4]

In response to this analysis, federal authorities promulgated a National Blood Policy in the early 1970s that sought to assure the existence of a blood supply that was adequate to meet medical needs and was safe and accessible. To oversee the implementation of this new policy framework, a private-sector American Blood Commission was established.

The National Blood Policy did not challenge the fundamental structure of the industry in which the American Red Cross, which collected about half of the whole blood donated in the nation, and other noncommercial local blood banks, which collected the remainder, "functioned as regional monopolies, protected from commercial competition, exempt from most consumer suits . . . [and were] free to divide geographical markets among themselves."[5] What it emphasized, however, was that volunteerism had to replace whatever payment continued to exist for whole blood. To drive commercial blood from the market, the FDA insisted that all whole blood and its components be labeled as derived from "paid" or "volunteer" donors.

The blood policy did not extend its assault on paid blood to plasma and its derivatives, which were collected and processed by pharmaceutical corporations, because it was widely assumed that the need could not be met by volunteers. It was such paid-for plasma that was the source of factor concentrate so central to the treatment of hemophiliacs, and that had freed them from the threat of crippling and life-shortening bleeding episodes.

It was into this bifurcated system of blood collection, regulated by the Food and Drug Administration in close collaboration with the industry that it was charged with overseeing, that HIV made its silent entry in the late 1970s.

The Making of an Iatrogenic Catastrophe: The Politics of Blood Safety

Apprehending the Threat of AIDS: Community and the Politics of Exclusion

With the CDC's July 1982 report on AIDS in three hemophiliacs as a threatening omen, the National Hemophilia Foundation sought to reassure patients dependent on factor VIII concentrate. "It is important to note that at this time the risk of contracting this immunosuppressive agent is *minimal* and the CDC is not recommending any change in blood product use."[6] This was a posture rooted in the assumption that nothing should be permitted to disrupt the use of factor concentrate that had so recently transformed the lives of hemophiliacs. It was this posture—one that the Foundation would maintain over the next three years—that would in later years be cited as evidence of an egregious paternalism, at best, and of a grand betrayal at worst. But despite these words of reassurance, there were those who believed that the three case reports were sufficient to warrant extraordinary concern about the safety of the blood supply. They also believed that it was appropriate to consider the option of identifying and excluding potential donors and sellers of blood who might possibly pose a risk.

For the political leadership of the gay community the potential for a socially catastrophic turn in public policy was all too easy to discern. Speaking on behalf of the Fund for Human Dignity, Virginia Apuzzo warned against a return to the "bad old days . . . when a recurrently scapegoated minority could be sweepingly restigmatized for the taint of bad blood."[7]

But for those who saw in the new threat of AIDS a matter of gravity requiring drastic measures, fears about invasions of privacy and the prospects of stigma paled as matters of significance. Though in its public posture the National Hemophilia Foundation remained silent about the desirability of pursuing the option of excluding all gay men from the donor pool, it quietly began to press for such a course within the blood banking community. On October 3, 1982, the Foundation's Board of Directors adopted a resolution put forth by its medical and scientific advisory council that urged "all sources of Factor VIII products to exclude from plasma donation all individuals who were homosexual, intravenous drug users, or recent residents of Haiti."[8]

And there was, indeed, increasing reason for concern. At a December 4, 1982, meeting of the Blood Products Advisory Committee of the Food and Drug Administration, a CDC official reported five additional cases of AIDS among hemophiliacs. He also reported an ongoing investigation of five AIDS cases that might well have been linked to blood transfusions received within the prior 18 months. In one case, an infant had received a donation from a gay man who, though apparently healthy at the time of donation, had developed AIDS seven months later. The official was especially pessimistic about the prospects for hemophilia patients because of the possible contamination of whole lots of factor VIII concentrate. In an observation that would prove to be uncannily prescient, he warned, "So if it is in the concentrate, and if it is transmissible in the concentrate, then you have a large proportion of the hemophilia population already exposed and you can expect that, no matter what you do at this point."

Six days later *Morbidity and Mortality Report* made public the additional cases of AIDS among hemophiliacs as well as the case of the 20-month-old child who had died of AIDS.[9] In its editorial comment, CDC stated, "This report and continuing reports of AIDS among persons with hemophilia A raise serious questions about possible transmission of AIDS through blood and blood products. The Assistant Secretary of Health is convening an advisory committee to address these questions."[10]

In the face of the accumulating evidence and the *MMWR* report of December 10, officials of the blood banking community responded with the voice of reassurance; that same voice was to characterize the public posture of some of the most prominent blood bankers over the next year. They also rejected the Hemophilia

Foundation's call for the exclusion of gay donors. Faced with scientific uncertainty, the blood bankers chose not to embrace so radical a proposal.[11] Gay men, especially in some parts of the nation, had become crucial to the donor pool. A loss of such donors would have had serious implications for maintaining the adequacy of the blood supply. While institutional concerns about the disruptive consequences of fashioning explicit exclusionary policies were at work, it was the language of stigma, privacy, and community that was called upon to justify a policy of restraint.

Just a week before the planned CDC conference that would become a defining moment in the history of the American epidemic, James Curran, head of AIDS activities at the Centers for Disease Control, expressed his fears about how divisive and volatile the session might become and cautioned the gay community that it might best respond to the challenge posed by the available evidence about the risk of AIDS in blood products by seizing the "political initiative with a call for voluntary withdrawal of all gay men from the donor pool. . . . The thing is, people are dying. The medical problem is more important than the civil rights issue."[12]

It was against this background of politically charged anxiety and a publicly announced decision on the part of the Alpha Therapeutics Corporation, a major supplier of commercial plasma products, that it would begin to exclude gay men and other high-risk individuals from its collection pool, that the CDC held its early January meeting.[13] Despite the presentation of CDC evidence about the risk of AIDS, prominent representatives of the blood banking community maintained their position that the data were insufficient. Most articulate in pressing the case for restraint were the eminent Dr. Aaron Kellner, president of the New York Blood Center, and Dr. Joseph Bove of Yale. Kellner argued, "Don't overstate the facts. There are at most three cases of AIDS from blood donations, and the evidence in two of the cases is very soft. And there are only a handful of cases among hemophiliacs."[14] Despite Bove's anxiety— expressed a month earlier at the FDA's blood products safety meeting— he dismissed as precipitate the call for action. "We are contemplating all these wide-ranging measures because one baby got AIDS after transfusion from a person who later came down with AIDS, and there may be a few other cases."[15] Kellner and Bove were not alone. At a closed meeting of the FDA's Blood Products Advisory Committee held the next month, prominent virologists would express their doubts as well.[16] Among them was Dr. June Osborn, who in later years would be named chair to the National AIDS Commission.

To the voices of skepticism at the January 4 meeting, CDC officials responded with a sense of dismay and urgency.[17] Donald Francis, who would in later years emerge as a sharp public critic of the lethargy of the early response to the threat of AIDS to the blood supply, and who would on retirement from the CDC offer his services as an expert to plaintiffs in litigation against blood banks and the industry, met the resistance with exasperation. "When will there be enough cases to act upon?"[18]

From the perspective of officials at the CDC, there were two options given the risks involved, both of which could be pursued in the name of safety: screen out donors who were at increased risk; adopt a surrogate screening test that could identify dangerous donations. One CDC official noted that more than 80% of gay AIDS patients carried hepatitis B core antibody. Although the introduction of such a test might not detect all who posed a risk, it could markedly reduce the threat of blood transfusion–associated AIDS.[19]

Representatives of the gay community forcefully opposed every suggestion that blood banks follow the lead taken by Alpha Therapeutics in questioning prospective donors about their sexual orientation and practices. Instead, many pressed for surrogate marker screening. It was blood, not donors, that should be subjected to scrutiny.[20]

For those who had hoped that a clear consensus would emerge from this meeting—which was widely reported in both medical and lay press—the day-long session was a profound disappointment. A decade later Dr. James Curran would note that the CDC's failure at the January meeting was rooted in its lack of credibility among blood bankers.

> We had followed every case of AIDS. We had a background in hepatitis B and sexually transmitted diseases. The emerging pattern looked very familiar. It came easy to us to understand the link between blood and AIDS. But we had few hematologists working with us. We were not part of the "club" on blood. We were viewed skeptically.[21]

Less than two weeks after the CDC meeting, the three major blood banking organizations—the American Association of Blood Banks, the American Red Cross, and the Council of Community Blood Centers—denounced proposals to exclude gay donors.[22] It was this position that compelled the American Hemophilia Foundation to make public its demand for the exclusion of gay men and others considered at high risk.

Stung by this announcement, the National Gay Task Force and more than 50 other gay political, social, and medical organizations issued a denunciation of the Hemophilia Foundation.[23] Explicit efforts to bar those at risk for AIDS from blood donation would, they asserted, be counterproductive. Those whose sexual orientation was still secret might feel pressured into donation in group- and especially workplace-based blood drives.

Despite the denunciation of either privately or governmentally imposed restrictions, gay physicians and medical groups began a tortured process of attempting to articulate a standard of social responsibility for protecting the blood supply that at the same time placed enormous emphasis on the importance of personal decisions by potential blood donors. Private discussions between the New York Blood Center and the medical leadership of the local gay community were begun to develop a method of self-exclusion that would permit those who, though subject to social pressure to donate, believed themselves at risk. The option of completing a confidential form would permit them to indicate that the blood they had given should be used "only for studies" rather than for transfusion."[24] Finally, in February, the American Association of Physicians for Human Rights adopted a statement advising those at risk for AIDS not to donate.[25]

The effort of gay leaders to prevent a governmental pronouncement on the exclusion of high-risk individuals from the blood donor pool was ultimately untenable, given the increasing frequency with which they themselves had sought to urge limited self-exclusion. On March 4, 1983, two months after the acrimonious CDC meeting on the risks of transfusion-associated AIDS, the Public Health Service issued its recommendations on the "Prevention of Acquired Immune Deficiency Syndrome (AIDS)."[26] The report noted that it appeared that "the pool of persons potentially capable of transmitting an AIDS agent may be considerably larger than the presently known number of cases."[27] In fact, because there was evidence that a latency period existed between exposure and the onset of illness, "physical examinations alone [would] not identify all persons capable of transmitting AIDS."[28] There was, therefore, no alternative but to treat all members of groups at increased risk for AIDS as posing a threat of transmission. Included were homosexual and bisexual men with multiple sex partners, as well as those who had sexual relations with such individuals. In carefully measured language and with full recognition that the blood banking community had expressly rejected the explicit screening of potential donors for sexual orientation, the Public Health Service put forth its "prudent" proposals. "As a temporary measure members of groups at increased risk should refrain from donating plasma and/or blood. This recommendation includes all individuals belonging to such groups even though many such individuals are at little risk for AIDS."[29] The precise method to be adopted to enforce such self-exclusion was not stipulated. Though specifying that laboratory tests, careful histories, and physical examinations be included among the approaches to be investigated, the recommendations carefully avoided any reference to the explicit use of questions about sexual orientation, the method proposed by the National Hemophilia Foundation but so opposed by gay leaders. Three weeks after the Public Health Service issued its statement, the Food and Drug Administration issued its implementation recommendations to those establishments involved in the collection of blood for transfusion and source plasma, as well as to manufacturers of plasma derivatives.[30]

However reluctantly, gay political leaders came tacitly to accept as a temporary measure the Public Health Service recommendations on exclusion. Ultimately, they believed, the development of a specific blood test would obviate the need for screening procedures—no matter how carefully designed—based upon sexual orientation.

A decade later, the issue of gay exclusion from the donor pool would resurface. Then, few would rally to the cause of reopening the donor pool to gay men—the issue was simply too hot to handle. For Haitians, who had also been excluded from the donor pool in the CDC's March 1983 recommendations, the struggle for re-incorporation into the community of blood donors would take on the characteristics of a broad-scale movement against national humiliation. Unlike their gay counter-parts, from whom they sought to distance themselves, they were to prove successful. Seven years after the initial bar was imposed, the FDA was compelled, under extraor-dinary political pressure, to rescind its exclusionary ruling.

Deepening Anxiety and the Search for Blood Safety: Beyond Donor Exclusion

Throughout 1983, the most forceful representatives of the blood banking commu-nity sought to minimize the risk and to allay public anxiety about the threat of transfusion-associated AIDS. Even after the publication of the PHS recommenda-tions on blood safety, they continued to cast doubt on the significance of the prob-lem. Thus in August 1983, Dr. Joseph Bove testified before the Congress that the risk of AIDS, *if such a risk existed*, was very small. In a statement that would be re-peated again and again and that would be cited in years to come as indicative of the grave misjudgment that then prevailed, Bove said, "If—and there is no evidence yet that this is so—but if all 20 cases under investigation by CDC finally turn out to be transfusion related, the incidence will be less than 1 in a million."[31] This was an extraordinarily remote risk when compared to more commonly encountered, and readily endured, social and medical hazards. In the face of such a minuscule threat from AIDS, what explained the sense of public anxiety and the rush to embrace unproven measures was, Bove declared, "the element of hysteria that surrounds the disease and anything even remotely related to it."[32]

But such efforts at risk minimization did not allay the fears of an increasingly anxious public. Perhaps the most significant indication of erosion in the faith in the safety of the blood supply, and an expression of the lack of credibility with which the spokespersons for the blood banking system were regarded, was the frequency with which those in need of blood insisted not only on the right to bank their own blood for use but on the right to designate friends and family whose blood they would rely on for transfusions. In a joint statement by the American Red Cross, the Council of Community Blood Centers, and the American Association of Blood Banks, issued in June 1983, the idea of directed donations was decried as an expression of "exces-sive concern." Blood bankers argued that there was no evidence that such donations would be safer. Indeed, they might be less safe because individuals so designated might feel compelled to donate blood despite a history of undisclosed high-risk activities. Finally, it was noted that a turn toward directed donations would seriously under-mine the nation's blood donor system. "Voluntary donation is essential for meeting our nation's needs for blood and blood products. There is a real concern that donors may refrain from routine blood donations while awaiting requests to provide directed donation."[33]

Deepening anxiety about the blood supply accompanied the publication in the *New England Journal of Medicine* in January 1984 of a major study of transfusion-associated cases of AIDS.[34] With the CDC's James Curran as lead author, the article was bound to affect the social climate. The completed investigations of donors whose blood appeared linked to the development of AIDS in recipients without known risk factors provided "circumstantial evidence that exposure to as little as one unit may result in transmission." But it was the clinical picture of these donors that was most disturbing. "The failure to identify definite cases of AIDS or even severe symptoms among donors examined suggests that affected donors with only mild or inapparent illness account for the majority of cases of transfusion-associated AIDS." Thus it was the asymptomatic carriers of the as yet to be identified infectious agent that posed the greatest risk.

Though Curran and his colleagues sought to provide some reassurance on the basis of the March exclusionary recommendations, the prospects for a marked rise in the number of transfusion-associated AIDS cases was acknowledged. Many AIDS-bearing transfusions had occurred before the first cases of AIDS were reported. In an accompanying editorial, Joseph Bove, who had so forcefully sought to oppose the effort to link blood and AIDS, noted that "Curran's data provides substantial evidence that transfusion-related AIDS does occur."

But while controversy surrounding the very existence of transfusion-associated AIDS came to an end, this was not true of the question of how to best secure the blood supply. On this central public health matter, debate continued most publicly over the matter of surrogate screening.

Surrogate Screening

Just as gay groups resisted the explicit questioning of donors about sexual orientation in the first years of the epidemic, blood bankers opposed proposals to initiate the testing of blood for indicators suggestive of a high risk for AIDS. In the absence of a serological test that could uncover occult disease in apparently healthy donors, those most convinced that the blood supply could serve as a vector of transmission argued that there was no alternative to the use of surrogate markers for those most at risk. The most obvious candidate was the hepatitis B core antibody test (anti-HBc). Not a diagnostic tool for uncovering hepatitis B itself, the test was an indication of past infection. But given the epidemiological similarity between those most at risk for hepatitis B and those most likely to have AIDS—drug users and gay men—the test could serve to identify individuals who should not donate blood.

For blood bankers, the proposal to undertake anti-HBc screening represented a potentially costly measure that would yield little public health benefit. Even for those who were willing to acknowledge that AIDS could be acquired through blood, the proposed surrogate test lacked scientific merit. The test was not specific enough to identify those at risk without including among those who would be identified individuals who could serve as healthy donors. The result of undertaking the proposed screening might well be shortages in the blood supply.[35]

Indicative of the state of confusion in this period was the response of federal officials in mid-1983 to a proposal from the Alpha Therapeutics Corporation to use anti-HBc testing in the production of clotting factor for hemophiliacs. Dr. John Petricciani, Director of the Office of Biologics at the FDA, wrote

> Such a proposal is presumably aimed at increasing the safety of the final product and indeed [your proposed] labeling as anti-core negative carries, in the current climate, the implications of a safer product. In the absence of some data indicating increased safety, we would feel any likely change to be unwarranted. We would also raise the possibility that in screening out all core antibody one might selectively remove protective antibodies such as those to hepatitis B.[36]

During 1983 the issue continued to fester as proponents of surrogate testing urged such a course as a matter or urgency and opponents portrayed their efforts as meritless. Indeed, when some blood banks initiated surrogate testing, their efforts were denounced by others as hysteria mongering. Finally, to bring closure to the issue, the FDA Blood Products Advisory Committee reluctantly entered the fray and decided in December 1983 to undertake a study of the issue. The results, three months later, did not resolve the issue but rather made even clearer the deep divide. A majority report opposed surrogate testing and warned, "Our current screening of high-risk donors could become less effective if high-risk donors heard that there was a screening test that could detect a hazard with their donation, related to AIDS transmission. Individuals might assume that, with the [surrogate] screening test in place they could continue to donate even if they fit into one of the high-risk groups. . . ."[37] A minority put forth the by now well-worn claim regarding the need to provide some measure of security beyond donor self-exclusion.

Remarkably the evidence adduced in the next decade did not resolve the controversy. Thus did Dr. James Goedert, Chief of the AIDS and Cancer Section of the National Cancer Institute state in 1994, when asked to identify the central events in the history of HIV transmission through blood products.

> In January 1983 throwing away a few percent of the donated blood units may have seemed terribly wasteful. . . . In retrospect, anti-HBc screening would have greatly reduced the number of transfusion-associated [although not clotting factor related] cases of HIV/AIDS. In my view the failure to screen . . . was a blunder that resulted from timidity and perhaps vested interests.[38]

Responding to the same inquiry, the president of the Council of Community Blood Centers stated

> In retrospect the decision not to implement anti-core testing was correct. The success of the swift action taken in preventing thousands, if not tens of thousands, of HIV in-

fections in blood recipients has, unfortunately, been lost in a popular retelling of the
AIDS experience that looks to assign blame for the epidemic and its consequence.
. . . Studies conducted in 1983 confirmed that anti-core had very little if any value in
protecting blood safety.[39]

To have responded differently at a moment when litigation sought to hold blood banks
accountable for their decisions a decade earlier would have been impossible.

Confronting Potentially Infected Clotting Factor: Product Recall and Viral Inactivation

Confronting Potentially Infected Clotting Factor:
Product Recall and Viral Inactivation

Unlike the controversy that surrounded anti-HBc testing, which bore on the interests of all persons dependent on the blood supply and which was intense and often
public, two issues bearing exclusively on hemophiliacs dependent on clotting factor—the disposition of lots of factor VIII thought to be potentially contaminated by
a single donor and the possibility of viral inactivation—received much more circum-
scribed attention. Both would, however, emerge in later years at the center of the
acrimonious and public conflict over whether corporations, the government, and even
the National Hemophilia Foundation had acted negligently, in utter disregard for
the most vital interests of hemophiliacs.

With the growing recognition in early 1983 that asymptomatic individuals could
transmit the as yet to be discovered etiologic agent responsible for AIDS, a number
of critical questions surfaced: Could a single individual infect a lot of factor concentrate composed of the plasma of thousands of individuals? Which individuals should
be considered as having posed a risk? Those who subsequently developed signs and
symptoms suggestive of AIDS? Or only those with a confirmed diagnosis?

As the National Hemophilia Foundation first began to consider this issue, it
exhibited extraordinary caution. In commenting on the decision of Hyland Therapeutics to withdraw a lot of clotting factor in May 1983, it declared

> It is not the role of the NHF to judge the appropriateness of corporate decisions made
> by individual pharmaceutical companies. However, we urge that patients and treaters
> recognize the need for careful evaluation of blood products.[40]

But by July, the Foundation's Medical and Scientific Advisory Council had taken a
much more aggressive posture: Lots of concentrate should be withdrawn not only if
they included material from an individual diagnosed with AIDS but also when such
concentrate included plasma derived from an individual who subsequently "in the
best medical judgment *of the manufacturers* has characteristics strongly suggestive
of AIDS."[41] (emphasis supplied)

When the FDA's Blood Products Advisory Committee met to confront this issue,
it was warned by pharmaceutical firms that a policy of automatic recall of all suspect
lots of concentrate would wreak havoc with the supply. Speaking on behalf of four

members of the Pharmaceutical Manufacturers Association involved in the manufacture of antihemophilic factor, Dr. Michael Rodel noted that a single frequent donor
could be represented in as many as fifty plasma pools in a given year. If such an individual were subsequently discovered to have AIDS and a decision made to withdraw
any concentrate linked to his donations, "the potential for serious disruption of supply
would occur."[42] A fellow representative of the pharmaceutical association warned that
a policy of imposed automatic recall of suspect lots would "establish a precedent leading to an eventual life-threatening short supply of . . . product; add to the fear and concern in the mind of the user . . . ; and cause the industry to make a critical [economic]
evaluation of whether it would continue producing their products."

Based on these warnings and threats, the committee chose to support the view
that recall of lots of concentrate be treated as "discrete events." The determination
as to whether a suspect lot should be distributed would need to consider "the degree
of specificity of the diagnosis, the time of onset of symptoms in relation to the time
of donation, the potential effect upon immediate supply of Factor VIII and the long
term production of this essential plasma derivative."[43]

Indicative of the extent to which some experts at the time believed that the decision to treat product recall in a conservative manner would pose no risk to hemophiliacs was the observation of the Chief of Infectious Diseases at the Georgetown
University Hospital in Washington, D.C. "I think the pooling and dilution [of any
infectious blood] will probably protect [virtually everyone who receives it]."[44]

At the end of the 1980s, when the dire consequence of factor contamination
was evident, and when the decisions made earlier in the decade were increasingly
being subject to scrutiny, June Osborn, then dean of the School of Public Health at
the University of Michigan and a prominent figure on federal advisory panels on
AIDS, would seek to capture the uncertainty of the times, treating the decisions made
with great charity.

> At the time of the debate . . . the trade-off was certainly a two-sided equation that needed
> discussion. . . . As it turned out . . . hemophiliacs certainly caught the fullest possible
> brunt of the HIV epidemic. But their well being was at instant issue in 1983, and the
> trade-off was, therefore, very much a proper subject for weighted discussion.[45]

Unlike the question of product recall, the issue of viral inactivation of clotting
factor was rooted not in the threat posed by AIDS but rather in the lingering problem of hepatitis transmission to hemophiliacs. Despite the availability of a screening
technique for hepatitis B, the possibility of transmission continued into the late 1970s
because of the virulence of the virus, which could cause infection at levels too low
for the screening test to detect.[46] Efforts to develop a process through which the lingering viral threat could be eliminated proceeded sluggishly. Many believed that
because a hepatitis B vaccine was on the horizon and most hemophiliacs had already
been exposed, little benefit would be obtained even were it possible to inactivate

hepatitis B virus. Furthermore, there was deep concern that a pasteurization process would render factor VIII concentrate a less effective treatment, one that would make the care of hemophiliacs more difficult. In sum, "hepatitis was viewed to be an acceptable risk for individuals with hemophilia because it was considered a medically manageable complication of a very effective treatment for hemophilia."[47] This was a judgment that would become the subject of acrimonious recriminations in the early 1990s, when hemophilia activists would charge that it was this attitude that ultimately permitted HIV to infect those dependent on clotting concentrate.

The difficulties that might attend the utilization of heat treatment of factor VIII were made clear by the licensing of the first such technique in Germany in 1981. Behringwerke's heat process, the company acknowledged, resulted in a loss of potency of 50%; others thought the decrease in effectiveness even greater. Because of such reduced potency it became necessary to obtain greater quantities of plasma, resulting in supply problems. And despite the increased cost — heated factor was priced at 10 times that of non-heated concentrate — it was unclear whether the new product inactivated hepatitis C as well as hepatitis B.[48]

Based largely on efforts to confront the hepatitis problem, U.S. fractionaters had continued to investigate the possibility of heat treatment. In fact, the first such process was submitted to the FDA for approval in June 1982, a month before the first reported case of AIDS in an American hemophiliac. That process was licensed in March 1983, and by early 1984 five companies had obtained licenses for heat treatment.[49]

By that time, there was obvious interest in whether such a process could protect factor VIII from the as yet undiscovered agent responsible for AIDS — it would be just a brief four months before federal authorities would announce the discovery of the retroviral etiologic agent. But it was not until October 1984 that the National Hemophilia Foundation's Medical and Scientific Advisory Council would declare

> Because heat treated products appear to have no increase in untoward effects . . . , we now recommend that treaters using coagulation factor concentrates should strongly consider changing to heat treated products with the understanding that the protection against AIDS is yet to be proven.[50]

General use of heat-treated factor began in 1985. It was a process that all but rendered clotting factor HIV-free. But because of limitations on the procedures then in use, about 20 additional hemophiliacs became infected from 1985 to 1988, when modifications in the process of viral inactivation rendered clotting factor safe.[51] By then HIV had already infected an entire generation.

Screening the Blood Supply for HIV: Ending the Threat of Infection

In April 1984, a little more than a year after the Public Health Service announced its donor exclusion recommendations, Secretary of Health and Human Services Margaret Heckler announced at a national press conference that HTLV-III (subsequently renamed HIV), a retrovirus, had been identified as the agent responsible for AIDS. Government officials were quick to announce that a blood test for the antibody to the virus would be commercially available within six months. Within a month of the announcement, the American Red Cross made public its plans to begin wide-scale trial testing of blood donations for antibody to the virus.

But no sooner had the prospect of the availability of such a long-awaited test been made public than concern about how it would be applied began to surface within the gay community. Thus, in early July, the National Gay Task Force expressed fears about the possibility that the antibody test would be used by insurers to make under-writing decisions, by employers to screen out workers and job applicants, by health care workers to identify those they would not treat, by the military to bar recruitment, and by the immigration and naturalization authorities as a barrier to entry into the United States. Their fears, which seemed exaggerated to some, were in subsequent years to prove remarkably prescient.

As part of the strategy designed to slow the rapid movement toward licensing of the antibody test, an effort was begun by gay political groups to argue that the test in preparation was inaccurate and might actually decrease the safety of the blood sup-ply by inadvertently undercutting the force of voluntary deferral guidelines. In a re-markable about-face, the long-sought objective blood test was cast as the threat and exclusion on the basis of risk group membership was portrayed as the more appro-priate strategy.

But gay groups were not alone in their concern about how the implementation of the new test would affect the safety and adequacy of the blood supply, especially if, as was anticipated, blood collection agencies would be required by federal offi-cials to notify donors of their test results. Blood bankers were also disturbed about the burden—in time, resources, and professional staff requirements—that the an-ticipated requirement for notification would place on them. Indeed, there was con-siderable resistance to the very notion that blood bankers had an obligation to as-sume such a role.[52] Finally, there was concern during the prelicensing period about the fact that the planned test would produce an unacceptably high level of false-positive findings in low-risk populations.

But to the Food and Drug Administration, licensing of the blood test was a matter of the highest priority despite the uncertainties associated with its implementation. On January 11, 1985, the Public Health Service issued its "provisional" recommen-dations for the screening of blood. All blood donors were to be told that their blood would be tested for antibody to the virus; if results were positive, donors would be notified in a confidential manner. Neither blood banks nor donors could elect to avoid such notification. Those whose blood tested positive would have their names placed on the blood collection agency's donor deferral list along with others deemed unacceptable as donors. Blood that was initially reactive to the antibody test was not to be used for transfusion or the manufacture of other blood products, even though it was admitted that the proportion of false positives among the general donor population on an initial test would be high. It was therefore recommended that no donor notification occur before at least a second test was done. Finally, the FDA made clear that the antibody test was to serve in addition to, rather than as a replacement for, donor self-deferral. Such an approach was necessitated by the small possibility of false-negative test results among those who had been infected by the AIDS virus, but had not yet developed sufficiently detectable levels of antibody. Indeed, because of the fear that large numbers of those at risk might seek to donate blood to determine their status and might go undetected because of the limits of the new assay, federal authorities quickly funded a network of centers where individuals could be tested anonymously.

Blood bank testing began in April 1985. Four months later, at a special July conference sponsored by the National Institutes of Health and the Food and Drug Administration, the first months of blood donor testing were evaluated. The conclusion: testing had been a success. The director of the Center for Drugs and Biologics of the FDA reported that "these tests are doing an extremely good job of screening potentially AIDS infectious blood units out of the blood supply."[53] Whatever the lingering risk, the initiation of antibody testing in mid-1985 had all but brought to an end the threat to the blood supply posed by HIV.

1978–1985: The Epidemiological Toll

In the seven years from 1978, when HIV first entered the blood supply and the moment when security was achieved, many thousands of hemophiliacs and blood transfusion recipients became infected.

Among hemophiliacs it has been estimated that 96% of high-dose factor VIII recipients, 92% of moderate-dose recipients, and 56% of low-dose recipients became infected.[54] Overall 75% to 85% of hemophiliacs treated in this period became HIV-positive.[55] The timing of those infections tells a remarkable story. In one study of selected hemophilia treatment centers, half of all infections occurred between September 1980 and October 1982, just three months after the CDC reported its first AIDS case among hemophiliacs. By January 1983, the date of the CDC's first public meeting on blood transfusion–associated AIDS, 62% to 89% of hemophilia A patients who would be infected had already become so. Because of the international dominance of American pharmaceutical firms in the production of factor concentrate, HIV infection among hemophiliacs was worldwide.

The only study that has sought to estimate the extent of infection among those who received transfusions between 1978 and 1984 concludes that approximately

29,000 individuals had been infected. Assuming that 60% of transfusion recipients die of their underlying disease within six months of transfusion, some 12,000 individuals survived with HIV infection. Just less than half of those who would be infected had become so by the end of 1982, the date of the first report of AIDS in a transfusion recipient.[56] These estimations are not too different from those reported by the Irwin Memorial Blood Center in San Francisco. There it was estimated that between 1978 and 1984, some 2135 surviving blood transfusion recipients were infected with HIV; 52% had become so by December 1982, 67% had been infected by June 1983, just three months after the Public Health Service issued its first recommendation on protecting the blood supply.[57]

These data would be of profound significance in the years to come as both political and legal battles emerged over the question of how much might have been done and when to prevent the spread of HIV infection through the blood supply. They also underscore the bitter irony of the effectiveness of the measures instituted to secure the blood supply in 1984–5. By then only 561 cases of AIDS in blood transfusion recipients and hemophiliacs had been reported. The seeds had been sown, however, for a fatal disease that would in the ensuing years take a toll that would dwarf those numbers. By the end of 1995, more than 12,000 cases linked to the blood supply would be reported (Table 1-1).

The Aftermath of Infection: The Politics of Restitution

Litigation

As transfusion recipients and hemophiliacs discovered that they were the victims of an iatrogenic catastrophe, they turned to the legal system for redress, seeking financial compensation for their suffering, for the cost of medical care and lost income, as recompense for foreshortened lives. But as they turned to the courts, they confronted a nearly insuperable barrier to successful litigation. In virtually every state, blood and blood products were protected by "blood shield laws" that carved out an exception to the principle of strict liability that prevailed in tort law for injuries resulting from defective products.

The origins of the blood shield exemption date to the early 1950s, when the New York Court of Appeals held that the provision of blood to a hospitalized patient who had acquired hepatitis as a result of a transfusion was not a "sale," because it was integral to the hospital's mission of caring. Hence blood and blood products were a service, and the standard of product liability did not apply. "The art of healing frequently calls for a balancing of risks and dangers to a patient. Consequently, if injury results from the course adopted, where no negligence or fault is present, liability should not be imposed upon the institution or agency actually seeking to serve or otherwise assist the patient."[58]

Table 1-1. AIDS cases among hemophiliacs and blood transfusion recipients, by year of diagnosis

	1981	1982	1983	1984	1985	1986	1987	1988	1989	1990	1991	1992	1993	1994	Total
Adults															
Transfusion	2	13	50	122	297	513	812	884	867	752	776	746	683	777	7294
Hemophilia	2	7	18	59	120	184	283	364	337	354	404	467	459	438	3496
Children															
Transfusion	2	5	9	18	47	33	46	43	38	31	24	27	26	16	365
Hemophilia	0	2	3	4	12	23	31	31	36	33	28	10	11	5	229
Total	6	27	80	203	476	753	1172	1322	1278	1170	1232	1250	1179	1236	11384

Source: Centers for Disease Control and Prevention, unpublished data.

In subsequent years most state courts across the country adopted the reasoning of the New York tribunal. Where there were exceptions,[59] blood banks pressed for legislatively defined shield statutes. In that effort they were singularly successful — only three states had not passed such legislation by the end of the 1970s.[60] Typical of such statutes was California's, which stated:

> The procurement, processing, distribution or use of whole blood, plasma, blood products and any blood derivatives for the purpose of infusing the same . . . shall be construed to be and is declared to be . . . the rendition of a service by each and every person, firm, or corporation participating therein, and shall not be construed to be and is declared not to be a sale.[61]

Although such statutes had been subject to challenge in the pre-AIDS era by critics who viewed them as providing unwarranted protection to both for-profit and not-for-profit entities, it was the AIDS epidemic that fostered the most far-reaching ideological challenge to the doctrine.

In the face of prevailing statutory and judicially crafted protective standards, plaintiffs could only rest their legal claims on arguments regarding negligence. Should the blood banks have more effectively screened donors at high risk for AIDS? Should surrogate testing have been implemented when transfusion-associated AIDS was first reported? When HIV antibody testing became possible in mid-1985, how should inventories have been treated? Should lots of clotting factor have been withdrawn when donors with AIDS or suspected of having AIDS were discovered to have contributed to the plasma pool? To each of these questions the courts would be asked to respond in the light of what was known or should have been known at the time when the understanding of AIDS was evolving. Perhaps most critically, they would be asked to determine the standard against which to judge the actions of defendants. Would it be the objective standard of what the reasonable individual could have been expected to do, or would it be the standard of professional conduct reflected in the general practice of those involved in procuring, processing, and distributing blood?

Throughout the 1980s, virtually all courts held that the standard against which blood banks and others associated with blood products should be judged was that of the profession. When trial courts on rare occasions held otherwise, they were invariably overruled on appeal. In the first trial verdict on behalf of plaintiffs involving an infant who had received a transfusion from an HIV-infected blood donation in January 1983, the court held the Irwin Memorial Blood Bank in San Francisco liable. But on appeal that decision was reversed. In addressing the question of whether Irwin should have initiated surrogate testing, the appeals court examined the practice of the industry in 1983 and concluded that an entire profession could not be negligent.[62]

Because of the complexity of the American judicial system involving both state and federal courts and the absence of any systematic mechanism for tracking lawsuits and those cases that result in out-of-court settlements, it is impossible to provide anything more than an estimate of the number of cases brought by individuals infected through the blood supply. Nor is it possible to determine, with any degree of certainty, the ultimate disposition of those cases. One analysis completed in 1993 suggested that upwards of 300 cases had been filed. Others have suggested the figure could be as high as 500.[63] In a major review of litigation involving approximately 150 cases, only 14 had resulted in decisions favorable to plaintiffs. In those successful lawsuits the awards had been substantial, totaling $75 million; the actual payments to plaintiffs, however, had been significantly lower.[64]

As the 1980s came to a close, legal commentators began to note a trend toward a more sympathetic reception to plaintiffs' suits.[65] That altered context would have an impact on the extent to which defendants—blood banks, hospitals, and physicians—would, in the future, seek to avoid costly litigation and the possibility of defeat by out-of-court settlements, some of which could be quite substantial.

The standard of professional practice that had served the industry so well was brought into question in the early 1990s by the Colorado Supreme Court. In *Quintana v United Blood Services*, the court held that compliance with the industry's formally articulated professional standards and with widely adhered-to practice was "not conclusive proof that additional precautions were not required." Were this new doctrine—an echo of an opinion rendered almost 60 years earlier by Judge Learned Hand, who had held that an entire calling could, in fact, be negligent—to become the standard against which blood banks and others would be judged, the course of litigation would be affected profoundly. The sense of alarm among the blood banks provoked by *Quintana* and other indications that the protective legal doctrines that prevailed in the 1980s might be unraveling was captured in observations made in 1992 by attorneys for the American Association of Blood Banks:

> Science and good medicine [will] become only part of the equation. Public perception often seen by the jurors as fact may actually control. The exercise of sound medical judgment may be inhibited and defensive medicine extended to the field of blood banking. The number of donors eligible to give blood may be unnecessarily reduced, with blood shortages becoming more severe. Scarce health care dollars may be spent inappropriately. The resolution of this issue will clearly have important ramifications for blood banks and the public they serve.[66]

Most striking about the 1980s was the fact that those affected by blood transfusions and blood products had sought redress as individual litigants. None of the collective action that had emerged within the gay community had occurred. This was true both of those who shared little but the fact that as patients they or their family members had received transfusions and hemophiliacs who because of the nature of their disease had developed important social networks involving entire families.

The Emergence of Hemophilia Activism

In the early 1990s, a sudden and dramatic change was to occur within the hemophilia community. Buffeted by knowledge of extraordinary levels of HIV infection among those with the most severe form of the disorder, the difficulties of seeking redress through the courts, the acts of discrimination that had so injured children seeking entry to school—the August 1987 burning of the home of the Ray family in Arcadia, Florida, because their infected sons had attempted to enroll in school was but the most egregious event—hemophiliacs began to embrace a new militancy. It was a militancy that borrowed from the AIDS activism that had emerged within the gay community, but that at the same time carried with it a perspective that was to set apart those who became infected through blood products. Finally, it was a militancy that would shake the relationship between hemophiliacs and their families on the one hand and the National Hemophilia Foundation on the other and would raise troubling questions about the extent to which physicians who had cared for hemophiliacs had betrayed their fiduciary responsibilities.

At roughly the same moment, organizations reflecting the sense of disaffection emerged on both coasts. In Massachusetts, Jonathan Wadleigh began to organize the Committee of Ten Thousand (COTT) as a support group for hemophiliacs who believed their needs had not been met by the National Hemophilia Foundation. On the West Coast, Michael Rosenberg took a more aggressive stance as he organized the Hemophilia/HIV Peer Association. It was Rosenberg's vision that would ultimately inform and shape the fury of those who would come to see their plight as the consequence of profound institutional failure, although it was COTT that would take on the more enduring organizational form.

"Causes and Effects of the Hemophilia/AIDS Epidemic" can be read as a manifesto of the new militancy. In it, Rosenberg laid bear his claims against those who had failed American hemophiliacs.[67] A "genocide" was occurring because of the "commercially driven practices of certain large pharmaceutical corporations." The "reckless disregard" of the manufacturers of processed plasma and the failure of the FDA to alter "unsafe medical industry practices" were responsible for the HIV epidemic among hemophiliacs.

> The hemophilia population is the only AIDS risk group that became HIV-infected because we consumed products sold at a profit by major corporations. And with the exception of persons who were transfused with contaminated blood, only our community has been brought down by AIDS precisely because we followed the advice of our doctors.

The roots of the problem went back to the 1970s when corporations had failed to respond to the threat of hepatitis B in clotting factor. Had they done so, "they would have prevented the transmission of HIV." Such a failure did not follow from the state of knowledge in the 1970s nor from the limited technical capacity to undertake viral inactivation. It was rather the "predictable consequence of a pattern of choices that consistently placed commercial considerations above the safety of consumers."

Rosenberg next turned his ire against the National Hemophilia Foundation, "presumably the advocate for America's hemophiliacs." Here too failure was rooted in the 1970s. "It is difficult to comprehend how the NHF could have failed to sound an alarm" about hepatitis B. And when in the early 1980s AIDS began to appear, the pattern of negligence persisted, this time with even more devastating consequences. "From the get-go the NHF and its Medical and Scientific Advisory Council advised hemophiliacs not to be alarmed and not to change their treatment methods. . . . That remained the advice we were given in 1983, 1984 into 1985. . . . In effect we were told by NHF to use [clotting factor] just as though there were no danger of AIDS."

The "colossal wrongheadedness" of the Foundation and its medical leadership was compounded by a failure to speak openly and honestly about the risks associated with factor concentrate. "There are few hemophiliacs who, had they known the truth about the dangers . . . would not have cut their AFC [antihemophilic factor concentrate] usage by 90%. True, there would have been an increase in the number of painful days, and treatment would have been more inconvenient. But when that option is weighed against AIDS, I suspect that many people and many physicians would have made different treatment choices."

In other contexts, but especially when underscoring the betrayal by physicians who testified in court against hemophiliacs seeking redress from concentrate manufacturers, the language used to describe the medical leadership of the NHF would be even sharper. Dr. Louis Aledort, whose career spanned the remarkable advances in the treatment of hemophilia, would be labeled the Mengele of the Hemophilia AIDS Holocaust.

In the face of such betrayal, it was only natural that hemophilia activists would seek to create new organizations to defend their interests.

> We—the alienated—do not identify with the hemophilia institutions. After all the debacle of the 80s, we do not need an organization that cozies up to the corporate factor makers; we do not need an organization that can be bought off cheaply with small grants [from those corporations] and PR gimmicks. We need an organization that demands—not in lip service but for real—that every person who needs it gets the safest factor available and that is affordable.[68]

The most comprehensive indictment laid down by the new militants was compiled by the Committee of Ten Thousand. *The Trail of AIDS in the Hemophilia Community* includes several hundred pages of documents, largely obtained during the course of discovery in legal proceedings, and stands as the "evidence that demands a verdict." It epitomizes the effort to revise radically the terms of debate over blood and AIDS. For much of the 1980s, as blood banks and others involved with the unfolding events that linked blood and AIDS sought to defend themselves against charges of negligence, they had successfully asserted that what was entailed was a tragedy, a series of awful events that could not have been avoided. It was the singular challenge of the hemophilia activists to shatter the hegemony of that characterization. The narrative of tragedy had to be displaced by the narrative of accusation.

The voice of protest was also a call to action, and in November 1992, in what they described as a turning point, dissident hemophiliacs brought their protest to the annual conference of the Hemophilia Foundation. At a sidewalk demonstration, protesters carried red-stained pickets declaiming, "AIDS, the Avoidable Tragedy." Inside the conference center, protesters wearing death masks confronted "the corporate mass murderers" in the commercial exhibit space. A "shame list" of physicians who had betrayed their patients by testifying on behalf of pharmaceutical companies in litigation on corporate liability for AIDS was presented. It was a list that was indistinguishable from the medical leadership of hemophilia treatment. Demonstrations like this would be repeated in the next years at NHF conferences. The hemophilia community had become a house divided.

Armed with this ideological perspective, the new hemophilia activists developed a three-pronged political strategy. They sought a congressional investigation to uncover the full extent of wrongdoing on the part of the blood establishments, launched a campaign for a publicly funded compensation scheme to make restitution to hemophiliacs and their families, and undertook a class action lawsuit designed to extract civil damages from those who were responsible for the plight of hemophiliacs. In each respect, the strategy set the Peer Association and the Committee of Ten Thousand against the Hemophilia Foundation, which was now viewed as shamefully complicit and compromised.

Demanding Truth

In May 1992, the Peer Association's *Action Now* called for a congressional investigation of the failures that had led to the infection of American hemophiliacs. "The full truth revealed by an investigation in the proper forum — Congress — is the very least the thousands of U.S. families of persons with hemophilia-related HIV deserve. We demand this. We will persist. We will not be brushed off. We will not take 'no' for an answer."[69] Within a year of that call, Senator Bob Graham and Representative Porter Goss, both of Florida (where the Ray family was so much a presence), were joined by the exponent of American liberalism Senator Edward Kennedy of Massachusetts in calling for an investigation by the Office of the Inspector General of the Department of Health and Human Services. Strikingly, in their letter to Secretary Donna

Shalala, it was the plight of hemophiliacs that was the exclusive focus of attention. No mention was made of those who had been infected through transfusions.[70] Two months later the Secretary responded by proposing that the Institute of Medicine undertake the inquiry. "Because a high level of scientific and medical expertise is required to conduct a thorough study, I have asked the [IOM], an external organization with proven experience in conducting studies of a similar nature, to undertake this task."[71]

The committee established by the IOM was, like other such committees, to have the aura of distinterested authority. The membership included respected scientists, medical, biological and social, as well as an ethicist. None was to have a history of having spoken out on the issues to be studied. That would have compromised the "objectivity" of the committee's work. The goal of the inquiry was not to make backward-looking, blame-attributing findings but to "describe the science and policy formulation processes as they evolved, to review subsequent changes to decision-making, and to provide guidance regarding approaches to policy development to be pursued in future efforts to protect the blood supply."[72]

The initial response of hemophilia activists was one of disappointment. The IOM committee would not have the power of subpoena; its inquiry would not have the political significance of an investigation by the Congress; it would not focus the nation's attention on the depths of the scandal. When, two years later, the committee issued its final and scathing report, these concerns were all but forgotten.

It would be hard to overstate the dramatic change that had occurred in the status of the American blood system over the decade that preceded the onset of and set the stage for the IOM committee's work. Investigative reports by journalists, congressional hearings, and the challenge of AIDS activists had rendered those who collected blood and manufactured blood products vulnerable. The aura that had surrounded the purveyors of the "gift of life" on the eve of the AIDS epidemic had vanished.

Randy Shilts' widely read *And the Band Played On*,[73] published in 1988, had pilloried blood bankers along with everyone else who had permitted the AIDS epidemic to take hold. In "AIDS, Blood and Politics," the Public Broadcasting System program *Frontline* presented an especially scorching attack on the vested interests that dominated the blood industry at the moment when the challenge of AIDS emerged. When, in mid-1993, FDA Commissioner Dr. David Kessler testified before a congressional committee that was yet again examining the safety of the blood supply, his carefully chosen words were designed to subvert whatever protective institutional myths continued to surround blood in America. Gone was the language of "service," so central to the legal framework that had informed the blood shield laws.

> Blood banking has become a manufacturing industry, an industry that must conform to high standards and quality control requirements comparable to those of the pharmaceutical companies and other regulated industries. That is how the FDA regards blood banking today, and that is how the industry must come to see itself.[74]

Addressing the failures of the blood banks and the American Red Cross against which he had taken "one of the strongest enforcement actions . . . during my tenure as Commissioner of the FDA,"[75] Kessler noted how pervasive the problems were. "This industry is not assuming adequate responsibility for putting in place and following the basic quality assurance programs and standard operating procedures required to assure the safety of the blood supply."[76] Lastly, Kessler was unsparing in his review of how the FDA itself had managed the blood system. A collaborative approach that did not reflect the regulatory dimensions of the FDA's protective mission had resulted in an inadequately monitored blood supply. Thus, in speaking of the saga of the Red Cross, he asserted that the FDA's belief "that a voluntary agreement with the American Red Cross would be sufficient was, I think, emblematic of our collegial approach to regulated industry at the time. Those days are behind us."[77]

None of this was lost on those involved in the American blood banking system. "The image of blood banks has been damaged. . . . Its image changed from that of a life-saving community service to one where motives and practices are viewed with skepticism and even hostility."[78]

As it began its work in the fall of 1993, the IOM committee received an emotionally riveting challenge from a day-long public hearing at which those whose lives had been affected by HIV-infected blood told their stories, laid bare evidence, made demands. For almost nine hours committee members heard testimony in a setting that more resembled a speak-out than a decorous hearing. Betrayal by physicians, the National Hemophilia Foundation, the fractionaters, and the government was the theme that united the voices of well-known activists and those who had rarely been heard before. They spoke of "murder" and demanded "justice." Hemophiliacs talked about their lives foreshortened, wives of their husbands dead and dying, sisters about their brothers, mothers about their sons. The anguish and rage were captured by Maxine Segal of Florida:

> I am here to tell you another story of the emotional pain of AIDS, how my two sons suffered and died, and how my suffering as a surviving mother never ends. I woke early on May 8, 1988, it was Mother's Day, the day I would bury my first born child, Scott. My second child, Doug, would stand beside me grieving for Scott, knowing that he would soon follow his brother. My despair was three-fold that day. The scorching in my heart at losing Scott, the anguish in my head from knowing I would lose Doug too, and the agony in my gut in realizing that soon no one would ever call me "mother" again.

This was not the cry of someone whose young children were taken from her. Each was 36 when he died. Rather, it was the bleak voice of a mother confronting the fact that she "could not protect her children. My torment is forever."

Her suffering, like that of so many others who testified that day, was transformed by a political vision:

Today I bring my anguish and my anger and my grief to this open forum. . . . Today [I] demand justice and shout to the world and to this committee, "How did you let this happen to us? Why did you do nothing to prevent this?"

If the victims of "greed and disregard for human life" were clear, so too were those responsible. Drs. Louis Aledort and Margaret Hilgartner, leading figures in the treatment of hemophilia in the early 1980s, corporations such as Cutter, the National Hemophilia Foundation and its Executive Director Allan Brownsten, and finally the FDA. All had to be "brought to justice."[79]

Not all the testimony was so emotionally raw, but enough was, and members of the Committee were visibly shaken.

The testimony ended nine hours after it had begun, with a statement by Louise Ray, the nationally known Florida mother of three boys with hemophilia. "You see," she said "the bumper sticker that says 'Blood, A Gift of Life'? That is such an atrocity. For us blood was a gift of death. You individuals who sit before us today, you hold the key to our future, one of hope that our country will at long last be protected, or you hold the key that opens the door of fear that the future generations of hemophiliacs will also be lost to neglect."[80]

That Louise Ray spoke last after a long list of less well-known speakers is indicative of the care with which the day's program was considered. It is all the more striking, therefore, that no one spoke as, or on behalf of, non-hemophiliacs who became infected through blood transfusions. The day, whether by design or lack of sustained effort to reach out to others, belonged to those with hemophilia.

Nine months later, on July 13, 1995, the IOM committee issued its report. Cautiously, even ponderously written, the report was nevertheless clear in its judgment that much, if not all, of the burden of AIDS in those dependent on the blood supply could have been avoided had those with clinical, corporate, and governmental authority acted differently in the early 1980s and late 1970s. In the struggle between those who had adopted the exculpatory narrative of tragedy and those who had embraced the narrative of accusation, the committee had clearly embraced the perspective of the latter. The committee chose not to emphasize the moral failings of venality and greed, but rather stressed the institutionally rooted inadequacy of the response of those who should have acted more aggressively in the face of the unfolding evidence. In that regard it differed little in posture from that of the Reagan-appointed Presidential AIDS Commission that had reported in 1988 "the initial response of the nation's blood banking industry to the possibility of contamination of the nation's blood by a new infectious agent was unnecessarily slow."[81]

On each of the matters that had emerged as a focus of litigation and of political dispute, the committee found that too little was done.

When confronted with a range of options for using donor screening and deferral to reduce the probability of spreading HIV through the blood supply, blood bank officials and federal authorities consistently chose the least aggressive option that was justifiable. . . . Among these options were asking male donors about sexual activity with other men and screening donated blood for anti-HBc antibody. . . . Both . . . were reasonable to require in January 1983.[82]

On the question of when factor VIII should have been subject to virus inactivating heat treatment, the committee argued that the tragedy of AIDS could have been avoided had action been taken to confront the challenge of hepatitis B in the 1970s. Prevailing institutional arrangements explained the failure.

Heat treatment processes to prevent the transmission of hepatitis could have been developed before 1980. Treaters of hemophilia and public health service agencies did not, for a variety of reasons, encourage the companies to develop heat treatment measures earlier. Strong incentives to maintain the status quo and a weak countervailing force concerned with blood product safety combined to inhibit rapid development of heat treated products by plasma fractionater companies.[83]

In failing to recall lots of clotting factor that might have been contaminated by donors suspected of having AIDS, the committee concluded that the FDA had been "cautious and inadequate."[84]

Finally, on grounds of medical ethics, physicians and the National Hemophilia Foundation were taken to task for their failure to fully disclose to patients the risks associated with the use of factor VIII concentrate.

Paternalistic assumptions about medical decision-making led to failures to adequately disclose the risks of continuing use of AHF concentrate and enable individuals to make informed decisions for themselves. Failure [to communicate] the possibility of widespread infection in the hemophiliac community led to ancillary failures to warn possibly infected individuals of the risks they might pose to others through sexual contact.[85]

In drawing its lessons for the future, the committee focused on the institutional weaknesses that might leave the nation vulnerable to future threats to the blood supply. It urged the establishment of a new, high-level, government position—that of a Blood Safety Director—responsible for coordinating the Public Health Service responses to new and emerging threats; the creation of a Blood Safety Council to evaluate current and potential threats to the blood supply; the adoption of a stringent regulatory approach by the FDA to the blood system; and a reshaping of the Blood Products Advisory Committee, which had exemplified the all-too-intimate collaborative relationship between the medico-industrial complex that surrounded blood and those responsible for its regulation.[86]

On none of these issues was there much dispute within the committee, and indeed the recommendations followed quite organically from the analysis that had preceded it. On the question of compensation for those who had been infected through the blood supply, however, the committee did experience internal dissension, and on that matter the recommendation that came forth was unusually cramped. This is all the more striking because the activist call for compensation—for justice— was integral to the call for a congressional investigation. The committee, with one dissenting vote, urged that the federal government consider the establishment of a no-fault compensation system for those who might in the future suffer harm from blood and blood products, but it was unwilling to recommend such a scheme for those who had become infected with HIV. "The no-fault principle . . . *might* serve to guide policy makers as they consider whether to implement a compensation system for those infected in the 1980s."[87]

What can account for the committee's timidity on a matter so close to the center of the debate over AIDS and the blood supply, especially since its analysis so painstakingly pieced together a tale of institutional failure? In part the answer is to be found in the confining definition of the committee's task—to examine the past with the purpose of making recommendations only about the future. When the issue of compensation of those who had been infected with HIV did arise in the committee's deliberations, the members were informed by the IOM staff that the question was beyond the scope of its mission; if the report broached the issue it would be excised in the review process.

The response by federal officials to the IOM report is indicative of how much had changed by mid-1995. In commenting on the study that she had commissioned, Secretary of Health and Human Services Donna Shalala declared

> In principle we accept the IOM recommendations; in practice, I believe we have already implemented many of them. We must continue to do everything in our power to see that similar tragedies will not occur again.[88]

The FDA, which had suffered the most striking criticism in the IOM report, and which did not want it thought that it had been pressured into reform in anticipation of the committee's report, asserted that it had quite independently begun to undertake regulatory changes designed to safeguard the blood supply. Most notably it had moved to thoroughly revamp the nature of the Blood Products Advisory Committee by excluding as members those whose institutional affiliations could compromise the capacity for independent judgment.

Ironically, the most enduring contribution of the IOM study was not its effort to chart a course for the future but its "establishment" of a narrative of the events of blood and AIDS in the first years of the epidemic. In many important ways it was a narrative not too different from that which had been provided years earlier by journalist-chronicler Randy Shilts in *And the Band Played On*. But because of its provenance, the account provided by the committee was viewed as objective, above the fray. As one writer noted in the *Washington Post*, "The value of this document is that unlike most of the reams of articles and books that have been written about AIDS, it is free of polemic and political rhetoric."[89]

Demanding Justice: The Struggle for Compensation

In the fall of 1991, Dana Kuhn, a hemophiliac with HIV infection who would in later years emerge as a leading proponent of the new militancy, wrote to then Secretary of Health and Human Services Louis Sullivan, calling on the U.S. government to create a compensation program for hemophiliacs and in so doing join in the "humane proceedings of at least 17 other countries." The cost of health insurance, the inability to purchase life insurance, the need to prepare for funerals and assure the economic well-being of families when work became impossible were cited as financial justifications. As important were the burdens associated with the death of children and spouses and the need to be compensated for the psychological effects of an impending doom brought on by someone else's negligence.

The call for compensation was ultimately to become a centerpiece of the demands articulated by hemophilia activists. It was not only a demand for financial relief, it was a demand for justice, a partial payment for the wrongs that had been done. What so infuriated hemophilia activists was that the National Hemophilia Foundation had opposed such a compensation scheme. In so doing, the NHF stood alone among the world's hemophilia associations, a number of which had successfully sought compensation in Europe, Canada, Japan, and Australia.

As early as 1988, the executive director of the NHF made clear his opposition to such a scheme. His arguments would inform NHF efforts even when, under pressure to change, it modified its posture. First, he asserted that in the absence of a strong welfare state ideology in the United States, it was unlikely that the notion of compensation would have much support. Second, he doubted that the Congress would be willing to establish the precedent of providing compensation for other groups that might be afflicted by mass iatrogenic injury. Third, an effort to obtain compensation would conflict with the more pressing agenda of obtaining government support for paying for safer but ever more expensive clotting factor. Fourth, and most arresting, he argued that an effort to obtain compensation for those infected through the blood supply would be dangerously divisive, separating "innocent victims" from others afflicted by AIDS.

> It is highly unlikely that compensation could ever be considered for all individuals exposed to HIV—this has not occurred in any of the other countries that have initiated or are considering compensation programs. Thus any compensation strategy . . . would be an ideological throw-back to Elizabethan Poor Laws, with notions of deserv[ing] and undeserv[ing] populations. . . . Further this notion of deserv[ing] innocent victim would . . . trigger a major outcry and declaration of war from the gay community.[90]

In short, the pursuit of compensation would be futile, counterproductive, and morally retrograde.

Nevertheless the NHF and its AIDS Task Force did study the issue of compensation in subsequent years.[91] But even as the organization itself began to inch away from its outright rejection of compensation, an important voice of resistance persisted. Don Goldman, a hemophiliac, who as a former president of the Foundation and chairman of its Board of Directors had helped to shape and guide the organization during the early years of the epidemic and who had served on the National AIDS Commission—its only hemophiliac member—was a strong advocate of unity among all those affected by HIV. He warned of the implications of compensation:

> The impact on future research is worth considering. If it turns out 20 years from now that rDNA products have a presently unknown side effect, will we then be demanding compensation? We have consistently argued that for a small population such as those with hemophilia, that if we wait for new products until they can be fully tested on thousands of people, no new drugs will be marketed.[92]

The infection of America's hemophiliacs was no one's fault. It was, after all, a medical tragedy.

Despite such resistance and under pressure from hemophilia activists, the NHF ultimately took on a commitment to a "financial assistance" program for hemophiliacs—based on contributions from blood fractionaters. But in so doing its efforts bore the mark of the great caution of prior years, a desire to avoid confrontation, and a commitment to avoiding offense to the gay community.[93]

The NHF strategy—which activists denounced as "seeking crumbs from the table"—all but collapsed in August 1993. The blood industry announced that because of both the magnitude of the NHF proposal—$125,000 for each person with hemophilia and HIV—and the anticipation of an inquiry to be undertaken by the Institute of Medicine, it was "questionable as to whether discussions should continue." The NHF responded furiously to this setback, and in language more typical of its militant critics, termed it "unacceptable and . . . an intentional and well-considered effort to undermine both the nature and spirit of cooperation." "Nothing," said the Foundation, "is more costly than a human life, yet industry has the audacity to imply that our proposal would cost too much money. . . . Given the magnitude of the tragedy and its direct link to factor use, can industry afford not to join in the endeavor?"[94]

This was the context within which the efforts of the Committee of Ten Thousand to generate Congressional support for a public compensation plan emerged and ultimately bore fruit. Although the extended process was beset with the (by now to be expected) clashes between the NHF and its more militant antagonists,[95] the result was the introduction of the Ricky Ray Hemophilia Relief Fund Act of 1995. Named for the 15-year-old son of Louise Ray who had died of AIDS in 1992, the

legislation would establish a $1 billion fund to pay an estimated 8000 infected hemo-
philiacs, their infected spouses or offspring, or their surviving families $125,000 each.
This payment was to represent "partial restitution to individuals who became infected
because of the failure of the government to secure the blood supply."[96]

Strikingly, the legislation did not extend its compensatory scope to non-
hemophiliacs infected through blood transfusions. Despite efforts on the part of
hemophilia activists and their political allies to justify the exclusive focus on those
who had been infected through clotting factor, it is clear that neither the facts involved in the transmission of HIV through the blood supply nor the moral logic
that undergirded the claim for restitution could explain this decision. Rather, it
was the unique result of political considerations. An aide to Representative Porter
Goss, a prime sponsor of the legislation and a conservative Republican committed
to budgetary restraint, simply noted, "If you increase the numbers you increase the
cost."

The Ricky Ray Relief Act did not receive the support of the most important and
effective AIDS lobbying coalition, the AIDS Action Council. Not surprisingly, many
within the organization were offended by the implicit distinction between those who
had been infected through blood and those infected through sex. Whatever support
did exist for the legislation within the AIDS Action Council vanished when Porter
Goss's press briefing on the bill seemed to cross the boundary of the tolerable in
making distinctions among those infected with HIV.[97] Despite the absence of support from AIDS Action, the early fears expressed by the NHF regarding the political
acceptability of a compensation scheme, and the studied silence of the Clinton
administration, the proposed legislation had by mid-1996 acquired the support of
more than half of the members of the House of Representatives. It fared less well
in the Senate and died before the Congressional session ended. The Ricky Ray Act
was re-introduced into the 105th Congress, supported by House Speaker Newt
Gingrich.[98] Indicative of the broad appeal of the legislation, despite the budget-
slashing mood in Washington, was that among the 151 initial cosponsors were those
spanning the political spectrum from the Republican right to the Democratic left.
Despite failed attempts on the part of some Senators to extend the scope of compensation to blood transfusion recipients, Congress finally passed the Ricky Ray
Act in October, 1998.

Holding Corporations Accountable: Class Action and Beyond

On September 30, 1993, hemophilia activists largely linked to the Committee for
Ten Thousand filed a class action lawsuit against the four manufacturers of factor
concentrate in the United States as well as the National Hemophilia Foundation.
The fractionaters had to be held accountable for their crimes. More than monetary
compensation "people wanted, *needed*, aggressive action against [the] huge multi-

nationals that so callously profited while filling our veins with deadly viruses." Such aggressive action was contrasted with the approach of the National Hemophilia Foundation, which had approached the corporations "with hand held out" in search of "assistance." With class action, COTT asserted, "We are now dealing from a position of strength."[99]

How far this class action suit was from the moment in 1985 when Don Goldman, then Chairman of the Board of the NHF could write, "So long as fractionaters have followed NHF recommendations concerning AIDS, NHF oppose efforts to impose strict liability for AIDS on manufacturers of clotting factor,"[100] and from the moment later in that year when the NHF Board would oppose the certification of a class action suit in California, at the urging of a fractionater, because such a legal action, it was asserted, would violate the confidentiality of hemophiliacs who might choose to remain anonymous.[101]

Indeed, the history of the NHF's opposition to or great caution about the desirability of bringing civil actions against the manufacturers of clotting factor would be cited in the 1990s as emblematic of its betrayal of those it purported to represent. Central to the explanation that would emerge in the activist critique was the extent to which the NHF had grown dependent on financial support from the corporations that had distributed infected clotting factor.

Prior to the filing of the class action lawsuit, some 300 cases involving 400 plaintiffs had been filed by hemophiliacs. The goal of the class action was not simply to consolidate these cases, which were at various stages of litigation, but to make possible the recompense of those who had failed to take action either because of the legal costs, the restrictions imposed by state statutes of limitations, or fears that their identities would become public.

Almost a year after *Wadleigh v. Rhône Poulenc* was filed in federal district court in Chicago, Judge John Grady granted class certification to the plaintiffs. In so doing he eliminated the central procedural hurdle in such cases. Seven months later, that victory was reversed when, on appeal, Richard A. Posner, among the most prominent Federal Appeals Court judges, took the unusual step of reversing the lower court's certification. In a 2 to 1 decision that rested, in large part, upon a complex series of technical considerations, Posner wrote, "With all due respect for the district judge's commendable desire to experiment with an innovative procedure for streamlining the adjudication of this 'mass tort' we believe that his plan so far exceeds the permissible bounds of discretion in the management of federal litigation as to compel us to intervene and order decertification."[102]

At base, Posner's decision represented a judicial policy determination driven by concerns for how class certification might affect an industry that had prevailed in 12 of 13 prior cases involving hemophiliacs heard in federal court. For the consensus that might emerge from the determinations of many tribunals the class action would substitute a single trial before a single jury instructed in accordance with no actual law of any jurisdiction—a jury that will receive a kind of Esperanto instruction merging the negligence standards of the 50 states and the District of Columbia. One jury, consisting of six persons . . . will hold the fate of an industry in its hand. This jury may disagree [with] the decisions of prior federal juries that have examined this issue] and hurl an industry into bankruptcy. . . . With the aggregate stakes in the tens or hundreds of millions of dollars, or even in the billions, it is not a waste of judicial resources to conduct more than one trial, before more than six jurors, to determine whether a major segment of the international pharmaceutical industry is to follow the asbestos manufacturers into [bankruptcy].[103]

Judge Posner was careful to note that in the light of such a prospect, the defendant firms might well be compelled to offer a settlement. Indeed, COTT's leaders had argued that on the eve of the filing of the class action lawsuit, a settlement offer, more robust than had ever been suggested before, was made precisely because of the threat of litigation. But Posner did not hide his concern about the equity of such offers made under conditions of economic duress. "Judge Henry J. Friendly," Posner wrote, "who was not given to hyperbole, called settlements induced by a small probability of an immense judgment in a class action 'blackmail settlements.'"[104]

In the aftermath of the decertification decision, tensions emerged between activist plaintiffs and their attorneys, the former pressing for an appeal to the U.S. Supreme Court, the latter preferring to focus on the hundreds of individual lawsuits that had been consolidated for some purposes of pre-trial discovery under special federal rules. For the activists such a strategy represented a "sellout" of the thousands of hemophiliacs who had been unable or unwilling to bring individual lawsuits. For their attorneys such a strategy was crucial to maintaining the pressure on the corporations to reach a settlement. So embittered did relations become that members of the Committee of Ten Thousand went to court to dismiss their lawyers who were litigating the consolidated cases. The court rejected their efforts, comparing it to a mutiny on an airline mid-flight.

Indicative of the free-for-all that emerged, Corey Dubin, president of COTT, entered into secret negotiations with Baxter International, one of the four firms involved in litigation, in an effort to wrest a settlement. In an argument that would have a profound impact on how far the plaintiffs would be willing to press and in an effort to underscore the extent to which there existed the basis for a common ground, Dubin reported, "I told [Baxter] they were going to have to live with us when all the high-powered litigators were gone." He also noted that hemophiliacs would, for medical reasons, remain dependent on the survival of the fractionaters. They could not drive them into bankruptcy. "If you buy a Pinto from Ford that blows up, you can tell Ford to go to hell. But I don't have that luxury."[105] This was indeed litigation very different from that described by Judge Posner.

The secret negotiations with Baxter were ultimately aborted, but in April of 1996 the four fractionaters, including Bayer A.G. of Germany, Rhône-Poulenc Rorer, a unit of Rhône-Poulenc of France, and Alpha Therapeutics, a unit of Japan's Green Cross, made an offer of $600 million to affected hemophiliacs and their families, with an additional $40 million to cover legal fees and administration. Were 6000 individuals to seek compensation, $100,000 would be available for each. Were larger numbers to seek compensation, the individual awards would be reduced.

Some saw the settlement offer, an effort on the part of the clotting manufacturers to resolve the ongoing threat of litigation without admission of fault, as a significant gesture. To others it represented an insult. Dana Kuhn, who had worked with the NHF for years before rebelling and becoming a leader of COTT, denounced the proposal: "To someone who took factor concentrate once and whose wife [was sexually infected by him and] died and left him with a three-year-old and a six-year-old, this is an insult."[106] That the Japanese, including the Green Cross, had just awarded $420,000 to each affected individual made the offer appear all the more inadequate.

Further complicating the offer was the fact that if 100 or more potential hemophiliac litigants opted out and sought to pursue their own cases in the belief that they could obtain larger awards, the companies would withdraw the plan. Hemophilia activists were confronted with the prospect of a divisive battle between those who viewed the most recent offer as good enough—given their life expectancies—and those who believed that in the name of justice, they deserved more. But in this instance the latter had, because of their capacity to opt out, the power to affect the interests of the former. Seeking to prevent such a split, COTT reasserted the importance of solidarity:

> The goal of COTT has always been to gain the greatest good for the largest number of people while ensuring that no harm is done to those with filed cases. This means that while we push for a global settlement, . . . we also protect the right of those with filed cases to . . . press their individual claims. . . . Some in the community have suggested that these two goals are mutually exclusive. We categorically deny this position. . . . Both must be obtained if we are to serve the ultimate interests of those harmed in this holocaust.[107]

When those eligible were polled by the court, 6200, approximately 95%, indicated that they would accept the proposed settlement.[108] When the federal court, which retained supervision over the negotiations between the litigants, held a hearing to evaluate the fairness of the settlement offer, two issues emerged as critical. Would those whose medical care had been paid for by Medicaid or private insurance confront demands for repayment? Would those currently receiving welfare benefits suddenly find themselves deprived of such support because of the $100,000 award? Judge

Grady made it clear that unless these issues were resolved in the interest of the plaintiffs, he would reject the proposed settlement.[109]

It took six months of complex negotiations with federal and state authorities, but in May 1997 the issues were ultimately resolved. The defendant corporations had agreed to increase the settlement by $30 million—paying $12.2 million to the federal government and $18 million to private insurers and state governments. A special-needs fund would be created for individuals receiving welfare payments— a fund that they could draw on without jeopardizing their eligibility for public assistance.[110]

In the end, the Committee of Ten Thousand, which had played such a crucial role in fostering the class action litigation, rejected the settlement as a profound betrayal. Like the National Hemophilia Foundation, the lawyers who had been engaged to defend the interests of hemophiliacs had danced to the tune of other masters.[111] Despite this disappointment, American hemophiliacs and their survivors had at last joined the ranks of those in other nations where some form of payment had been made to those injured by HIV-contaminated factor concentrate. With the passage of the Ricky Ray Act, entailing a promise of about $100,000 in federal payments to each infected hemophiliac or surviving family member, long years of activist struggle had finally born fruit. In stark contrast was the state of affairs that prevailed with regard to individuals who had become infected through blood transfusions. Their infections were no less the consequence of an iatrogenic castrophe; yet isolated and without organizational voice, each had to stand alone before the courts in the search for justice.

Conclusions

The past decade has witnessed remarkable improvements in the safety of the American blood supply. The tragic consequences of the transmission of HIV through blood and blood products in the late 1970s and early 1980s has been of overriding importance in fostering those improvements. So too has the subsequent litigation that has threatened what had been the near-invulnerability of those involved in the collection and distribution of blood and blood products.

Blood safety has been radically enhanced by the introduction of screening tests, the use of direct donor questioning about risk factors, increased reliance on autologous blood transfusions, and the more judicious use of blood transfusions—which, it is now understood, may entail an irreducible level of risk. With regard to HIV, it has been estimated that 1 in every 450–600,000 donations of screened blood is contaminated.[112] For hepatitis B, the risk has been estimated at 1 in 63,000; for hepatitis C, 1 in 103,000. These lingering risks are rooted in the limits of current tests to detect viruses soon after infection occurs, the so-called "window period."[113] As a result of such progress, researchers from the National Institutes of Health concluded in

1995 that, "Blood has become one of the safest medical therapies."[114] That view was echoed two years later by a report from the U.S. General Accounting Office, which found "the blood supply is safer today than at any time in recent history."[115]

Indicative of the extent to which concerns regarding blood safety had come to dominate public policy was the FDA decision to introduce p24 antigen screening for HIV infection. Because of its capacity to reduce the risks associated with the "window period," it has been estimated that such testing would identify 5 to 10 units of infected blood per year, at an estimated annual cost of $60 million.[116] Because each infected unit may be broken down into its components and transfused into several individuals, it has been estimated that the additional screening will cost approximately $2.3 million per quality-adjusted life-year saved, a figure far in excess of the standard used in making public health determinations.[117]

Given this record of achievement it is not surprising that the current period is characterized by an odd mix of self-congratulation and anxiety. A tone of assurance had, after all, prevailed when blood bankers had asserted that the risks of acquiring AIDS through the blood supply were minuscule, perhaps 1 in a million. It is within this context that Harvey Feinberg, then Dean of the Harvard School of Public Health, warned that a "simple-minded focus on safety is no longer the appropriate [approach] for those concerned with sensible use of the blood supply." With the very high levels of security already attained, incremental improvements would come at very high costs and would produce only marginal benefits. "Today," he concluded, "the harder kind of question is how can we define and attain a desirable balance among the goals of safety and adequate supply and benefit to patients—all while maintaining our ethical responsibility to donor, to the patient, and to society at large?"[118]

These are not new questions. Indeed, they were the questions first posed in the 1970s when the National Blood Policy was formulated, at a time when the prospect of a catastrophe like AIDS was all but unimaginable. Having experienced the HIV epidemic, and aware that as many as 20,000 men, women, and children will die as a result of their use of blood and its derivatives, we are compelled to consider Feinberg's questions. Newly chastened, we now know that at some moment in the future the blood supply will be threatened by a new pathogen. The recent debate over p24 antigen screening makes clear what the cost of additional safety may be, and the public appears ready to pay the price of enhanced safety. When told that the risk of acquiring a serious or fatal transfusion-related malady was one half of one percent, 60% of those polled in a 1997 survey reported that more money should be spent to reduce those harzards.[119] Concerns over blood safety may thus presage irresistible pressures that will require the expenditure of public resources that might well be applied to other, more critical, public health threats. But blood is, after all, different.

In the wake of the disaster of AIDS and blood, we are left with two broad questions: Will the experience of the 1980s and the debate of the 1990s have prepared us to better respond to protect the public health? And will we be better prepared to meet the economic and social needs of those who will, despite the best of efforts, fall victim? How we answer those questions will depend not simply on the science that will be available to us but on the conceptions of justice that will guide our actions. If the history of AIDS and the blood supply has taught us anything, it should be that both the effort to protect the blood system and to compensate those who may be its victims entail, at base, political determinations regarding the distribution of the social burdens of risk and uncertainty.

NOTES

1. Centers for Disease Control (CDC), "Pneumocystis Carinii Pneumonia among Persons with Hemophilia A," *Morbidity and Mortality Weekly Report* (July 16, 1982), pp. 365–367.

2. T. Murray, "The Poisoned Gift," *A Disease of Society: Cultural and Institutional Responses to* AIDS, eds. D. Nelkin, D. Willis and S. Paris (New York: Cambridge University Press, 1991).

3. H. Sapolsky and S. N. Finklestein, "Blood Policy Revisited: A New Look at the Gift Relationship," *The Public Interest* (Winter 1977), pp. 15–27.

4. The Office of Technology Assessment, *Blood Policy and Technology*, 1985.

5. H. M. Sapolsky and S. L. Boswell, "The History of Transfusion in AIDS: Practice and Policy Alternatives," *AIDS The Making of a Chronic Disease*, E. Fee, D. Fox eds. (Berkeley, CA: University of California Press, 1992), p. 176.

6. National Hemophilia Foundation, *Hemophilia Newsnotes*, "Hemophilia Patient Alert #1" (July 14, 1982).

7. *New York Native* (August 2–15, 1982), p.11.

8. Charles Carman and Louis Aledort, letter to William Dolan, November 2, 1982.

9. "Update on Acquired Immune Deficiency Syndrome (AIDS) Among Patients with Hemophilia A," *MMWR* (December 10, 1982), 644–652, and "Possible Transfusion-Associated Acquired Immune Deficiency Syndrome (AIDS) — California," *ibid.*, pp. 652–654.

10. *Ibid.*, p. 654.

11. William Dolan, letter to Louis Aledort, December 20, 1982.

12. *Advocate* (February 17, 1983), p. 9.

13. William Check, "Preventing AIDS Transmission: Should Blood Donors Be Screened," *Journal of the American Medical Association* (February 4, 1983), p. 569.

14. *Ibid.*, p. 568.

15. *Ibid.*

16. FDA Blood Products Advisory Committee, February 7–8, 1983.

17. James Allen, Interview, Briarcliff Manor, NY, March 31, 1988.

18. *Philadelphia Inquirer* (January 9, 1983), p.1.

19. R. Shilts, *And The Band Played On* (New York: St. Martin's Press, 1988).

20. *Philadelphia Inquirer* (January 9, 1983), p.1.

21. Interview.

22. American Association of Blood Banks, American Red Cross, and Council Community Blood Centers, "Joint Statement on Acquired Immune Deficiency (AIDS) Related to Transfusion," January 13, 1985, mimeo.

23. National Gay Task Force, press release, January 27, 1983.

24. Johanna Pindyk, interview, November 17, 1986.

25. American Association of Physicians for Human Rights. "The AAPHR Statement on AIDS and Blood Donation," February 19, 1983, mimeo.

26. CDC, "Prevention of Acquired Immune Deficiency Syndrome (AIDS) Report of Interagency Recommendations," *MMWR* (March 4, 1983), pp. 101–103.

27. *Ibid.*, p.102.

28. *Ibid.*

29. *Ibid.*

30. Director, Office of Biologics, National Center for Drugs and Biologics, Memorandum to All Establishments Collecting Blood for Transfusions, March 24, 1983.

31. Subcommittee of the Committee on Government Operations, House of Representatives, 98th Congress, First Session, August 1 and 2, 1983, pp. 162–163.

32. *Ibid.*

33. Joint Statement of the American Red Cross, Council of Community Blood Centers, American Association of Blood Banks, June 22, 1983.

34. J. Curran, et al., "Acquired Immunodeficiency Syndrome (AIDS) Associated with Transfusions," *New England Journal of Medicine* (January 12, 1984), pp. 69–75.

35. R. Parloff, "Tainted Tort," *The American Lawyer* (September, 1992), pp. 76–81.

36. John C. Petricciani, letter to Marietta Carr, May 8, 1983.

37. See M. Rodell "Hepatitis B Core Antibody Testing Study Group," *Plasma Quarterly* (Fall 1984).

38. James J. Goedert, letter to Lauren Leveton, August 22, 1994.

39. William M. Coenen, letter to Lauren Leveton, August 10, 1994.

40. Hemophilia Newsnotes Medical Bulletin, Chapter Advisory 7, May 11, 1981.

41. Hemophilia Information Exchange, AIDS Update, Advisory 11, November 2, 1983.

42. FDA Blood Products Advisory Committee, July 19, 1993, minutes, p. 106.

43. Dennis Donohue, memorandum to John C. Petrucciani, "Results of the Blood Products Advisory Committee Meeting Related to the Safety of Plasma Derivatives," July 21, 1983.

44. "Donor Restraint Urged; Recall of Tainted Blood is Opposed," *Washington Post* (July 23, 1983), p. A6.

45. June Osborn, "Public Health Considerations and Trade-Offs," *Proceedings, the Nation's Blood Supply: Is Absolute Safety Achievable?*" November 1, 1989, National Academy of Sciences.

46. Institute of Medicine, *HIV and the Blood Supply* (Washington D.C: National Academy Press, 1995), p. 85.

47. *Ibid.*, p. 93.

48. *Ibid.*, p. 87.

49. *Ibid.*, p. 92.

50. Hemophilia Information Network, Medical Bulletin 15, Chapter Advisory 20, October 13, 1984.

51. J. Epstein testimony, hearing before the Subcommittee on Oversight and Investigation of the Committee on Energy and Commerce, House of Representatives, 103rd Congress, First Session, July 18, 1993, p. 34.

52. "Conference on AIDS, Ethics and the Blood Supply," *Proceedings* eds., R. Bayer, N. Holland, E. Simon (American Blood Commission, 1985).

53. C. Marwick, "Blood Banks Give HTLV III Test Positive Approval at Five Months," *Journal of the American Medical Assocation* (October 4, 1985), p. 1681.

54. D. Korner, P. Rosenberg, L. M. Aledort, et al., "HIV-I Infection Incidence Among Persons with Hemophilia in the United States and Western Europe, 1978–1990," *Journal of Acquired Immune Deficiency Syndrome*, 7 (1994):279–286.

55. C. E. Stevens, "Human Immunodeficiency Virus Transmission Through Blood, Blood Products and Tissue and Organ Donation" *AIDS: Biology, Diagnosis, Treatment and Prevention*, 4th Ed., eds. V. T. DeVita, S. Hellman, and S. A. Rosenberg (New York: Lippincott-Raven 1996).

56. T. A. Peterson, K. J. Lui, W. Lawrence and J. R. Allen, "Estimating the Risks of Transfusion- Associated Acquired Immune Deficiency Syndrome and Human Immunodeficiency Virus Infection," *Transfusion*, 27(5) (Sept.–Oct. 1982), pp. 371–373.

57. M. P. Busch, M. J. Young, S. M. Sanson, et al., "Risk of Human Immunodeficiency Virus (HIV) Transmission by Blood Transfusions Before the Implementation of HIV-I Antibody Screening, *Transfusion*, 31(14) (1991), p. 11.

58. P. T. Westfall, "Hepatitis, AIDS and the Blood Product Exemption from Strict Product Liability in California," *Hastings Law Journal* V. 37, p. 1109.

59. D. L. Russo, "Blood Bank Liability to Recipients of HIV Contaminated Blood," *University of Dayton Law Review*, 18(1) (1992), p. 92.

60. R. D. Eckert, "The AIDS Blood-Transfusion Cases: A Legal and Economic Analysis of Liability," *San Diego Law Review* (Spring 1992).

61. IOM, *op. cit.*, p. 48.

62. J. R. Talavera, "Quintana v. United Blood Services: Examining Industry Practices in Transfusion-Related AIDS Cases," *Cornell Journal of Law and Public Policy*, 2 (1993), p. 495.

63. C. Kelley and J. P. Barber, "Legal Issues in Transfusion Medicine: Is Blood Banking a Medical Profession?" *Selected Topics in Laboratory Medicine*, 12 (4), (1992), p. 832.

64. J. M. Kern and B. B. Croy, "A Review of Transfusion-Associated AIDS Litigation, 1984–1993," *Transfusion*, 34:6 (1994), pp. 484–91.

65. D. Stevens, "Negligence Liability for Transfusion-Associated AIDS Transmission," *Journal of Legal Medicine*, 12 (1991), pp. 221–241.

66. Kelly and Barber, *op cit.* p. 819.

67. M. P. Rosenberg "Causes and Effects of the Hemophelia/AIDS Epidemic" *Action Now* (May 1992).

68. M. P. Rosenberg, "Addressing Alienation in the Hemophilia Community: The Time for Business as Usual Has Passed," mimeo [ND].

69. M. P. Rosenberg, "It is Time for an Investigation by Congress," *Action Now* (May 1992).

70. Senator Edward M. Kennedy, Bob Graham, Porter Goss, letter to Secretary Donna Shalala, April 27, 1993.

71. Donna Shalala, letter to Porter Goss, July 1, 1993.

72. Institute of Medicine, "Study of HIV Transmission to Hemophiliacs Through Blood Products," work statement, mimeo.

73. R. Shilts, *op. cit.*

74. *Blood Supply Safety*, "Hearing before the Subcommittee on Oversight and Investigation of the Committee on Energy and Commerce, House of Representatives, 103rd Congress, First Session, July 28, 1993, p. 20.

75. *Ibid.*, p. 21.

76. *Ibid.*, p. 21.

77. *Ibid.*, p. 22.

78. J. McCullough, "The Nation's Changing Blood Supply System," *JAMA* (May 5, 1993), p. 2239.

79. Transcript of meeting September 12, 1994—Committee to Study HIV Transmission Through Blood Products, U.S. Department of Commerce, National Technical Information Service.

80. *Ibid.*, p. 153.

81. President's Commission on the Acquired Immune Deficiency Syndrome Epidemic: Final Report (Washington, D.C., 1988), p.78.

82. IOM, *op. cit.*, p. 6

83. *Ibid.*, pp. 95–96.

84. *Ibid.*, p. 208.

85. *Ibid.*, p. 23.

86. *Ibid.*, pp. 218–222, 230.

87. *Ibid.*, p. 224.

88. "Statement of HHS Secretary Donna E. Shalala: Release of Report on H.I.V. and the Blood Supply." *HHS News.* July 13, 1995.

89. Abigail Trafford, "Second Opinion," *Washington Post* (September 19, 1995).

90. Alan Brownsten, memorandum to Charles Carman, March 21, 1988.

91. NHF Hemophilia/AIDS Financial Relief Plan: Guide, April 24, 1992, mimeo.

92. Don Goldman, memorandum to Ad Hoc Committee on Compensation, June 13, 1992.

93. Memorandum of the Ad Hoc Committee on Compensation adopted by the NHF Board of Directors, November 22, 1992, Atlanta, Georgia.

94. "Coburn Angry at Industry Rejection of SAC," *Action Now* (September 1993), p. 3.

95. "An Open Letter to the Hemophilia Community from the Community Advocacy Working Group, *The Common Factor* (April 1995), pp. 24–26.

96. Ricky Ray Hemophilia Relief Fund Act of 1995.

97. Mark Barnes, interview.

98. D. Shaw, "Gingrich Backs Bid to Pay $900 Million to HIV Infected Hemophiliacs," *Philadelphia Inquirer* (March 21, 1997).

99. "Certification: Moving Toward Social and Economic Justice," *The Common Factor* (September 1994), p. 33.

100. Deposition of A. Brownsten.

101. National Hemophilia Foundation, Board of Directors, October 31, 1985.

102. In the Matter of Rhane-Poulenc Rorer, Inc. 51 F.3d 1293 (7th cir. 1995), p. 1297.

103. *Ibid.*, p. 1300.

104. *Ibid.*, p. 1298.

105. *New York Times*, "Blood, Money and AIDS: Hemophiliacs are Spent, Liability Cases Bogged down in Dispute" (June 11, 1996), p. D1.

106. *New York Times* (April 19, 1996), p. D2.

107. Committee of Ten Thousand, *COTT Communiqué 11*, Legal Update, "Litigation or Settlement, What is in our Best Interests?"

108. "U.S.A. Hemophilia Settlement Garners 95 pct. Approval," Reuters, November 25, 1996.

109. Memorandum from David S. Shroger, head counsel to members of the hemophilia community participating in the settlement, December 18, 1996.

110. "Makers of Blood Products Settle U.S. HIV Suit," *The Lancet*, 349 (1997) p. 1459.

111. D. Shaw, "Settlement is Approved in Hemophiliacs Suit," *Philadelphia Inquirer* (May 7, 1997).

112. E. J. Lackritz, G. A. Salten, J. Aberle-Grasse, et al., "Estimated Risk of Transmission of the Human Immunodeficiency by Screened Blood in the United States, *"New England Journal of Medicine*, 333;26 (1996), pp. 1721–1725.

113. G. B. Schreiber, M. P. Busch, S. H. Kleinman, "The Risks of Transfusion-Transmitted Viral Infections," *New England Journal of Medicine*, 334;26 (1996), pp. 1685–1689.

114. E. M. Sloand, E. Pitt, H. G. Klein, "Safety of the Blood Supply," *Journal of the American Medical Association*, 274;27 (1995), pp. 1368–1373.

115. U.S. General Accounting Office, *Blood Supply Transfusion-Associated AIDS* (February 1997).

116. J. P. au Buchon, J. D. Birkmeyer, M. P. Busch, "Cost Effectiveness of Expanded Human Immunodeficiency Virus: Testing Protocols for Donated Blood," *Transfusion*, 37 (1997), pp. 45–51.

117. M. Busch, H. J. Alter (letter), *Transfusion*, 36 (1996), p. 382.

118. H. V. Fineberg, "Summation and Interpretation—Where Do We Go From Here?" *The Nation's Blood Supply: Is Absolute Safety Achievable?* Proceedings from a national conference held on November 1, 1989, at the National Academy of Sciences, Washington, D.C.

119. "Nations Blood Supply 'Never Been Safer' Though Survey Finds Wide Support for Greater Safety Measures," PRNewswire, July 10, 1997.

2

HIV and Blood in Japan
Transforming Private Conflict into Public Scandal

Eric A. Feldman

I n his classic 1971 book, *The Gift Relationship*, the English social theorist Richard Titmuss wrote:

> . . . in all cultures and societies, blood has been regarded as a vital, and often magical, life-sustaining fluid. . . . Men have been terrified by the sight of blood; they have killed each other for it; believed it could work miracles; and have preferred death rather than receive it from a member of a different ethnic group.[1]

The profound importance of blood, the symbolic weight and social meaning that Titmuss identifies as shared in all cultures, is illustrated by the fierce controversy caused by the distribution of HIV-contaminated blood products in Japan.

In July 1996, the Tokyo and Osaka District Courts supervised an out-of-court settlement that transformed Japanese hemophiliacs from the victims of corporate malevolence and greed into victors who achieved the most lucrative HIV/blood settlement in the industrialized world. The Ministry of Health and Welfare (MHW) and five pharmaceutical companies agreed to apologize for the HIV infection of 1800 Japanese hemophiliacs, and to pay each plaintiff 45 million yen (US$ 375,000).[2] That figure went well beyond the money paid to infected hemophiliacs in France, where government officials were jailed for their role in the HIV/blood scandal; it made the absence of any compensation in the United States look even more anomalous. What had once appeared to be a hopeless lawsuit by a group of marginalized and dying hemophiliacs became one of the most volatile medical and political scandals of the postwar era.

In many countries, the scapegoating of particular actors, the search for blame, and the identification of villains and victims are familiar reactions to conflicts over injuries caused by modern medicine. Examining such conflicts provides a window through which to observe the reactions of bureaucracy, the media, legal institutions, the public, and affected individuals. Conflicts over HIV-tainted blood are particularly revealing. They combine the symbolic freight of blood, the stigma of AIDS, the victimization of clearly identifiable groups, the power of big business, the regulatory responsibility of the state, and the risk and uncertainty of a new viral threat to public health policy.

Four aspects of Japan's HIV/blood scandal highlight its distinctiveness, and point to general tendencies in how contemporary conflicts over health are managed and resolved. They are the emphasis on the foreign causes of domestic crisis; the official focus on individual blame rather than on institutional failure; the perception that there is something unique about Japanese conflict; and the political inability to extract useful policy lessons from public conflicts. Each of these will be discussed in the conclusion, after the history of Japanese blood policy, and the complex contours of the conflict over HIV and blood, have been fully explored.

The Origin of Japan's Blood System

After Japan's defeat in World War II, Americans working as officials in the General Headquarters of the Allied Powers (GHQ) undertook the reform of many Japanese institutions. One of those reforms centered on the Japanese Ministry of Health and Welfare. Among the ordered changes at the MHW was the establishment of guidelines for blood safety, in part because of concern about syphilis infection from blood transfusions. In addition, GHQ officials pressed the Ministry to put the Japanese Red Cross Society (JRC), formed during the Meiji Period (1868–1912), in charge of blood services. An agreement between the MHW, the JRC, and the Japanese Medical Association (JMA) in 1949 affirmed that the JRC should be at the center of Japan's blood system, in part to emulate the role of the Red Cross in European countries.[3] Administrators of the JRC visited blood banks in the United States, and in 1952 the Japanese Red Cross Society Tokyo Blood Bank was opened.[4] Using a system of blood deposit and return, the JRC sought to make Japan self-sufficient and wholly dependent on non-remunerated donation. But an immediate conflict emerged with a new and rapidly growing industry: commercial blood banks.

Japan's commercial blood banks emerged from military contact with China. Occupying Manchuria before and during World War II, Japanese army units conducted research on biological and chemical warfare. As part of that research, it is well documented that Japanese scientists used human subjects in a series of experiments aimed at understanding the properties of blood. Most notorious among the army units was Unit 731.[5]

Manchuria served as a training ground for many of postwar Japan's elite scientists. Murata Ryosuke, for example, who conducted medical experimentation in Nanjing, went on to direct the National Institute of Health.[6] One scientist who rose to prominence was bacteriologist Naito Ryoichi, who returned to Japan after the war, was (like most of his colleagues) granted immunity in the Tokyo War Crimes Trials, and founded a company called the Nippon Blood Bank in 1950.[7] At almost the same time, commercial blood banks were opened in Yokosuka and Hiroshima. By 1957, 32 blood banks were operating in Japan.[8]

These blood banks operated as for-profit enterprises with paid donors. Newspapers at the time regularly described the pale and unhealthy individuals who made a living from selling their physical resources. Stories were told of long lines of the unemployed waiting to sell their blood, often weary, sometimes fainting because they had sold too frequently. The poorest lived beneath Tokyo's bridges, sleeping in straw baskets; those who died were thrown into the river.[9] The blood they sold, thin and lacking nutrients, came to be called "yellow blood." Such stories did not dampen enthusiasm for blood-selling, and the amount of blood collected in commercial centers increased dramatically in the 1950s.[10] Naito's technical knowledge of blood helped to make the Nippon Blood Bank a financial success. He continued his re-search during the 1960s at the University of Tokyo, where one of his assistants was Abe Takeshi, who would become leader of the AIDS Task Force.[11] In 1964, the Nippon Blood Bank changed its name to the Green Cross Company, which became Japan's largest pharmaceutical company.

Blood collection centers operated by the Japanese Red Cross, opening two years after the first commercial enterprises, found it difficult to compete with companies that paid blood donors. In 1952, the JRC's first year of operation, only 507 donations were received.[12] A conflict soon emerged between the JRC and the Nippon Blood Bank over whether blood should be treated as a pharmaceutical product by the MHW. Nippon Blood Bank pressed the ministry to consider blood a pharmaceutical, so that the ministry would reimburse physicians for the cost of whatever blood they used. As for all pharmaceuticals, the reimbursement rate would be higher than the cost, and blood would become a source of profit to doctors and hospitals. The alternative, pro-moted by the JRC, was to consider blood a body part, not a pharmaceutical product. This would erase the possibility of profiting from the purchase and sale of blood, and make the JRC the only feasible institution for blood collection and distribution.[13] Nippon Blood Bank prevailed, donations to the JRC decreased to 130 annually, and in 1955 it too began to purchase blood on a limited scale. Tension between the JRC and the Green Cross Company has continued to the present.

By 1960, when the 8th Congress of the International Society of Blood Transfu-sion and the 2nd International Conference of the Red Cross were both held in Tokyo, almost the entire blood supply in Japan was obtained commercially. Participants from abroad were openly critical of Japan's reliance on purchased blood.[14] At about the same time, students at Waseda University, an elite private school in Tokyo, organized in order to promote blood donation.[15] In 1964, Edwin Reischauer, U.S. ambassador to Japan, was attacked by a deranged youth in Tokyo and lost a considerable amount of blood from a stab wound. Rushed to a hospital and given an emergency transfu-sion, Reischauer contracted hepatitis. The embarrassment this caused in Japan led to a cabinet decision of August 21, 1964, that pressed for a nonremunerated, domes-tic blood system.[16] Only five years later, almost all whole blood used in Japan was obtained through donation.[17] Having thrived in the 1950s and early 1960s, commer-cial blood banks declined precipitously from the mid-1960s, and were almost gone by 1970.[18] The last commercial blood bank in Japan closed its doors in 1989.

The Japanese Red Cross may appear to have triumphed over the for-profit blood banks, but its victory was not complete. Just as the commercial blood banks were becoming obsolete in the domestic whole-blood market, advances in blood technol-ogy created a new niche for the blood companies. Like the Green Cross, those enter-prises had transformed themselves into pharmaceutical companies. They soon took control of products manufactured from blood for which the non-remunerated blood supply in Japan was inadequate. One of those products, cryoprecipitate, was approved by the MHW in 1970. Blood concentrates received ministry approval in 1978.[19] Each of these products changed the lives of Japanese hemophiliacs. Both were isolated from plasma collected primarily in the United States, where a commercial market ensured an adequate supply. Having moved away from a for-profit blood system domestically, Japan became wholly dependent on international, commercial sources for its supply of blood products. That fact would come to play a central role in the conflict over HIV-tainted blood in Japan.

The MHW gave its blessing to a blood system divided between whole blood and blood products by agreeing to consider blood products as pharmaceuticals. Like all other Japanese pharmaceutical products, products manufactured from blood are reimbursed at a price that is determined every two years by the Central Social Health Insurance Council (*Chuikyo*) of the MHW.[20] Physicians and hospitals are payed based on the cost of Japanese-made blood products. Because domestic products were significantly more expensive than imported products, this meant that inexpensive imported blood products were reimbursed at a generous level. And because a large percentage of the operating funds and profits of health care providers comes from their ability to reap the difference between the list price of medicine (reimbursed by the government) and the amount they actually pay for drugs (negotiated with pharmaceutical companies),[21] foreign blood products were a source of large profits for Japanese private-practice physicians and hospitals.[22]

Japan's First AIDS Case

In a nation where the phrase "Number One" (*ichiban*) has a moral connotation, the announcement of the first AIDS case became a symbol of how Japanese policy-makers regarded the victims of this new disease. During several closed-door sessions of the Ministry of Health and Welfare's AIDS Task Force (*AIDS Kenkyu Han*) in 1983, there was extensive discussion over how the symptoms of an ill hemophiliac should be interpreted. The question before the Task Force was whether the hemophiliac was Japan's first AIDS patient.

Dr. Abe Takeshi was the hemophiliac's physician and chairman of the Task Force. Abe believed that his patient displayed a number of AIDS-like symptoms, and these were discussed at a Task Force meeting. Because of various medical complications with the case, the Task Force consulted with scientists from the U.S. Centers for Disease Control (CDC). The CDC experts reviewed the medical records and were unanimous; they believed that Abe's patient had died of AIDS.[23] When the Task Force discussed the case a second time, it still could not reach a consensus that AIDS should be declared the cause of death.

Never did the ministry acknowledge that it had considered but rejected a hemophiliac candidate as Japan's AIDS case number one.[24] Nor did the ministry issue a warning that Japanese hemophiliacs may have been at risk for getting AIDS from the blood products they used to control their clotting. The Task Force's failure to acknowledge that AIDS was infecting Japanese hemophiliacs helped to ignite the controversy over HIV and blood in Japan that emerged over the following decade.

Not until March 1985 did the MHW announce Japan's first AIDS case. The patient was an artist, not a salaried worker; a Japanese national living in the United States, not Japan; an "outsider," not a "normal" Japanese.[25] The "foreign" nature of HIV in Japan was emphasized.

There is some irony to the outcome of the Task Force's decision to demur from identifying a hemophiliac as the first Japanese with AIDS. If the intended result was to draw attention away from government policy, place blame for AIDS on individual behavior, and delay the recognition that many Japanese hemophiliacs were infected because they used contaminated blood products, it succeeded, but only temporarily. Ultimately, the decision returned to haunt the MHW. It exposed the ministry to criticism that those with decision-making power were indifferent to the value of hemophiliac lives. It lent credence to claims about the close relationship between the ministry and pharmaceutical companies, which were profiting from the sale of contaminated blood products. It underscored the importance of reevaluating a wide range of accepted practices, such as the ministry's supervision of clinical trials and its use of external advisory committees. The failure to identify a hemophiliac as Japan's first AIDS victim—whether intentional or unintentional—was the spark that eventually led to a torrent of criticism that caused the transformation of a medical tragedy into a political scandal.

The "Coming Out" of Hemophiliacs

Of the approximately 5000 hemophiliacs in Japan, about 40%, or 2000, are HIV-positive.[26] With fewer than 2000 reported cases of AIDS in Japan, and under 5000 people who have tested HIV-positive, hemophiliacs represent the largest group to be affected by the disease. For hemophiliacs, a high rate of HIV infection is only their most recent burden. In addition to the physical pain and disability hemophilia can cause, hemophiliacs have also long suffered from social prejudice resulting from their medical condition. Before the era of AIDS, hemophiliacs were often excluded from schools and jobs.[27] AIDS has exacerbated such tendencies. Teachers have demanded that hemophiliac children bring evidence to school stating that they are not HIV-positive. Classmates have taunted those with hemophilia, saying "you are an AIDS patient."[28] Some employers have required adults to provide copies of HIV test results. Neighbors have shunned hemophiliacs whom they previously accepted.[29] A survey by the Friends of Hemophilia Society in Kyoto found that hemophiliacs are routinely turned away by dentists, internists, surgeons, and pediatricians.[30]

Before and since the onset of AIDS, such adversity served as a unifying factor. Special camps operated for children. Newsletters provided information about health and recreation. Organizations like the Friends of Hemophilia Society offered a friendly refuge from social prejudice. Like hemophilia groups in many nations, these associations for Japanese hemophiliacs were once led by physicians and pharmaceutical companies that promoted medication and new treatment techniques at gatherings they helped to finance. But as evidence mounted internationally about the possible transmission of AIDS through blood and blood products, and hemophiliacs perceived the medical and social threat of AIDS, they decided that their interests were no longer served by medical leadership.[31]

By the late 1980s, hemophiliacs discovered that many among them were infected with HIV. They surveyed the landscape for appropriate villains on whom to blame their misfortune. Some may have felt anger at their private physicians, but accusations against individuals were limited by the fact that hemophiliacs remained deeply dependent on them for continuing medical care. More easily vilified were officials at powerful medical institutions like the MHW and pharmaceutical companies. In addition, hemophiliacs, their physicians, and blood policy officials identified a common culprit; blood products imported from the United States. There would ensue violent disagreement among these parties about the culpability of Japanese actors. But none questioned the conclusion that Japanese dependence on foreign blood products was a fundamental policy misstep that led to a domestic iatrogenic tragedy.

The quick-to-mobilize hemophiliacs stood in stark contrast to the lack of political organization that has characterized gay groups in Japan. There is a long history of homosexuality in Japan, but it is relations between individuals, not group action, that prevails. Membership in gay organizations is small, and most such groups operate without budgets or publicity.[32] Therefore, unlike the gay population in the United States, for which the emergence of HIV/AIDS served as a call to arms, in Japan the gay community has not become politicized as a result of HIV. In part, this results from the epidemiology of HIV in Japan, in which gay men are far less prominent than hemophiliacs. Japanese hemophiliacs, not men who have sex with men, came to be identified with AIDS.[33] The Japanese gay population took refuge behind the many HIV-infected hemophiliacs; their organizations forged an identity that emphasized Japaneseness, not sexual preference. For many, safe sex came to mean relations among Japanese men only, and avoiding "unsafe" Westerners was the "prevention" strategy of choice. By the early 1990s, nine of the ten gay saunas in Tokyo's most active gay entertainment district prohibited entry to foreigners.[34] Apparently less alarmed by the medical than the social risks posed by HIV, gay men and their organizations have been almost invisible in debates over Japanese AIDS policy.

The absence of gay groups in the policy-making arena made the activities of hemophilia groups especially visible. Even before AIDS legislation was announced in February 1987, a preliminary draft was leaked to the press, and hemophilia groups editorialized in Japan's mass circulation *Asahi Shimbun* that the legislation would violate the rights of those who were already victims of pharmaceutical products.[35] On February 19, 1987, a MHW draft law was distributed to the press.[36] It included a reporting requirement for all people with HIV or AIDS, and penalties for individuals with AIDS or HIV infection who engaged in unsafe sexual acts or donated blood.[37]

Hemophilia groups quickly criticized the bill as failing to protect the right to privacy of AIDS sufferers.[38] Groups representing hemophiliacs also claimed that the bill would bolster the general public prejudice and discrimination against those with genetic defects, especially hemophiliacs. Three weeks later, the Social Affairs Subcommittee of the Liberal Democratic Party approved an amended version of the AIDS law.[39] Hemophiliacs again aggressively attacked the bill.[40] Matsuda Juzo, professor of medicine at Teikyo University, stated:

> I am afraid the legislation would be targeted 99.9 percent at hemophiliacs. In addition to the congenital handicap, they may even be ostracized from society.[41]

When the AIDS Prevention Law was finally discussed in the Diet in 1988, one change made in committee stood out as particularly significant. It read: "[C]ases of HIV-positive persons infected through blood products (hemophiliacs) do not have to be reported to the government." The exemption in part resulted from the relationship forged between hemophiliac groups and the MHW official largely responsible for writing the legislation. He was consulted by the Social and Welfare Committee during its hearings, and suggested reforms to the proposed AIDS law to make it palatable to hemophilia groups but acceptable to the government.[42]

Exclusion from most provisions of the bill, however, did not appease hemophiliacs. To a great extent, exclusion failed to address their most import concerns: financial compensation, better medical care, and freedom from discrimination. Before the bill was passed, many HIV-positive hemophiliacs had received treatment at health care facilities, where their identities became known and their HIV status was reported to prefectural health authorities. Invisibility was no longer a viable option.

More significantly, hemophiliacs increasingly emphasized that the AIDS Prevention Law specified no distinctions between individuals with AIDS, despite hemophiliacs being the "innocent" victims of bad blood. Such a view was reinforced by two prominent members of the 1983 MHW AIDS Task Force. Shiokawa Yuichi put the matter baldly: "[Y]ou don't get infected [by HIV] if you live a sound life."[43] Abe Takeshi expressed a similar view: "[H]emophiliacs keep their lives very nice."[44] When Shiokawa and Abe were called to testify before the Diet in 1996 about their roles in the decision to continue importing unheated blood products, they were no longer so vocal in their praise of hemophiliacs.

The "Fourth Route"

During the decade following the announcement of the first case of AIDS in Japan, not a single case of HIV transmission through whole blood was reported. It was an anomalous statistic, and one that highlighted the relative safety of domestic whole blood in contrast to imported, contaminated blood products. In the United States and many other countries, the proportion of HIV-infected hemophiliacs was similar to that of Japan, but in gross numbers there were far more non-hemophiliacs infected with HIV through whole blood. But in Japan, with a 40% rate of infection among hemophiliacs, the first non-hemophiliac case of HIV infection through blood was not announced until June 1994. Even then, it was blood products, not whole blood, that were to blame.

Only weeks before the 1994 International AIDS Conference in Yokohama, the case of a Japanese infant infected by unheated blood products used to treat hemorrhaging was reported.[45] The MHW commissioned a study to explore the extent of such cases, and sent questionnaires to 1300 hospitals with pediatric wards. Of the approximately 700 that responded, the ministry learned that 37 of them had given unheated, imported blood products to at least 188 hospital patients.[46] By June 1995, only three HIV cases were confirmed, all the result of blood products administered to infants. The following month, an adult treated with blood products during surgery joined the short list of victims. When he died several months later, his family filed suit against the government and Green Cross, the supplier of his contaminated blood product, in the Osaka District Court. They contended that he was infected in April 1986, when heated products were already available.

These four cases were dubbed by the media "fourth route" (*dai yon rūto*) infections. Along with unprotected sex, mother to fetus, and hemophilia-related routes of HIV transmission, infection through blood and blood products administered as part of medical treatment or surgery in Japan claimed its own epidemiological category.[47] Within a month, the number of recognized fourth-route victims had increased to 17. Four of them were infected by blood collected domestically, presumably before November 1986, when blood screening was introduced.[48] The ministry reissued its questionnaire to more hospitals, and revealed that 91 used unheated blood products to treat far more patients than was previously believed. One was a woman treated after ovarian surgery. She promptly sued the government and pharmaceutical companies for 145 million yen (US$ 1.2 million). Other cases will undoubtedly emerge. As a MHW committee continued to investigate fourth-route infections in spring 1996, 1200 hospitals were found to have used imported, unheated blood products. For the first time, the ministry discussed identifying the consumers of such products and implementing measures to limit further transmission from those unknowingly infected.

Compensating Hemophiliacs

Persistent lobbying by the hemophilia associations helped them to create a working relationship with MHW officials and others involved with the AIDS bill. Hemophiliacs understood that they would be unable to prevent the eventual passage of the legislation. But they continued to assert their right to compensation, in order to gain concessions from the government. In turn, the government was searching for a way to partially satisfy, and thus silence, the group most critical of the proposed law. What resulted was a system through which hemophiliacs affected by AIDS would be given financial relief as a way to lessen the sting when the AIDS bill became law, a method of carrot-and-stick compromise called *ame to muchi*, literally "candy and a whip."

On April 16, 1988, the Ministry of Health and Welfare announced the establishment of a relief scheme (*HIV Kansen Higai Kyusai Seido*) for hemophiliacs, to be implemented January 1, 1989. Payments to the fund were gathered by a section of the MHW's Pharmaceutical Affairs Bureau, Biologics and Antibiotics (*Seibutsu Seizaika*), responsible for the management of blood clotting factor. Bureaucrats in that section approached the companies selling imported blood products in Japan and persuaded them to contribute. This was not difficult, given the close ties between the MHW and the pharmaceutical industry.

The relief system was modeled after a scheme designed to compensate those who suffered from iatrogenic diseases such as SMON (subacute myelo-optico neuropathy, a neurological disorder). SMON's etiology was eventually attributed to a stomach medication, and litigation from 1971 into the 1980s resulted in a finding that the government and pharmaceutical companies had been negligent in permitting its use.[49] One result of the SMON litigation was to emphasize the MHW's duty—moral and legal—to confirm the safety of medication. Another result was the creation of an Adverse Drug Reaction Fund, which operates with drug company donations.[50] By 1995, for example, the Fund had paid 4.7 billion yen (US$ 37.5 million) in compensation to 1714 victims of thalidomide.[51] The Fund explicitly excluded liability for injury caused by blood or blood products.

Beneficiaries of the blood compensation scheme were separated into two general groups. One, HIV-positive people who were infected by blood-clotting drugs, had AIDS-related symptoms, and had stayed in the hospital for more than eight days received 29,000 yen/month (US$ 242.00) for an indefinite period of time. The other, those with a diagnosis of full-blown AIDS, received varying amounts. Persons under 18 years old received 85,600 yen/month (US$ 713.00), and those over 18 got 208,900 yen (US$ 1740.00) monthly. Families who lost a hemophiliac family member to AIDS received a flat sum of 5,648,400 yen (US$ 47,070) if the victim was not the primary breadwinner, and 156,900 yen/month (US$ 1307.50) for up to 10 years, less the time the person received money as a patient, if the person was the primary breadwinner. Initially, asymptomatic HIV-positive individuals received no compensation.

In late 1993, after a series of negotiations, the MHW agreed to pay a subsidy to HIV-positive spouses of people infected by imported, tainted blood products. Beginning in April 1994, the approximately 30 affected spouses who qualified for the program received the same compensation as HIV-infected hemophiliacs with AIDS-related symptoms, 33,000 yen/month (US$ 275.00).[52]

Immediately following passage of the AIDS Prevention Law, and implementation of the compensation scheme, hemophiliacs intensified their demands for an official apology. They viewed financial relief as small consolation for having been infected with HIV. Hemophiliacs had tried unsuccessfully to have the government admit its culpability in the distribution of tainted blood, insisting that the ministry describe the payment scheme with the Japanese words *isharyo* or *hosho*, implying an admission of fault and an apology, rather than *kyusai*, which lacks a moral dimension.

The ministry steadfastly denied its responsibility for infecting hemophiliacs, and hemophiliacs intensified their claims of rights infringement, and their demands for an apology. They then went to court, in two groups that eventually included almost two hundred plaintiffs, claiming that the Ministry of Health and Welfare, and five pharmaceutical companies, had been negligent in distributing HIV-tainted blood. The hemophiliacs demanded an apology, as well as a large cash settlement.

Blood in the Courts

The Claim

On October 27, 1989, a group of HIV-positive hemophiliacs and family members of hemophiliacs who died of AIDS filed a lawsuit in the Tokyo District Court. Over the next several years, additional plaintiffs were added, and a similar case was presented to the Osaka District Court.[53] Plaintiffs were organized into several associations (*HIV Sosho o Sasaeru Kai*, for example) modeled on Japanese citizens' movements of the 1970s. Emphasizing the importance of effective legal and political action, and of mobilizing a large citizens' movement, an attorney presenting oral arguments in the Tokyo District Court harkened back to SMON and stated, "I think that we have learned on other occasions that rights will not be bestowed from above if we are silent."[54] At the helm of the Tokyo attorneys' group was Suzuki Toshihiro, a central figure in the movement to legislate patients' rights. Defendants were five pharmaceutical companies—Green Cross Corporation, Cutter Japan, Baxter Corporation, Bayer, and Nippon Zoki Pharmaceutical Corporation—as well as the Ministry of Health and Welfare.[55]

The central issue in the litigation was whether the defendants were negligent in importing and distributing blood concentrates that led to the seroconversion of many Japanese hemophiliacs. Plaintiffs highlighted the long period between the emergence of technical knowledge in the United States about the connection between blood and HIV, and the termination in Japan of the distribution of unheated, contaminated blood products—in July 1985 for factor VIII, and in November 1985 for factor IX.[56] Each plaintiff demanded 115 million yen (US$ 958,333), including a 15 million yen (US$ 125,000) attorney's fee. Damages were sought for being infected with HIV, suffering from AIDS, and social discrimination. In the pleadings, several major elements of negligence—causality, foreseeability, and avoidability—were vigorously contested.

Causality

The skeleton of the plaintiff's claim was (1) there was a high risk of HIV infection from imported U.S. blood products; (2) the injured parties used those products; and (3) after using them, plaintiffs became infected.[57] Unfortunately for the plaintiffs, their claim was complicated by the existence of five corporate defendants, each of which sold almost identical blood concentrates. Most plaintiffs used the products of different companies at different times. The defendants thus claimed, for example, that if the products of companies x and y were used in 1979 and 1980, and those of company z were used in 1983, since the first AIDS case was reported in 1981, only company z is responsible for the HIV infection.

In response, plaintiffs argued that the HIV virus is complex and unpredictable, but that should not absolve x and y of responsibility. Although AIDS was not recognized until 1981, the virus was surely present in the late 1970s. They pressed the court to accept a theory of multiple infection, or alternative liability, under which all companies supplying blood concentrates from the late 1970s would be held responsible for any subsequent infection. A critical question before the courts, therefore, was how to handle the possibility of multiple infection, and how to parcel out fault, at a time when AIDS was not yet a known disease.

Foreseeability

The most vexing issue in the litigation was whether the defendants could have foreseen the injury caused to the plaintiffs. Even the plaintiffs concede that in the 1970s no one could have foreseen the possibility of HIV infection, because HIV was unknown. Instead, they highlighted the inherent dangerousness of non-Japanese blood products, underscoring the tendency of Japanese blood authorities to focus on the "foreign" causes of HIV contamination in Japan. Conditions inherent in the collection and distribution of American blood products, they claimed, made it foreseeable that some disease-causing virus would be transmitted.[58] At the very least, they asserted that "with regard to HIV contamination specifically, they [drug companies and the MHW] could have forecasted in July 1982 [when the CDC identified three hemophiliacs with AIDS] the risk that the [imported] concentrates might have contained a new life-threatening pathogen, which was afterwards called HIV."[59]

One attorney for the plaintiffs pointed out a blood collection center in San Francisco's Castro district. It was described as a despondent, unsanitary gathering place where 10% of donors were "homos,"[60] many others black or Mexican. Similarly, a Japan National Broadcasting (NHK) report emphasized that some blood plasma used to make concentrates in the United States came from centers in South and Central America, where different blood samples were combined in plastic bags and left on dirty floors.[61] In addition, it was claimed that imported blood is more infectious than local blood, because a virus that is dormant in one area can become infectious somewhere else.[62]

Even before the plaintiffs filed their legal papers, both houses of the Diet passed Resolutions calling for domestic self-sufficiency in blood products in 1988, and the MHW initiated the New Committee for the Study of the Promotion of the Blood Program in 1989. One result of the Ministry investigation was its directive to the Japan Hospital Association and two other hospital organizations to give priority to blood products manufactured domestically, despite the greater profits from using foreign-made blood.[63] The Japanese Red Cross concluded that "this dependence on importation for plasma derivatives presents problems from the standpoints of ethics, safety, and stability of supply. . . . "[64] Still, in 1991, only 24.4% of plasma derivatives used in Japan came from domestic blood. The remainder continued to be imported from the United States until the mid-1990s.

Avoidability

Even if HIV infection could have been foreseen, the question remains whether it could have been avoided. Here, the disagreement between plaintiffs and defendants was technical. All parties agreed that hemophiliacs required a steady supply of blood-based medication for their disease, so that defendants could not have stopped distributing all blood products. But there was disagreement about what constituted effective medication. Plaintiffs contended that cryoprecipitate, manufactured from Japanese blood supplies, was an adequate treatment, particularly because HIV infection and the death of many people was a foreseeable consequence of distributing concentrates made from imported blood. Medical experts were divided, though several testified on the plaintiffs' behalf.[65] Plaintiffs argued that the MHW should have stopped importing and using concentrates at the latest by July 1982, and instead should have utilized domestic cryo supplies.

The Response

Defendants in the litigation, joined by their role in a common human tragedy, had deeply divided interests. Tension between the pharmaceutical companies and the Ministry of Health and Welfare, for example, resulted from the funding of the 1989 compensation scheme for hemophiliacs. While the ministry had obtained financial donations from the five pharmaceutical company defendants, the government itself made no financial contributions. Instead, the MHW considered the administration of compensation claims and payments an in-kind contribution that obviated the need for government funding.

Another source of tension, between foreign and domestic pharmaceutical companies, resulted from the different technology they possessed for heat-treating blood products. Baxter, the first company to receive FDA approval to market heated products in the United States (in 1983), was also the first to apply to the MHW for permission to sell heated products in Japan. In the early 1980s, Baxter's share of the Japanese factor VIII market was, on average, less than 20%, whereas the Green Cross controlled over half of the market. Companies like the Green Cross that did not yet manufacture heated product were not anxious for the MHW to allow Baxter's application. It is possible that their desire to retain market share and use up their stockpiles of unheated blood products may have led them to lobby against Baxter's application.

Linked by the lawsuit, however, defendants made a strategic decision primarily to present a unified defense. In doing so, they relied on two general arguments. First, pharmaceutical companies emphasized that scientific knowledge in the early 1980s of the as-yet-unidentified etiologic agent that caused AIDS was ambiguous, so it was justifiable to continue importing and distributing foreign blood products. Second, the MHW highlighted aspects of the regulatory system designed to safeguard the Japanese public from dangerous products, and claimed that the delays caused by the system were intended to ensure the safety of heated products.[66]

With regard to limited scientific knowledge, defendants emphasized that in July 1982, when the first cases of hemophiliacs with a new and deadly disease were reported by the U.S. Centers for Disease Control, no one in the world knew how the disease was spread, whether or not it was a virus, whether it was always deadly, or how to detect it. Not until April 1984 was HIV identified; only in March 1985 was a test developed that could detect HIV in blood.[67]

It was argued by the defendants that they kept apprised of, and participated in, the work of the international scientific community with regard to identifying HIV and developing techniques to secure the safety of blood products. When convinced of product safety, they began using them in Japan.[68] As explained by a ministry official in the late 1980s,

> With regard to the danger posed by imported blood products, there was really nothing else that could be used for the medical treatment of hemophiliacs. If we stopped importing and using it, there was the possibility of a real disaster . . . AIDS was discovered in America in 1981. Before that, even in Japan, there was the AIDS virus. We didn't know that blood products were a cause of AIDS, we didn't even know about AIDS.[69]

From this perspective, the distribution of tainted blood products to Japan's hemophiliacs was a tragedy, but an unavoidable one, given the state of scientific knowledge.

In addition to knowledge limitations, defendants also highlighted the legal and regulatory system as presenting reasonable limits to ministry action. In the early 1980s, as evidence accumulated in the United States of a new disease, possibly a virus, possibly spread through blood and blood products, responsibility for blood in Japan was divided. The Japanese Red Cross collected and distributed whole blood in Japan, while blood products were under the control of the Green Cross and other pharmaceutical companies. Since pharmaceutical companies were importing and distributing blood products purchased from donors in the United States, responsibility fell to the MHW to oversee and license their activities.

Even after the U.S. FDA approved the sale of heat-treated blood products, Japanese regulators remained cautious. Ministry officials claimed that research on the heat-treating of blood in the United States was inadequate. They analogized blood factors, which are proteins, to eggs, also proteins. After an egg is boiled, explained one bureaucrat in the Pharmaceutical Affairs Research Bureau, the outside retains a shape identical to a raw egg, even though the inside has changed. Concern that blood could go through a similar transformation was said to have led the ministry to conduct its own extensive tests before approving heat-treated products.[70]

What would be described by critics as the ministry's excessive caution emanates in part from its legal responsibility to ensure the safety of all drugs it approves for distribution, sale, and use, and the numerous accusations that Japan leads the industrialized world in "drug-induced tragedies."[71] The SMON incident, for example, contributed to a general public distrust of the Ministry of Health and Welfare, and the ministry's awareness of its public relations troubles. One plaintiff stated that he joined the HIV litigation because of the hypocrisy of the MHW, which claimed to keep AIDS out of Japan with the AIDS Prevention Law but in fact imported it via tainted blood.[72] Like swine flu in the United States, which contributed to a cautious institutional culture at the CDC and affected its actions toward HIV and the blood supply,[73] SMON and other iatrogenic diseases in Japan were partially responsible for the hesitancy of the MHW to move quickly in approving heated blood products.

Like the U.S. FDA, the Pharmaceutical Affairs Bureau of the MHW is charged with responsibility for overseeing the safety of pharmaceutical products.[74] Before 1967, most drugs could be imported and marketed in Japan without domestic clinical trials. Foreign products did not require trials because such products were not considered "new drugs" and could be rapidly approved.[75] Revision of the Pharmaceutical Affairs Law in 1979, a consequence of the many lawsuits filed because of drug side effects, resulted in the establishment of a compensation system and articulated a domestic approval process for pharmaceutical products. From 1979 until 1986, when the law was again revised, foreign clinical trials to demonstrate the safety and efficacy of new drugs were not accepted; all trials had to be conducted in Japan, on native Japanese.[76] Exceptions could be made for drugs that were not "new." But ministry officials limited such exceptions to cosmetic changes in the packaging or presentation of a pharmaceutical. While plaintiffs asserted that the heating of blood products did not make them different from unheated products, MHW bureaucrats insisted that heated products were "new" and required evaluation.[77]

Determining the level of scientific evidence required for a drug to be deemed safe and effective, oversight of research and testing protocols, regulating the pricing and dispensing of drugs—all stretched the level of manpower and expertise of the MHW. The Biologics and Antibiotics Division of the MHW, for example, which had authority to make decisions about blood products, employed fewer than a dozen professionals. Highlighting these various institutional features, the defendants in retrospect justified waiting until testing was completed in 1985 to approve heated blood products.

Plaintiffs countered that the MHW delayed the approval of heated blood products in Japan for reasons that had nothing to do with ambiguous information about HIV transmission through blood, or with a regulatory process designed to protect the public. Rather, they claimed that the ministry and the private sector negligently distributed contaminated blood because of a corrupt relationship between MHW officials and the companies they were entrusted to regulate. That relationship featured a reliance on advisory committees (*shingikai*) dominated by individuals who had a financial interest in the outcome of ministry decisions; employment patterns that led many former government officials to accept lucrative positions in the pharmaceutical industry; and bureaucratic norms that encouraged the MHW to consider the market share of domestic companies a relevant factor in regulatory decisions. Each of these became increasingly contentious as the lawsuit proceeded, slowly, through the courts.

The Settlement

Plaintiff Pressure and a Court Proposal

The institutional framework of litigation in Japan, particularly the protracted court process, made it unlikely that the 1989 HIV lawsuits would be decided in less than a decade. As the legal process continued, strains and tensions began to take their toll; bickering between the Osaka and Tokyo plaintiffs over strategy and goals threatened to undermine the solidarity of the litigants. Many plaintiffs were HIV-positive and could not endure a lengthy lawsuit; almost one third of the original plaintiffs had died by 1995. Arguments in the Tokyo and Osaka District Courts ended in May and July, 1995, respectively; decisions were expected six months later. There was little doubt that any verdict would be appealed immediately.

As the Tokyo District Court judges prepared their opinion, the activities of the plaintiff's support groups escalated. Suddenly, shifts in national politics, brought about by the Liberal Democratic Party's (LDP) 1993 loss of a majority of seats in the Diet for the first time in over three decades, became a factor in the bad blood controversy. Until 1995, the coalition government had maintained a hard line, and was able to keep control of the MHW. The entire HIV-tainted blood episode took place during the rule of the LDP, and politicians from that party were predictably wary of accepting responsibility for spreading HIV infection. But that position softened when a new Health and Welfare Minister, Mori Churyo, was appointed in August by Prime Minister Murayama of the Social Democratic Party of Japan (SDP), formerly the Socialist Party.

Mori wasted little time in announcing that he would consider a compromise solution to the litigation if it were recommended by the courts.[78] Soon after, in October 1995, what had seemed a typically lengthy legal battle took a turn. The Tokyo and Osaka District Courts jointly recommended an out-of-court settlement in which each plaintiff would receive 45 million yen (US$ 375,000), with payment divided 60/40 between the pharmaceutical companies and the government. In comparison to settlements in the SMON and thalidomide cases, where the government was ordered to pay one third and the drug companies two thirds, the allocation of payments suggested that the court considered the government particularly culpable.[79] The recommended payments would be the largest ever in a Japanese pharmaceutical-related case, more than HIV-infected hemophiliacs received in any other nation.[80]

In the written settlement proposal, the courts justified their recommendation by declaring their sympathy for infected hemophiliacs. As victims of discrimination, unable to receive care for HIV infection, fearful of disclosing their names and addresses, the courts wrote that hemophiliacs were dying from a tragedy for which they bore no responsibility.[81] Under the Pharmaceutical Affairs Law, the Ministry of Health and Welfare was responsible for protecting Japanese citizens from drug side effects, and the manufacturers of pharmaceuticals were responsible for selling safe products. Together, according to the courts, the ministry and the companies should have undertaken at least one of three possible interventions: provide information about the potential danger of unheated blood products; promote alternative therapies, such as cryoprecipitate, imported heated products, or the emergency manufacture of domestic blood products; or stop selling unheated products.[82] Because the defendants knew the risks posed by contaminated blood but pursued none of these options, the courts suggested that they accept responsibility and voluntarily settle the case.

It did not take long for each defendant to agree to participate in settlement negotiations. Although the Tokyo and Osaka Courts had not rendered a specific opinion on the plaintiffs' negligence claim, the language of the courts' proposal made clear its substantial agreement with the plaintiffs' position. Refusing to negotiate would have been unthinkable. Neither the plaintiffs, the defendants, nor the court, however, could have anticipated the political developments that pushed the HIV-contaminated blood litigation into its final phase.

Blood, Bureaucracy, and the Political Process

Political observers predicted that Prime Minister Murayama's rule would be short-lived because he headed a transitional government founded by an unlikely coalition. Although his tenure lasted much longer than expected, Murayama resigned in 1995, and his successor, former minister of finance Hashimoto Ryutaro, took control. Lacking a majority of seats in the lower house of the Diet, Hashimoto's Liberal Democratic Party was unable to form a single-party government. Hashimoto was consequently dependent on the same coalition behind Murayama; the LDP, former prime minister Murayama's Social Democratic Party, and a recently formed party called New Party Sakigake.

Sakigake was by far the smallest of the coalition partners. But it was credited with having brokered the political compromise between the parties that allowed Hashimoto to become prime minister, and its participation in the coalition would be rewarded. The form of the reward was not in question—appointment of a Sakigake member as the head of one ministry—but which ministry was not yet decided. As Hashimoto configured the cabinet, his first choice for leading the Ministry of Health and Welfare unexpectedly pressed for a different appointment, and the post of Minister of Health and Welfare became available. A political opportunity for some, a peril for others; Sakigake's Kan Naoto stepped forward.

Kan entered politics in the 1970s by working on the campaign of Fusae Ichikawa, one of the first women to serve in the Diet. During his student days at the Tokyo Institute of Technology, he was active in the anti–Vietnam War protests, and he carried the image of an outside reformer into his political work with the publication of his book, *A Citizen Guerrilla Challenges the Parliament.* Kan's affiliation with the Social Democratic Union, a small splinter group, ended in 1994, when he joined Sakigake.

The opportunities presented by the HIV/blood conflict were not lost on Prime Minister Hashimoto. It was Hashimoto who as Minister of Health and Welfare in 1979 tearfully apologized on behalf of the Japanese government for the SMON incident. He promised that the government would prevent future drug-related disasters, and the Pharmaceutical Affairs Law was revised to make the ministry responsible for drug safety. Hashimoto used the affair to political advantage, taking credit for being more open than ministry bureaucrats about the damage caused by the ministry-approved drug. Hashimoto's experience may in part explain why his first choice to head the MHW was a member of his own party. The controversy over HIV and blood was potentially volatile. Managed by a member of the LDP, it could be treated cautiously and quietly; in the hands of a politician not dependent on the largesse of the LDP, it could be used to embarrass the dominant party and bring into public view the internal workings of the MHW. Kan was clearly a risky choice.

Within weeks of taking control of the ministry, in January 1996, Kan transformed the conflict over contaminated blood. No longer was it hemophiliac plaintiffs against the MHW and pharmaceutical companies. Health and Welfare Minister Kan turned against the corps of career bureaucrats in his ministry, and elevated the dispute over HIV-tainted blood into the most volatile political scandal of the 1990s.

Documents Lost . . . and Found

In August 1983, hemophiliacs had questioned the MHW about the safety of blood products and requested information from the ministry that would assist them in making treatment decisions. They were met with assurances that "changing the medical treatment and the method of blood collection and distribution for hemophiliacs is unnecessary," and "blood concentrates are safe, so the blood system does not have to be changed."[83] Without the equivalent of the U.S. Freedom of Information Act or other means of obtaining government documents, hemophiliacs had no way to obtain more detailed information.[84] At a November 6, 1983, meeting of the Friends of Hemophilia Association, Abe Takeshi, then chair of the MHW AIDS Task Force that debated Japan's AIDS case Number One, presented a "Proclamation of Safety." It said in part:

> Presently, the need to worry about AIDS is slight, so to worry about stopping blood imports from the U.S. is probably excessive. Imports will continue to be approved so hemophilia treatment will not be disrupted. Within the subcommittee, I have heard that there are some who think the importation of unheated products should be stopped, but those are remarks from doctors who don't really know hemophilia. For me, this is inconceivable. All of you are being saved because of blood products.[85]

Kan's first public act in the HIV-contaminated blood conflict was to order bureaucrats in his ministry to produce the files long requested by the plaintiffs. If they were "missing," as was claimed, it was time to investigate and find them. In mid-January, less than one week after taking office, he met with his vice-minister and the director of the Pharmaceutical Affairs Bureau to discuss the formation of a committee charged with finding the relevant documents. They reportedly were cool to the idea, arguing that the documents were no longer available, and that even if they could be found, new information would complicate the court's efforts to settle the litigation.[86] Kan likened the state of affairs at MHW to the Monju incident, when a government ministry covered up information relevant to the leak of a nuclear power plant. He ordered the creation of an HIV Infection Investigation Project Team, and in only three days their search was rewarded. On February 9, 1996, Kan held a press conference to announce that nine long-missing files had been located.[87] They included detailed meeting minutes and information related to the 1983 discussions of Abe's AIDS Task Force, and similar material from its Subcommittee on Blood Products, chaired by Abe's disciple, Kazama Mutsuyoshi. Explaining the sudden appearance of the files, the current director of the Pharmaceutical Affairs Bureau stated:

> We looked so many times. This is the result of a conscious effort of investigation . . . I am surprised [by the timing of the discovery], and it [the timing] is very unfortunate.[88]

Secretly, however, some of the documents had already been circulated to plaintiffs and other interested parties within and outside the ministry. It was only the public that remained uninformed. Over the next months more documents were uncovered, and in a carefully orchestrated series of events, the "discovered" documents were slowly released to the press.

The Kan-Kan War: Old Documents, Continuing Tensions

In his late forties, articulate, intelligent, and politically savvy, Minister Kan was on the verge of becoming a national hero. On February 16, 1996, he met with 200 HIV-infected hemophiliacs and their families at the Ministry of Health and Welfare, and offered the apology that had for so long eluded them.

> Representing the ministry, I make a heartfelt apology for inflicting heavy damage on the innocent patients. I also apologize for the belated recognition of the ministry's responsibility for the case. I understand that the delay has tormented the victims.[89]

In what became known in Japan as the Kan-kan war, a pun on the fight that developed over HIV and blood between Minister Kan and ministry bureaucrats, known as kanryō, the minister had won a decisive battle. He apologized for the ministry, but there was no confusion about the meaning of his apology. Kan had no link to the 1983 MHW, no influence on decisions about blood products, no responsibility to protect hemophiliacs from HIV. By apologizing, he simultaneously won the support of the public, and declared the career bureaucrats in his ministry venal and corrupt. Accustomed to closed-door decision making, controlling information, and covering up mistakes, bureaucrats watched as the internal workings of their ministry were revealed to the public.

Information that emerged from the first publicly released file, a file that was prepared by Mochinaga's then subordinate, also fanned the flames of scandal. The file, turned over to the press on February 21, contained information about three Task Force meetings between June and August 1983. Designated the "Gunji File" after the director of the Biologics and Antibiotics Division of the Pharmaceutical Affairs Bureau during that period, Dr. Gunji Atsuaki, the file consisted of material indicating that the Task Force had discussed the potential danger of imported, unheated blood products.

Most contentious were notes written by Gunji in preparation for a July 4, 1983 meeting of the AIDS Task Force. Titled "Handling of Blood Products and AIDS," the document clearly outlines a possible MHW response to HIV and blood in three points. First, recommend the use of heated products; second, encourage foreign pharmaceutical companies developing heated products to seek approval from the ministry as soon as possible; third, use administrative guidance in instructing pharmaceutical companies not to use unheated blood products. The document also acknowledges that these actions could have an impact on domestic pharmaceutical companies.

Nonetheless, after a second meeting of the AIDS Task Force one week later, a decision was made to continue importing unheated blood products. Who made that decision? On what basis? Why didn't the ministry communicate its concern about blood products to consumers? Many have demanded to know exactly what happened on July 11, 1983, at the Task Force meeting. That line of investigation is unlikely to be productive. There is no reason to believe that the process of decision making within the Task Force was different from the normal method through which consensual decisions are reached on Japanese committees. Rather than a vigorous, direct, animosity-filled confrontation, discretion and silence are used to great effect. No verbal confrontation about whether or not to continue using unheated products was necessary. So long as the status quo was maintained, Gunji's preparatory memo could have easily been presented, discussed, and then ignored. The decision to continue importing unheated blood products, in effect, would have been no decision at all.

Whereas Gunji was vilified by the press for drafting the July memo but failing to act on its recommendations, Abe Takeshi, the chair of the Task Force, was accused of pressuring the Task Force to allow the continued use of unheated products for his own financial gain. Plaintiffs long asserted that Abe delayed the approval of heated blood products "so that a Japanese company which lagged behind in developing the blood product could catch up with rival firms."[90] A delay would allow the Green Cross to make large profits on unheated, foreign blood products that it had purchased (or could obtain at a discount), while developing competitive heating technology. Abe was accused of accepting a bribe from Green Cross in exchange for the delay, and at the same time demanding money from rival firms in exchange for approving the clinical testing of heated blood products.[91]

Other members of the AIDS Task Force who treated hemophiliacs may have been equally self-serving in supporting the continued use of unheated products. As the price of imported products fell, a consequence of the introduction of heated products into the U.S. market, physicians and other sellers of unheated products experienced increased profitability because the margin between their purchase price and reimbursement price increased. Profits also swelled because of increased consumption, due to the approval of self-injection of blood products in March, 1983.[92] Physicians advising the ministry on blood policy thus had a financial interest in continuing current policy. Understaffed, lacking independent oversight, reliant on outside experts for policy expertise, the MHW failed to craft a blood policy that served the public interest.

Equally distorting of decisions about blood products were the strong bonds resulting from the practice of *amakudari*. Literally "descent from the heavens," *amakudari* describes the career path of a bureaucrat who retires from a position of regulatory authority and accepts a lucrative position in the private sector.[93] There are rules that regulate the employment of former officials, but they are mostly honored in the breach. For MHW officials, particularly those in the Pharmaceutical Affairs Bureau, the lure of a high pharmaceutical company salary can blunt the edge of what might otherwise be a discriminating regulatory posture.[94] Moreover, those in positions of responsibility within the ministry inevitably work with company officials who were formerly one's colleague or boss. Matsushita Renzo, for example, a former director of the Pharmaceutical Affairs Bureau, assumed the presidency of the Green Cross Corporation. One of his colleagues in the Bureau was Mochinaga Kazumi, Gunji's superior, now a member of the Diet (Gunji, in a less usual career move, left the government for an academic post at the University of Tokyo). Abe was installed in a lucrative position at one of the Green Cross's affiliated foundations. Over just a few years, four other senior officials from the Pharmaceutical Affairs Bureau followed Matsushita to the Green Cross. Other pharmaceutical companies selling blood products, and the association representing them, the Japan Blood Product Association, adhered to similar personnel practices.[95] The strong ties created between government and industry through this practice raise doubts about the underlying motivations of MHW blood policy, and give credence to accusations that the MHW allowed the continued use of unheated blood products in order to protect domestic companies from foreign competition.

A Second Proposal

On March 7, 1996, the Tokyo and Osaka District Courts announced a second version of their proposed October settlement. It did not increase the lump-sum payments from 45 million yen (US$ 375,000) to 60 million yen (US$ 500,000), as plaintiffs had demanded. But it did recommend that in addition to the basic payment, every hemophiliac with AIDS receive 150,000 yen monthly (US$ 1500), and that the current MHW-administered compensation scheme continue. The court also suggested that a medical care system for victims of contaminated blood be established, whereby the government would pay for all medical care provided to HIV-positive hemophiliacs and 40% of the care provided to those with AIDS, with pharmaceutical companies paying the balance. As in the first recommendation, the court emphasized that the government and pharmaceutical companies were responsible for the distribution of tainted blood, and urged them to apologize. And it set a settlement deadline of March 29, leaving the parties only three weeks to settle differences that had simmered during six years of litigation.

It did not take long for the pharmaceutical corporations to echo the sentiments expressed by Minister Kan. The plaintiffs assembled into five groups on March 14, 1996, and visited the offices of the five pharmaceutical companies they held responsible for their HIV infection. At each location, presidents and top executives of the companies offered their apologies, emphasizing that hemophiliacs were innocent victims of HIV. In Tokyo, Bayer President Wolfgang Plischke stated: "We would like to apologize from the bottom of our heart for the suffering of hemophiliac patients and their family members, who are unwitting victims of a terrible tragedy."[96] At the Japanese headquarters of Baxter, President Bob Hurley announced:

> On behalf of Baxter employees worldwide, I would like to extend a sincere and deep apology to the HIV infected victims including the plaintiffs and their families. You are the innocent victims of a terrible disease and we deeply regret that the early versions of the therapies that were designed to save lives, carried the virus that causes AIDS.[97]

In Osaka, Green Cross President Kawano Takehiko read from a prepared statement, saying, "We deeply regret that our products created a serious situation that resulted in pain and grief." Those in the room became indignant, accusing him of offering superficial and insincere words. Kawano then accepted responsibility on behalf of his company, got down on his hands and knees, and bowed so deeply that his forehead touched the floor. It was the defining moment of the conflict; a display of physical and psychological vulnerability from the president of Green Cross, the company that had its start in blood banking, dominated the domestic pharmaceutical industry, exerted enormous influence on the government, and was accused of importing contaminated blood products and inflicting a fatal disease on thousands of vulnerable Japanese citizens. New revelations and further outrage would keep the nation focused on the blood scandal. But nothing could supplant the image of a rumpled President Kawano that flashed on every front page and television news in the nation.

One day later, Minister Kan reiterated his apology, and signaled the government's intention to settle the HIV litigation. At a ceremony on March 29, all parties to the conflict signed a settlement agreement prepared by the court, which stated:

> Each of the defendant Government and Pharmaceutical Companies hereby apologizes from the bottom of its heart for the fact that enormous damage, physically and mentally, has been caused to the HIV infected victims including the Plaintiffs.[98]

Litigation over HIV-contaminated blood products came to a close.

The Aftermath

Settling the litigation did not end the search for answers to the many questions plaintiffs and others raised about HIV-contaminated blood in Japan. In spring 1996, in an effort to bring to light further information about HIV-contaminated blood, the Health and Welfare Subcommittee of the Lower House of the Diet held a series of hearings. The Subcommittee summoned the central actors responsible for blood policy in 1983 to testify as unsworn witnesses (*sankonin*), bowing to strong opposition in the Diet against requiring those testifying to take an oath (*shonin*). Among those called to the Diet were Abe Takeshi, head of the MHW 1983 AIDS Task Force; Gunji Atsuaki, former director of Biologics and Antibiotics, MHW; Kazama Mutsuyoshi, Abe's associate who chaired the blood products subcommittee of the AIDS Task Force; and Mochinaga Kazumi, director of the Pharmaceutical Affairs Bureau from 1981–1983 and currently an LDP Diet member. They were questioned through a procedure whereby representatives from each political party were allotted time based on their party's representation. The LDP, for example, was allowed 45 minutes of a three-hour session; the Communist Party was limited to 15 minutes.

The hearings provided an opportunity for politicians to voice their outrage and display scorn of bureaucratic behavior. Former bureaucrats had a chance to express their sincere regret—with the exception of Abe, who refused to acknowledge the possibility that he failed his many hemophiliac patients. The mass media could satisfy the news-hungry public with stories of formerly high-ranking bureaucrats taken to task by politicians. Issues of profound importance were discussed at the hearings, such as the limits and exercise of power possessed by the AIDS Task Force, an issue at the heart of studies on the role of advisory groups (*shingikai*) in Japanese politics. But the structure of the proceedings made it impossible to conduct the authoritative investigation promised to plaintiffs in the settlement agreement. A second set of hearings several months later, with sworn witnesses, covered little new ground.

With the announcement of a court-recommended settlement in October 1995, and public attacks on the ministry by a new, politically appointed minister without allegiance to Japan's long-ruling Liberal Democratic Party (LDP), the Office of the Prosecutor abandoned its reticence to investigate accusations made against certain actors years earlier, and began sifting through evidence of possible criminal wrongdoing.[99] They examined complaints filed by hemophiliacs against Dr. Abe, who was accused of failing to reveal to his patients their actual medical diagnoses.[100] Like other physicians who treated hemophiliacs, Abe feared that if hemophiliacs were told they were HIV-positive, they would commit suicide or intentionally infect others. He also claimed that many hemophiliacs did not want, or need, to know their test results. According to Abe, "I have all the information on their [HIV-positive hemophiliacs'] behavior. They have no opportunity to give the infection to other persons in most cases."[101]

Despite such confidence, some spouses of hemophiliacs who were infected joined a group of hemophiliacs in accusing Abe of murder. They alleged that Abe knew the blood products he administered to hemophiliacs could infect them with HIV. In August, 1996, the Tokyo police arrested the 80-year-old Dr. Abe Takeshi. According to the prosecutor's office, the nation's most illustrious hemophilia expert had ignored scientific evidence of blood product contamination when designing the blood policy of Teikyo University Hospital, where he was once vice-president. Abe's failure, prosecutors claimed, caused hemophiliac patients treated with blood products at the hospital in the 1980s to become infected with HIV.[102] He was released on 100 million yen bail.

Murder accusations were also filed against Matsushita Renzo, former director of the MHW's Pharmaceutical Affairs Bureau, who left that position to become president of the Green Cross Company. The first non-hemophiliac adult to be reported HIV-infected from a blood transfusion died in December 1995. His relatives claim that he was given HIV-tainted blood products in April 1986, and that those products were sold by the Green Cross long after the danger of unheated products was known. Matsushita, another former Green Cross president, and Kawano, the Green Cross president who apologized to the hemophiliacs, have all been arrested. Gunji Atsuaki, director of Biologics and Antibiotics at the ministry in 1983, was also investigated, accused of perjury while testifying during the negligence litigation because he had "no recollection" of certain events at the MHW in 1983. He has not been arrested. Pharmaceutical firms that sold unheated products and physicians who used them have also been investigated by prosecutors.

Prosecutors have uncovered enough evidence of wrongdoing in some of these cases to bring them to trial. But the investigations are in some ways an unfortunate distraction, deflecting attention from the more serious structural problems at the root of the HIV/blood tragedy.

Conclusion

The HIV/blood scandal provides an opening through which to observe how Japanese social, political, and legal institutions respond to conflicts involving scientific uncertainty, medical injury, and a public search for blame. Four aspects of the Japanese response stand out; foreign causes of domestic crisis are emphasized; institutional failure is minimized while individual responsibility is highlighted; national conflict is treated as unique; and issue-specific response is valued over general policy learning.

Blaming Foreign Blood

Japanese folk beliefs treat blood as the template of identity. A, B, AB, and O are not simply regarded as biological indicators; they are thought to describe the character of different types of individuals, similar to how zodiac signs are considered by some to be a way of classifying personalities. Families also have identities, captured in the concept of bloodlines. More social than biological, bloodlines are created through patterns of marriage and procreation. Even the Japanese state is in part defined through the metaphor of blood. During the slow death of Emperor Hirohito in 1989, the media published daily reports of his oral (*toketsu*) and anal (*geketsu*) bleeding, a second reminder (after Hirohito's postwar renunciation of divinity) that the Emperor, the embodiment of the state, is sustained by the most human and magical of substances.[103]

The identification of blood with identity, family, community, and the state in Japan leads to a sharp distinction between "our" blood and "their" blood, an echo of policies of national blood self-sufficiency found in many nations. Fueled by the political economy of blood products in Japan, almost all of which were imported from the United States until the 1990s, *foreign* blood, more than Japanese bureaucrats, or politicians, or corporations, or physicians, has been highlighted as the primary cause of Japan's HIV-tainted blood tragedy. The media, infected hemophiliacs, even the government itself have regularly intoned that had only Japanese blood been used, rather than impure American products, there would have been no HIV-infected hemophiliacs in Japan. The conflict over HIV and blood in Japan has thus strengthened traditional prejudice and xenophobia about the undesirability and impurity, metaphorical and biological, of foreign blood.[104]

Individual, Not Institutional, Failure

Throughout the conflict over HIV and blood, critics ridiculed the MHW's system of clinical trials; cited examples of a long history of iatrogenic tragedies as evidence that dangerous drugs were regularly distributed; denounced the close links between the ministry and the pharmaceutical companies it regulates; and claimed that entire sections of the ministry, like the Pharmaceutical Affairs Bureau, were incompetent or flawed. Leaders of the health and welfare bureaucracy moved rapidly to deflect attention from general structural malignancies at the ministry to particular individuals who could be held accountable for the spread of HIV through blood. In a climate of accusation and animosity, Dr. Abe Takeshi emerged as the villain, the most visible and the least sympathetic character in Japan's national tragedy over HIV and blood.

As chair of the early-1980s AIDS Task Force responsible for making key decisions about blood policy, Abe had been an important government adviser. Because he was not a state employee, however, his ministry connections were not sufficiently strong to inspire the unconditional support of career bureaucrats. More important to those at the ministry was the need to manage the firestorm caused by the recent public release of previously concealed documents that detailed government blood policy making in the 1980s. Like the Japanese expression *tokage no shippo kiri* — dropping a piece of its tail, the lizard creates a diversion for the pursuer and is able to survive fundamentally intact — the ministry abandoned its most vulnerable part and collectively ran for cover.[105] Instead of undertaking a careful examination of the institutional factors that made possible the distribution of HIV-contaminated blood, individual actors, and their actions, became the central focus of official blame for the HIV tragedy. Those outside the government have continued to point out the pathologies of institutional failure, and those inside the MHW sometimes admit that "the system" was faulty. Nonetheless, the actors, faults, and remedies related to "system" failure remain abstract, whereas individual behavior has been pinpointed and prosecuted.

Treating Japan's Conflict as Unique

One aspect of what has rapidly become the conventional wisdom about HIV and blood in Japan is that the incompetence and/or malevolence of the Ministry of Health and Welfare and pharmaceutical companies caused the HIV infection of at least 40% of Japanese hemophiliacs. This is contrasted to events elsewhere, particularly in the United States, where blood products were made safe by heat treatment 18 months before they were in Japan. Such actions, it is claimed, could have saved Japan's hemophiliacs. A unique set of institutional and social conditions, combined with individual decisions, is therefore cited as causing the distribution of HIV-contaminated blood in Japan, which in turn caused a unique conflict. However compelling, this tale is wrong; it confuses the explanation of the *cause* of distributing HIV-tainted blood in Japan with the *consequences* of doing so.

It may be true that Japanese policy-makers and corporate actors were irresponsible or evil; perhaps they ignored their duty to ensure public safety or product effectiveness and were ruled by narrow self-interest. That may provide the basis for censure, condemnation, even imprisonment. But even if the government and pharmaceutical companies had acted impeccably, and had adhered to the highest ethical and legal standards, they could not have avoided infecting many Japanese hemophiliacs with HIV. In short, they were faced with the same tragedy as blood policy experts everywhere.

It is extremely difficult to say with any reliability when particular individuals were infected with HIV, and there are no medical studies that provide data that pinpoint the time when hemophiliacs were infected in Japan. But it is revealing to compare the date when heated blood products were available in countries outside Japan with HIV seroprevalence among hemophiliacs in those countries. In the United States, for example, cited with approval by Japanese hemophiliacs and their supporters because heated blood products were first approved in 1983, about 50% of hemophiliacs are HIV-infected. In Germany, where heated products were first approved in 1982, approximately 40% of hemophiliacs were infected. In fact, throughout western Europe, infection rates among hemophiliacs are close to 50%, even in countries that approved heated products more quickly than Japan. This is because HIV-tainted blood products were distributed from the late 1970s, well before the first cases of AIDS were recognized. It is impossible to say with certainty how many lives would have been saved if the Japanese government had acted more quickly. Yet even immediate, responsible action by the government and pharmaceutical companies would not have averted a tragedy. This is not a justification for the delay, nor does it provide a reason to overlook whatever malfeasance occurred. Still, it is imperative to be clear about the consequences of the timing of heat treatment in Japan, and to understand that the Japanese conflict, while distinctive, is not unique.

Lessons Not Learned

Almost every nation that has experienced conflict over HIV in the blood supply has sought to learn about, and to learn from, the controversy. The U.S. Department of Health and Human Services, prompted by Congress, charged the Institute of Medicine with investigating the causes, consequences, and lessons to be learned from blood contamination in the United States. The Kreever Commission had a similar charge in Canada, as did national commissions in Germany, Australia, and elsewhere. In Japan, there is no mechanism for establishing independent investigatory bodies, so those authorized to make recommendations for the improvement of blood policy are from within the Ministry of Health and Welfare (MHW). This has limited the depth of criticism and reform of the current system.

A small number of concrete policy consequences of the conflict over blood can be identified.[106] Whereas in the 1980s Japan imported more than 90% of its factor VIII, domestic manufacture of factor VIII began in 1991, and by 1995 Japan was self-sufficient.[107] The Japanese Red Cross finally began, in 1995, to distribute questionnaires to blood donors asking about HIV risk factors. A long-debated Product Liability Law, which went into effect on July 1, 1995, may be useful to those who suffer future injuries caused by blood products.[108]

Some attempts at institutional reform have been made, but they have not been terribly meaningful. Administrative reform at the MHW was advertised as creating a structure that would minimize the likelihood of future blood-borne pathogens, but there is little evidence to suggest that this has been accomplished. Meetings at the MHW are now public, so groups like Abe's AIDS Task Force now gather in public and have open discussions. Parts of the ministry have been abolished or renamed—

the Biologics and Antibiotics Division, for example, was renamed the Blood Enterprise Countermeasures Office (*Ketsueki Jigyo Taisaku Shitsu*). Such developments will not change the close government-business relations, bureaucratic behavior, or financial incentives that may have contributed to the distribution of tainted blood.

A full and fair investigation of the HIV/blood scandal requires an examination of the institutions that made it possible: the Ministry of Health and Welfare, *amakudari*, the Japanese Red Cross, pharmaceutical companies, and profit-making by physicians who rely on sales of prescription drugs for part of their income. These are likely to receive only superficial attention; MHW officials with investigatory power have little interest in making structural changes to the comfortable arrangement they now enjoy, and Minister Kan, who switched political parties prior to the October 1996 election, is no longer at the MHW. A single, simple, solution has thus come to the fore as the most desirable foundation for the future of Japanese blood policy; self-sufficiency of all blood products. Ideology has replaced safety, and sensible public health has become the final victim of public scandal.

NOTES

Research for this chapter was supported by the Robert Wood Johnson Foundation Scholars in Health Policy Research Program, The Toyota Foundation, and the Center for Global Partnership. I am grateful to Ronald Bayer, Robert Bullock, Christine Harrington, Chalmers Johnson, Dorothy Nelkin, Douglass Starr, Frank Upham, Mark Ramseyer, Shinichi Sugiyama and David Wolff for helpful comments, criticisms, and suggestions on an earlier draft.

1. Richard Titmuss, *The Gift Relationship* (New York: Vintage, 1971), pp. 15–16.

2. An exchange rate of ¥120/$1.00 will be used throughout this chapter.

3. Nihon Sekijyuji-sha, *Ketsueki Jigyō no Ayumi*, (Tokyo: Kozaido, 1991) p. 52; Ikeda Fusao, *Shiroi Ketsueki*, (Tokyo: Ushio, 1985), p. 124.

4. Blood Services Department, The Japanese Red Cross Society, "Blood Services 1995," p. 2.

5. In recent years, a number of books have addressed the ethical, medical, and legal dimensions of those events. See, for example, Sheldon Harris, *Factories of Death* (New York: Routledge, 1994).

6. "Japan: International HIV Blood Sales Expose War Guilt," *Daily Telegraph* (London), March 11, 1996.

7. Matsūra Yasuhiro and Suzuki Ishi, *Gisō—Chōsa Hōdō: Midori Jyūji Jiken* (Tokyo: Mainichi Shimbun-sha, 1983).

8. Naito, Ryoichi, "Ketsueki Ginkō: Sono 15 Nenkan no Ayumi," *Igaku no Ayumi* (July 5, 1958), 305–310, 307.

9. Ikeda, *Shiroi Ketsueki*.

10. Naito, p. 307.

11. Takasugi Shingo, "Abe Takeshi: Watakushi wa AIDS . . ." *Gendai* (October 1987), pp. 250–265, 262.

12. Ikeda, p. 125.

13. *Ibid.*, p. 126.

14. "Blood Services 1995," p. 3.

15. Ikeda, pp. 135–140; Nihon Sekijyūji-sha, p. 125.

16. That decision stated: "In view of the present state of the blood program and in order to establish a system that will secure an adequate supply of stored blood through voluntary donations as quickly as possible, the Government shall work for the propagation of the concept of blood donation and the formation of organizations for blood donation by national and local authorities and, at the same time, promote the improvement of the receiving system for donated blood by the Japanese Red Cross Society and/or local authorities." See "Blood Services" 1995, p. 4.

17. While this eliminated individual blood sellers who profited from giving blood, it did not eliminate all financial incentives in the whole blood system. For the Japanese Red Cross and others, whole blood is a lucrative enterprise.

18. It is remarkable that within a few years, the quantity of donated blood in Japan increased so rapidly. One possible explanation is that there had always been people willing to donate whose altruism had not been tapped. Once the Japanese Red Cross began recruiting donors by appealing to their community spirit, those who were not previously associated with the blood system stepped forward to replace those only willing to sell blood.

19. Cryoprecipitate comes from the third step in a process in which blood is first collected, plasma and red blood cells are separated, and cryoprecipitate (cryo), a mixture of various blood-clotting elements, is extracted. A more complex procedure in which individual clotting elements such as factor VIII and factor IX can be isolated and concentrated (hence the name concentrates) was developed later. Concentrates are the most effective way to treat hemophilia and have fewer side effects than cryo. But concentrates are made from the pooled blood of many, sometimes thousands, of donors, and are therefore more susceptible to contamination.

20. Naoki Ikegami and John C. Campbell, "Medical Care in Japan," *New England Journal of Medicine*, 333 (19) (November 9, 1995), p. 1297.

21. A more detailed description of the pharmaceutical industry can be found in Margaret Powell and Masahira Anesaki, eds., *Health Care in Japan* (New York: Routledge, 1990), pp. 179–186.

22. This system is inherited from China. Practitioners of traditional medicine (kampo) had to find a way to make a living from their work. They therefore needed to justify imposing a charge for their services. The actual consultation, however, was not deemed worthy of compensation, and a practitioner who demanded payment for a visit would have been quickly put out of business. Instead of a per visit or time-based fee, they earned a salary by charging for medication.

23. "AIDS Researcher Hid Hemophiliac's Death," *Japan Times* (February 26, 1996), p. 1.

24. Iida, Takaaki, "Nihon no EIZU wa Koko Made Kakusareteiru," *Gendai* (October 1987), pp. 236–265.

25. Such behavior is consonant with a common perception in Japan that foreignness, the "outside," is dangerous and contagious. A cartoon in an educational pamphlet for high school students, circulated by the Ministry of Education, for example, pictured cartoon images of black figures holding spears in a boat sailing from Africa to Japan, with the word "AIDS" emblazoned on the side of the boat.

26. "Ketsuyūbyō Kanja no 4 Wari," *Asahi Shimbun* (September 18, 1987).

27. Kyoto Chapter of Friends of Hemophilia Society, "Yunyū Ketsueki Seizai Higai Jitai Chōsa Ankēto" (Survey of the Actual Damage from Importation of Blood Products), February 1989.

28. "Hemophiliacs Targets of Abuse, Poll Shows," *The Daily Yomiuri* (April 12, 1988), p. 2.

29. *Ibid.*

30. *Ibid.*, note 49.

31. Shohei Yonemoto, draft paper on hemophilia associations in Japan, unpublished.

32. Japanese gay groups include AIDS Action, part of the International Lesbian and Gay Association, which spawned the AIDS Care Project, O.C.C.U.R., and Osaka Gay Community. International Friends is a support group for gay men.

33. It is interesting to note that hemophilia affects men almost exclusively, so that in both Japan and the United States the groups most identified with AIDS were virtually all male.

34. *Ibid.* Personal communication with Jim Frederick, International Friends, October 6, 1990.

35. Ishida Yoshiaki, "AIDS Taisaku no Hoseika ni Hantai," *Asahi Shimbun* (February 9, 1987).

36. "AIDS Reporting Plan Proposed in Drafts of Prevention Bill," *The Japan Times* (February 19, 1987) 2; "LDP Has Draft AIDS Bill," *Mainichi Daily News* (February 21, 1987) 12. For a more detailed discussion of the law, see Eric A. Feldman and Shohei Yonemoto, "Japan: AIDS as a Non-Issue," in David L. Kirp and Ronald Bayer, *AIDS in the Industrialized Democracies* (New Brunswick, NJ: Rutgers University Press, 1982).

37. While the draft did not explicitly limit penalties to those who engaged in *unsafe* sexual acts, this limitation can be implied from the language of the bill.

38. See, for example, Jocelyn Ford, "Innocent Victims of AIDS Worry that Government Ignores Their Rights," *Daily Yomiuri* (March 1, 1987), p. 2.

39. "LDP Panel Approves Ministry's AIDS Bill," *The Japan Times* (March 7, 1987), p. 2.

40. See, for example, Ishida Yoshiaki, Chairman of the Kyoto Branch, Japan Friends of Hemophilia Association, open letter regarding the AIDS Prevention Law, May 11, 1987; Yayoi Uchiyama, "Draconian AIDS Legislation," *Mainichi Daily News* (May 15, 1987), p. 6; Jiyū Jinken Kyōkai, "*AIDS Taisaku*" Wa Dō Aru Beki Ka, Tokyo (March 10, 1988).

41. *Ibid.*

42. The exemption did not include non-hemophiliacs infected through blood products, nor those infected through whole blood, though until 1996 there were no cases of either type reported by the MHW. Hemophiliac exceptionalism in AIDS policy is not unusual. In the United States, for example, the Ricky Ray Hemophilia Relief Fund Act of 1996, which seeks a one billion dollar congressional appropriation for HIV-infected hemophiliacs, does not compensate others infected through blood products.

43. "Number of AIDS Sufferers Reaches 371," *The Japan Times* (April 24, 1991), p. 2.

44. "Doctors Keep Hemophiliacs in the Dark," *Mainichi Daily News* (March 24, 1987), p. 12.

45. Japan is one of a small number of countries where blood products are administered to non-hemophiliacs.

46. "Ketsuyūbyō Igai Demo Shisha," *Yomiuri Shimbun* (July 7, 1995).

47. The World Health Organization does not recognize such infections as a distinct epidemiological category.

48. "17 Nin, Ketsueki Kansen no Utagai," *Yomiuri Shimbun* (August 21, 1995), p. 3.

49. Powell and Anesaki, pp. 185–186.

50. *Ibid.*

51. "Makers of Pharmaceuticals Taking Steps to Prevent Improper Use of Medication," *Yomiuri Shimbun* (August 24, 1995), p. 13.

52. "Ministry Will Help Tainted Blood Victims," *Japan Times* (October 17, 1993), p. 2.

53. For an overview of the litigation, see Kamei Masateru, "HIV Soshō no...," *Hougaku Semina* 481 (January 1995), pp. 22–26; Iwao Ikoma, "Tokyo HIV Soshō no Mezasumono," *Nihon no Kagakusha* 28 (July 1993), pp. 388–393.

54. Tokyo HIV Soshō Genkoku Dan, HIV Soshō o Sasaeru Ketsuyubyo no Kai, "Ima, Inochi no Omosa wa," pamphlet with selections from the oral arguments in the Tokyo District Court regarding litigation over distribution of HIV-contaminated blood. The argument here was presented in the Tokyo District Court, March 4, 1991.

55. Absent from the list of defendants was the Japanese Red Cross (JRC). This to some extent reflects the fact that the JRC had no active role in importing, distributing, or approving blood products used by hemophiliacs. Nonetheless, zealous plaintiffs could have included the JRC in their pleadings, at least for symbolic purposes. Taking the JRC to court in Japan, however, is considered bizarre, unnatural, and undesirable. The honorary chair of the JRC has since the Meiji period been a member of the Japanese royal family, which has bestowed a peculiar kind of sanctity on the organization. Attorneys, journalists, and government officials speak in hushed tones when discussing the JRC and its links to contaminated blood. In short, suing the JRC is taboo, and all parties to the conflict over HIV and blood have made sure to exclude it from the controversy.

Yet included in MHW files released in 1996 were notes indicating that the MHW in 1983 approached the Japanese Red Cross about the possibility of using the domestic, non-remunerated blood supply as the source of blood products for hemophiliacs. The Red Cross insisted throughout the HIV/blood conflict that although it had no policy-making power, if approached by the MHW, it would have gladly cooperated in creating a domestic supply of blood products. If the information in the documents is correct, however, it appears that the JRC was not receptive to the ministry's request to do so.

56. A detailed chronology of the important dates and events surrounding the importation and distribution of tainted blood can be found in Katahira Kiyohiko and Sato Tsugumichi, "Eizu Hassei no Shoki ni Okeru Nihon no Ketsuyubyo-Ketsueki Seizai Kankeisha no Ninshiki to Taiyō," *Nihon no Kagakusha*, 28 (306) (July 1993), pp. 17–22. Throughout the court conflict over HIV and blood in Japan, the United States has been used as a reference point. The United States was perceived as experienced with AIDS treatment, prevention, and education; possessed the best technical knowledge about possible routes of transmission; was the first country to heat-treat blood; and was the site of the invention of the ELISA test that screens blood for antibodies to HIV. It was thus treated as the "gold standard" for appropriate HIV policy. Don Francis and Bruce Evatt, formerly of the CDC, testified in the Japanese courts, as did a variety of other American experts. Meetings, reports, and recommendations of the CDC, the FDA, the American Association of Blood Banks, and other organizations have all been used as evidence of what Japanese officials knew, or should have known, about HIV and blood. Japanese involved in the blood litigation have traveled to the United States to obtain information and evidence.

Although the Pharmaceutical Affairs Law grants the Minister of Health and Welfare the authority to recall drugs, that authority was not exercised. Instead, the minister warned companies of the danger of unheated products, and suggested that they undertake a voluntary recall. Ministry officials long contended that unheated factor VIII was off the shelves by November 1986, and factor IX by the beginning of 1986. But it now appears likely that the Green Cross, Nippon Zoki, and others continued selling unheated blood products after the ministry suggested a recall. One case of a hemophiliac who was infected by HIV through contaminated blood products in April 1987 has already come to light. More are likely to follow.

57. The best description of the legal points at issue in the litigation, albeit from the plaintiff's perspective, is "HIV Soshō Benkyō Kai," 44 Ki Shihō Shushusei Natsu no Shukai Hōkokushū, Kyoto (April 27–28, 1991), pp. 96–117. It provides a framework for the following discussion.

58. "HIV Soshō Benkyō Kai," pp. 98–99.

59. Katahira Kiyohiko and Sato Tsugumichi, "AIDS as Drug-Induced Suffering in Japan," in S. Araki, ed., *Behavioral Medicine: An Integrated Biobehavioral Approach to Health and Illness* (Dortrecht: Elsevier Science Publishers, 1992), pp. 229–234.

60. The term "homo," written in a Japanese syllabary used for foreign words, is what some Japanese continue to call men who have sex with men, although the word "gay" is now common and less stigmatizing.

61. It is important to remember that these events occurred at a time of strained United States–Japan relations, when the term "Japan basher" was coined and an influential book titled *The Japan that Can Say No* was published.

62. The arguments made by the plaintiffs illustrate the degree to which issues of race, xenophobia, and nationalism can influence "legal" and "scientific" argument. Lest such concern about blood seem uniquely Japanese, it should be recalled that during World War II, under the approval of the Red Cross, the secretaries of War and the Navy, and the surgeon generals of the Army and Navy, plasma of white and black American soldiers was segregated. Historian John Dower quotes John Rankin, Congressman of Mississippi, who in support of this policy decried mixing blood as a Communist plot to "mongrelize America," and accused those who supported mixing of wanting "to pump Negro or Japanese blood into the veins of our wounded white boys regardless of the dire effect it might have on their children." John Dower, *War Without Mercy: Race and Power in the Pacific War* (New York: Pantheon, 1986), p. 348, fn. 40.

63. "Ministry Hits Use of Imported Blood," *Daily Yomiuri* (May 15, 1990), p. 2.

64. Blood Services Department, Japanese Red Cross Society, *Blood Services* (Tokyo: Japanese Red Cross Society, 1993), pp. 29–30.

65. Katahira and Sato, at p. 232, which describes the testimony of Dr. Kaneo Yamada, Marianna University School of Medicine, June 7, 1991, Tokyo District Court.

66. These views are summarized in Ministry of Health and Welfare, "Saiban no Jyoukyou," unpublished, 1995.

67. It took until 1989 for the U.S. Food and Drug Administration to ban the use of non–heat treated blood products, but well before that date U.S. corporations had voluntarily stopped using them. Institute of Medicine, *HIV and the Blood Supply* (Washington, D.C.: National Academy Press, 1995).

68. See the legal briefs of defendants in the litigation, on file with the author.

69. Takasugi Shingo, "Abe Takeshi: 'Watakushi wa . . . teki . . . .'," *Gendai* (October 1987), pp. 250–265, p. 261.

70. Interview with Sasaki Hiroshi, Pharmaceutical Affairs Bureau, Ministry of Health and Welfare, July 22, 1993.

71. A review of such incidents can be found in Katahira Kiyohiko et al., "Improvement of the Law and Procedures to Relieve Drug-Induced Suffering and to Prevent its Occurrence: Lessons from the Clioquinol Lawsuit and Other Cases in Japan," Proceedings of the Kyoto International Conference Against Drug-Induced Suffering, April 14–18, 1979, Inter-

national Congress Series 513. A recent case, deaths caused by the antiviral sorivudine, is discussed in Mark Robinson, "Making a Killing," *Tokyo Journal* (December 1994), pp. 32–37.

72. HIV Soshō Benkyō Kai," p. 108.

73. Institute of Medicine, *HIV and the Blood Supply* (Washington, D.C.: National Academy Press, 1995).

74. For a comparison of how clinical trials are regulated in the United States, France, and Japan, see Nudeshima Jiro, "Rinshō Shiken no Kisei no Ari-ho," *Shakai Hoken Jyunpō* 1904 (March 11, 1996), pp. 6–12.

75. Michael R. Reich, "Why the Japanese Don't Export More Pharmaceuticals: Health Policy as Industrial Policy, *California Management Review* (Winter 1990), pp. 124–150, 129.

76. Rosemarie Kanusky, "Pharmaceutical Harmonization: Standardizing Regulation Among the United States, The European Economic Community, and Japan," *Houston Journal of International Law*, 16 (1994), p. 686.

77. Personal communication with Gunji Atsuaki, April 26, 1996. There were similar concerns in the United States about the extent to which heat-treating blood products would reduce their efficacy.

78. "Courts to Push Settlement in HIV Suits," *Japan Times* (October 4, 1995), p. 2.

79. "HIV Suit Settlement," *The Nikkei Weekly* (October 9, 1996), p. 2.

80. Two attorneys for the plaintiffs discuss the proposed settlement in Iizuka Tomoyuki and Ito Toshikatsu, "Wakai Kankoku o Dō Miru Ka," *Hōgaku Semina*, 492 (December 1995), pp. 17–20.

81. "Wakai Kankoku ni Atatte no Shoken," *Hō to Minshushugi*, 303 (November 1995), pp. 6–7.

82. *Ibid.*

83. Suzuki Atsushi, "Tokyo HIV Sosho ni tsuite," February 1, 1992, unpublished report by an attorney representing hemophiliac plaintiffs.

84. I am grateful to Mr. Sugiyama Shinichi for his explanation of the chronology of events in this section.

85. Tokyo HIV Soshō Genkokudan, *Yakugai AIDS: Genkoku Kara no Tegami* (Tokyo: Sanseido, 1995), p. 20. Translation by Yamada Kaori.

86. "HIV Meguri 'Kan-Kan Sensou,'" *Yomiuri Shimbun* (February 18, 1996).

87. "83 Nen Tōji Shiryo Hatsugen," *Yomiuri Shimbun* (February 10, 1996), p. 1.

88. "Chōsa San Nichi De Mitsuketeta," *Yomiuri Shimbun* (February 10, 1996), p. 27.

89. "State Admits HIV Guilt," *Japan Times* (February 17, 1996), p. 1.

90. "Hemophiliac Group to Seek Compensation," *Mainichi Daily News* (February 5, 1988), p. 3.

91. "Blood Product Marketing Thought Willfully Delayed," *Mainichi Daily News* (February 7, 1988), p. 12.

92. For many years, hemophiliacs had fought for the right to intravenously administer their medication without physician supervision, and were allowed to do so beginning in 1983. This led to an increase in the importation, and consumption, of blood products.

93. This practice is most common in the Ministry of Finance and other powerful ministries. A recent survey reported that in 1995, one third of 444 former ministry officials who held the post of bureau chief or a higher position accepted lucrative positions in the private sector. "Lucrative Jobs Await Third of Finance Retirees," *Japan Times* (April 23, 1996). Officially there is a two-year waiting period before former government employees can accept private employment. Unlike the "revolving door" in the United States, employment patterns in Japan flow in only one direction.

94. For a discussion of some aspects of *amakudari* at the MHW, see Sakurai Yoshiko, "Shi to Kettaku: Koseisho to Midori Jyūji," *Bungeishunju* (May 1996), pp. 208–215.

95. "Seiyaku Gaisha ni OB 17 Nin," *Yomiuri Shimbun* (April 9, 1996); "Drug Firms Hired Ministry Officials," *Japan Times* (February 24, 1996).

96. Press release, Bayer Yakuhin, March 14, 1996.

97. Statement released to plaintiffs, Baxter, March 14, 1996.

98. Tokyo Chihō Saibansho, Wakaicho shō Kisaijiko, Hatasawa preliminary translation, April 5, 1996.

99. The Japanese criminal law provides that in particular situations, individuals not directly injured may notify investigating officials that they would like a particular matter prosecuted. This first stage, the complaint, carries no official weight, and ordinarily gives rise to an investigation of the alleged offense by the police or public prosecutor. After the investigation is conducted and the evidence evaluated, a decision is made as to whether a case will be prosecuted. Shigemitsu Dando, *Japanese Criminal Procedure*, translated by B. J. George (South Hackensack, NJ: Fred B. Rothman & Co., 1965), pp. 95, 323.

Because the Criminal Code does not specify a time within which investigations must be completed, response to complaints can be indefinitely prolonged if the investigating officials say that the investigations are ongoing.

100. Out of 454 hemophiliacs who responded to a survey in 1988, 106 were not informed of the results of their HIV tests.

101. "Doctors Keep Hemophiliacs in the Dark," *Mainichi Daily News* (March 24, 1987), p. 12.

102. Hemophiliacs, almost all men, suffer from a condition in which their blood does not spontaneously clot. The severity of the disease depends on the exact element missing from one's blood. For years, hemophiliacs were forced to limit their daily activities to avoid the possibility of excessive blood loss and death. The burden of hemophilia was greatly lightened when medical science isolated clotting factors VIII and IX, coagulant proteins, from blood.

103. Norma Field, *In the Realm of a Dying Emperor* (New York: Pantheon, 1991), pp. 19–20.

104. Because of the epidemiology of HIV, it is true that blood products from the United States carried a greater risk than those from Japan and many other nations. But that epidemiological fact does not support a distinction between domestic (safe) and foreign (unsafe) blood. It is the underlying prevalence of a pathogen in a population, not the national origin of blood, that is relevant.

105. I thank Mr. Yonemoto Shohei for teaching me this expression.

106. Sugiyama Shinichi, "Wakai to Sono Go no Tembō," *Hougaku Semina* 498 (June 1996), pp. 4–8, discusses post-settlement issues from the perspective of an attorney for the hemophiliacs.

107. There is now international tension over the exclusion from the Japanese market of imported factor VIII, particularly focused on the alleged refusal of the MHW to approve or even test a recombinant product (made from synthetic rather than organic material) manufactured by Baxter. It is an issue that company spokespersons have suggested could be put before the U.S. Trade Representative as an example of a nontariff trade barrier.

108. Statute 85 of 1995. For a discussion of the law, see Takahashi Fumitoshi, "Japan's Product Liability Law: Issues and Implications," *Journal of Japanese Studies*, 22 (1996), pp. 105–128.

3

The Nation's Blood

Medicine, Justice, and the State in France

Monika Steffen

The early years of the AIDS epidemic coincided in France with significant social, economic, and political change. But despite living in such turbulent times, the French continued to share a unanimous conviction: their national blood transfusion system was, without doubt, the world's finest example of scientific achievement and social solidarity. The public was thus dumbfounded when the *scandale du sang contaminé* (the contaminated blood scandal) erupted in the early nineties. The fact that half of all French hemophiliacs were infected with HIV and that France accounted for close to 60% of all recorded cases of post-transfusion AIDS in the European Union[1] was surely the result of corruption, dirty money, bad blood, doctors who murdered, state secrets, and conspiracy. These were the elements of the massive press campaign focused on tracking down the guilty parties.

In a television program watched by millions, Georgina Dufoix, one of three cabinet ministers accused by the press as accountable for the catastrophe, pleaded, *"responsable mais non coupable,"*[2] responsible but not guilty. The perceptions of 1991 were not the understandings of the mid-1980s, she declared. Dufoix sharply criticized the press, which, she asserted, had sensationalized and exploited a problem of extreme gravity involving extensive human suffering.

The former minister's words roiled the waters. The *Association Française des Hémophile* (AFH) declared its dismay, the *Association des Polytransfusés* accused the former minister of "discrediting journalists," and the opposition political parties called for charges to be brought "at the highest political level"[3] against the Minister of Social Affairs and against Laurent Fabius and Edmond Hervé, Prime Minister and Secretary of Health, respectively, in 1985. By the mid-1990s, former executives of the blood system would be sentenced to prison, and 24 blood sector experts, ministerial advisers, and others who had held the highest political offices would be subject to investigation pending prosecution.

Why were the waves of the "blood scandal" deeper and more violent in France than in other European countries, where the contamination rate of hemophiliacs is similar or even higher?[4] The story of contamination raises questions of a special kind in France given the hierarchical structure of its public administration and the strong powers of the Executive, which endows national decision makers with a high degree of authority. Why did the French political system not deploy its resources and mechanisms to avoid or limit contamination? If national expertise and problem-solving capacities proved insufficient, why did France not turn to foreign examples and international learning?[5]

The lethargy of the French administrative response and the sense of shock reflected in public opinion are linked in a way that reveals the profound significance of blood and the special status of the blood transfusion system. Involved was something more than a public health accident involving medical services. It was not solely the special nature of blood that made swift intervention so difficult and that provoked the paroxysms of outrage when that failure became known. Particular features of the organization of the French blood transfusion system and its legal[6] and policy-making systems contributed to what came to be considered a national calamity.

The Roots of HIV-Contaminated Blood

Background

The AIDS years coincided in France with unusually frequent elections and political change. The rise of the Socialists in 1981 led to political "cohabitation," first during 1986–88 and then again in 1993–95 between a Socialist president and a right-wing parliament—something unprecedented in French history. The Communist Party, associated with the first left-wing government, lost its influence, and a new extreme right-wing party, the National Front, gained a substantial number of votes. This led to growing electoral competition between conservatives and Socialists, which has dominated political life ever since.

The political context was to influence the HIV/blood story in three ways. First, forthcoming elections delayed decision making. Second, political alternation favored the growth of "ministerial cabinets," increasing the number of personal counselors surrounding new ministers. These "shadows of the ministers" had no specific status, but their influence, albeit tacit, was considerable.[7] They filtered access to the minister and information submitted to him or her, prepared files and decisions, gave orders to top civil servants, and cooperated with the cabinets of other ministries. Neither politically accountable to the president of the Republic, as are ministers, nor professionally accountable to administrative jurisdiction, as are civil servants, they were answerable to no authority.

Third, the electoral climate helped to politicize the AIDS issue via the *Front National* (the extreme right-wing party), which won its first seats in parliament in the spring of 1986. The National Front's campaign[8] centered on "national decline," in which immigration, delinquency, drug abuse, and AIDS were all considered part and parcel of the same problem. The unanimous and forceful response of the major political parties and opinion leaders was to defend freedom,[9] individual rights, and solidarity with AIDS victims against the risk of stigmatization and segregation. Therefore, AIDS became the ideological battlefield where political values of equality and universalism were to be demonstrated against a threat from the extreme right, thus diverting attention from the public health problem.[10] The result was a political and social consensus on minimizing the risks of AIDS. Further, during the entire decade, police repression against drug abuse was reinforced under all the governments, both left and right wing, so as not to leave this politically sensitive field open to the National Front. As a direct result, the concentration of drug addicts—potential HIV carriers—continually grew in prisons. This, in turn, would have profound, if unanticipated, implications for the French blood system.

It was the commitment to universalism in the face of right-wing challenges that led to a social and political consensus[11] that barely took account of the specific profile of the epidemic. The refusal to take into consideration the existence of "at-risk groups" (the term was even banned and replaced by "at-risk individual behavior") would make any effort to take steps to protect the blood supply through the exclusion of classes of at-risk donors extraordinarily difficult.[12]

In addition, economic difficulties contributed to shaping the HIV blood story. During 1981–83, the Socialists tried to stimulate economic growth with a program based on national production, the stimulation of domestic consumption, and an increase in social expenditure, reflected in the popular slogan "buy French," which, of course, implied producing French as well. The biomedical industry featured among official priorities, which helps to explain the emphasis in the early 1980s on national self-sufficiency for blood clotting concentrates relied on by hemophiliacs. A radical policy shift—henceforth maintained by all subsequent governments—followed in 1983. It focused on severe restrictions on public spending, primarily in social fields, which led to budget ceilings for public hospitals on which half of the blood transfusion centers depended. These policies also led to power shifts inside the Health Ministry, marginalizing even further the already weak General Department of Health (DGS, *Direction Générale de la Sante*),[13] which had central responsibility for the blood supply.

Organization of the Blood Transfusion System

Until the *scandale du sang contaminé*, the blood transfusion system in France was held in high esteem, enjoying the confidence of both the medical world and public opinion. The HIV/blood conflict signaled a discrepancy between the system's powerful ethical principles and its organizational structures, and brought attention to the negligence of the transfusion sector. Governed by an anachronistic 1952 law, the system lacked a structure that could be adapted to the industrial production of blood-based pharmaceuticals. AIDS arrived in a legal and regulatory vacuum.

Historical Roots[14]

The first transfusion center was created in a Parisian hospital in 1923. At the time, transfusions were carried out from "arm to arm." Those who provided blood were paid for their "donations." Private doctors as well as public hospitals developed networks of professional donors who would provide blood on demand. Until the 1950s, before national health insurance was fully operational throughout the country, transfusion recipients paid for their treatment.

The principle of voluntary donation is of fairly recent vintage in France. The good volunteer appeared as an outcome of World War II when injured partisans from the Resistance received free blood donated in secret places under the threat of arrest. With enthusiastic mass collections, voluntary blood donation became a widespread social movement as the Liberation army advanced. The legacy of this "*Route du Sang,*"[15] which followed the Allied armies, was twofold: the decentralization of the system, initially placed under the authority of the prefects of liberated territories, and the voluntary donor who entered history as a national hero.

After the war, the political forces of the Resistance strove to generalize the war-born innovation into a national public blood service. Protracted competition and political struggle set them in opposition to the medical advocates of the private model with professional donors organized into an extensive network with professional associations and collectively defined obligations as to lifestyle, contracts, tariffs, and publicity. In this competition the voluntary donor was presented as a courageous patriot, ready to sacrifice his life for the nation, whereas the professional donor was condemned for being a selfish blood seller, taking advantage of others' misfortunes.[16] The medical promoters of the voluntary model were actively supported by the Communist Party, its allied trade union, militant Catholics, and all Resistance-linked organizations.

A changing administrative structure and health care system provided an institutional context that all but assured the success of those who pressed for an end to the sale of blood. The newly created Social Security scheme and the development of public hospitals left little space for a private blood system, and the decree in 1952 legalized the triumph of the voluntary militants. It proscribed not paid donation but, rather, any commercial profit from the manufacturing and distribution of blood and derived products. A 1958 judgment by the State Council, in a case initiated by the Pharmacists' Council, prohibited the sale in pharmacies of any product derived from human blood. Their distribution was placed under the authority of medical doctors and was thus reserved for blood centers and hospitals. In the absence of institutional structures that might have made the sale of blood possible, paid donation disappeared. It was, however, only in 1993 that remunerated donation was legally prohibited.

A firm belief in its moral virtues bathed voluntary blood donation in a quasi "religious" aura, according to the American observer Jane Kramer.[17] It rested on the "dogma of the unassailable morality of the voluntary donor."[18] Because such blood was assumed to be pure, it was difficult to develop donor screening in France. Indeed, when the first hepatitis B test was introduced (HBS antigen) in 1976, donor screening was discontinued, replaced by biological assays that tested blood samples, not people.

Until 1991, when they moved into the shadows, blood donors retained a fighting spirit, organizing into more than 2000 local associations, which together formed a powerful national federation with more than 800,000 active members. Generously subsidized by the blood centers and local authorities, the associations enjoyed considerable political influence at both the local and national levels.[19]

A Heterogeneous Sector without Regulation

Before the 1993 reform, which in the aftermath of the AIDS disaster was to reorganize the entire sector, France had 170 blood centers (CTS) of which 163 were so-called transfusion centers—in other words, an average of at least one per department. The centers were responsible for collecting blood and plasma and for preparing labile products that could be stored for short periods. They supplied hospitals and the seven plasma fractionating centers. The latter prepared stable products (albumin, coagulation concentrates), which they then resold to hospitals and transfusion centers, which, in turn, supplied patients. The so-called regional centers, of which there were about 30, were affiliated with the major university hospitals. No hierarchical relationship existed among the various centers, which were all legally and financially independent. Half of the blood centers were public bodies, and the other half not-for-profit private organizations, depending on their initial setup and affiliation with hospitals, local authorities, or associations. All, however, functioned in the framework of blood transfusion as a public service.

The *Fondation Nationale de la Transfusion Sanguine* was entrusted with regional and interregional coordination of transfusion policies, with the task of advising the Minister of Health and undertaking research, international missions, and certain technical tasks such as keeping a national list of rare blood group donors. Despite the existence of the *Fondation*, the blood system was fundamentally heterogeneous. When in the 1990s the senate commission established to investigate the blood system in the aftermath of the AIDS disaster sought to characterize its essential features, it noted that the missions of the blood centers were "confused and ill-defined," constituting a conglomeration in which the only link was blood.[20]

Within the Ministry of Health, the General Department of Health (DGS) was formally charged with the responsibility of overseeing the full range of activities involved in the collection and distribution of blood: approving the CTS's and monitoring their activities; controlling the preparation, conservation, and quality of blood products, as well as the conditions under which they were delivered; and fixing the official prices for blood products, which were uniform throughout France.

Given these responsibilities, it is striking that no office within the DGS had the responsibility of executing this mission. Indeed, the range of tasks was merely part of the administrative duties of a single nonmedical official. Furthermore, the DGS depended on advisory bodies made up of blood sector specialists—those who came from the very sector the DGS was to oversee. Finally, the existing administrative rules and standards were utterly inadequate to meet the requirements of effective control over blood products and activities.[21]

In 1980, just prior to the onset of the AIDS epidemic, the National Health Laboratory (LNS), the Ministry's technical arm, was given responsibility for approving technical procedures and verifying the quality of blood products. These all-important functions were entrusted to two officials. It was the LNS that would be called upon, in 1985, to authorize the marketing of the first HIV antibody test.

The weakness of the supervisory authority and the resulting confusion of roles had two sources. The first involved the "legal vagueness" that surrounded the responsibilities of the various levels of the blood system.[22] The CTS's were looked upon as self-governing bodies because they were directed by doctors who were professionally independent. Officials from the Ministry of Health were never sure of their prerogatives, and they simply recorded sectoral policies. The second source of weakness was linked to general features of French health policy where the Ministry of Health functioned as an "administrative dwarf"[23] and where blood policy in particular provided an example of "republican feudalism"[24] combining the autonomy of local overlords with a public service lacking State authority.

Technical progress confronted the system with issues for which it was ill prepared. Conceiving a coherent policy of investment and technological choices was difficult in the context of a not-for-profit ideology, independent agents and administratively fixed prices. During the 1970s, many of the CTS's produced antihemophilic drugs (i.e., frozen and lyophilized cryoprecipitates). Factor VIII concentrates were imported until national production was launched in the early 1980s. Although seven centers engaged in the production of factor VIII clotting concentrates, two of them, the *Centre National de Transfusion Sanguine* (CNTS), one of the two constituents of the Fondation Nationale de la Transfusion Sanguine, and the Lille Center, accounted for nearly 80% of the national production in 1985. National self-sufficiency was attained in 1987.[25] By contrast, the production of factor IX concentrates, developed by the CNTS as early as 1959, adequately met national requirements from the outset.

The development of plasmapheresis was viewed by the donor associations as a threat to the symbolic value of blood donation.[26] Instead of collective donation near the homes or work places of donors—in most instances, a social occasion—plasmapheresis required donors to make individual appointments and to go to the blood centers, which also had to invest in appropriate facilities. The centers and the donors feared that plasmapheresis would undermine the monopoly of voluntary donation. The slow development of plasmapheresis resulted in intensified collection of full blood[27] and, consequently, in the overuse of transfusions in hospitals. So-called "comfort" and "safety" transfusions were common.[28] Indeed, only when the tragedy of AIDS in the blood supply emerged would the consequence of such profligacy become clear.

Blood Transfusion and Blood Product Recipients

The French Hemophiliacs' Association (AFH) was founded in 1955 by Professor Jacques Soulier, then the director of the CNTS, together with one of his hemophiliac patients. A close relationship with doctors remained a permanent feature of the hemophiliac associations. The latter lived in symbiosis with the CTSs that accommodated and funded them. The national association was instrumental in fostering the development of regional associations linked to regional blood centers. They in turn fostered the development of local groups. Their initial goals were to structure the milieu, inform hemophiliacs of available treatment, and pressure the authorities for free access to treatment. In the 1970s, the associations served to teach patients home care and self-injection. They informed families about the four specialized boarding schools for hemophiliac children, where they were taught to treat themselves and, in the 1980s, to take their own prophylactic drugs. "All young hemophiliacs went to these schools, where they formed networks and learned to live normally." The philosophy of the hemophiliac's autonomy and his right to live normally was formulated in these associations and schools. The perspective was a reflection of the commitment in social policy during the 1970s and early 1980s to promote autonomy and normal lives for all handicapped individuals, the elderly, and the mentally ill.[29] Against the image of the crippled hemophiliac, the new ethos promoted an athleticism: "All hemophiliacs to the summit of Mont Blanc." National self-sufficiency in clotting concentrates, it was believed, was to make possible the realization of the commitment to normalization.

France has about 40 centers specialized in the care of hemophiliacs. According to the AFH, half of all severe hemophiliacs are treated, often from childhood, in the CTS where they feel they are known. In 1971, hemophilia was added to the list of diseases covered 100% by health insurance. Treatment of the first patients with imported factor VIII concentrates started in 1975–76. After several years of observation, the doctors and the AFH promoted the large-scale use of these new products. At its annual congress in May 1980, the AFH called for the production in France of factor VIII concentrates to by-pass the fickleness of the international market and to conform to the principle of voluntary donation. Both the CNTS and the public authorities supported the proposition. In 1982, funds were made available by the ministry and health insurance to convert the CNTS facility located at Ulis for national production, which started in mid-1983 and increased by 60% in 1984.[30] However, the new production unit had no purification capacity; at the very moment that France embarked on a policy of rapid—and badly controlled—manufacture of factor VIII concentrate, AIDS came on the scene.

HIV in the Blood System

At the start of 1983, only 60 hemophiliacs were undergoing prophylactic treatment with factor VIII clotting concentrate,[31] although wide-scale use had been on the policy agenda for two years. In an editorial in the AFH journal *Hémophile* (November 1982), the president of the association criticized those running the French blood system for not meeting French hemophiliacs' needs and demanded increased imports of concentrate. Professor Soulier, of the AFH and the CNTS, responded in an "Open Letter to Hemophiliacs," which warned against a premature reliance on the new concentrates. The production of these new agents necessitated twice as much plasma, and therefore twice as many donations, aş the production of cryoprecipitates. More critically, "mysterious viral diseases could possibly be transmitted by fractions of commercial plasma. . . ."[32] Hence he urged hemophiliacs to revert to traditional local cryoprecipitates and proposed a two-year moratorium on the consumption and production of factor VIII.

Soulier's warning went unheeded. The final motion adopted at the AFH General Assembly in May 1983 stated that "the potential risk due to AIDS objectively evaluated is not likely to modify current prophylactic treatment," that "it is not necessary to interrupt nor to reduce the treatments. . . . Importation has to continue [and] national production increase." The Health Minister was asked to take steps toward developing a system that would increase the collection of plasma and enhance the prospect of the development of coagulant factors through genetic engineering.[33]

At this crucial juncture hepatitis B served as a conceptual model for understanding the threat of AIDS, a disease that still seemed nothing more than a theoretical danger. Unfamiliar with the risk of HIV, hemophiliacs were loath to "step backward." The president of the AFH, fully convinced of the benefits of prophylactic treatment, played an important part in promoting its use. The AFH was thus caught up in a dilemma with no exit.[34] The parents of hemophiliac children, in particular, were anxious not to revert to a former life of discomfort and social handicaps. The prescribing doctors and medical counselors of the association passed on reassuring messages. Outsiders were ignored:

> I tried in the early 80s, together with Doctor H, to lower pooled production in France, but we were confronted with a twofold opposition: the hemophiliac association, and their doctors. It was like a family, a solid front of opposition. The treating doctors underestimated the risk; they defended their patients, which is, of course, understandable. The problem was that none of us was sitting on the *Comite National*

d'Hemophilie, composed entirely of renowned specialists in hemophilia. (confidential interview)

Fueling the resistance to a return to older forms of treatment was a deep suspicion about the motives underlying such a course. "We didn't believe there was a serious risk, but rather that it was a way to cut health expenses . . . , because a severe hemophiliac costs a lot of money every year, and life expectancy is growing. We didn't want to be the ones that were sacrificed to save the health bill."

Where physicians did not embrace the use of factor concentrate, patients ultimately escaped the full brunt of HIV contamination. Thus hemophiliacs treated at the St. Antoine hospital in Paris, the most AIDS-affected area in France, had a far lower contamination level than the national average.[35] They were spared because an old doctor, wary of the new "miracle products," continued to use cryoprecipitate.

Screening Donors

The first official step toward AIDS risk reduction in the blood supply was taken with the DGS Circular of June 1983 asking all blood centers to practice donor selection. This ministerial initiative followed by one month that of the CNTS, which had implemented donor screening and confidential self-exclusion in May. The CNTS initiative generated strong protest from the sole existing gay organization at the time. The *Comité d'Urgence Antirepression Homosexuelle* addressed an open letter to the prime minister denouncing "anti-gay racism and the use of a biological phenomenon for moralizing purposes." The headlines in the left-wing daily *Libération* read, "Bad Blood: Gays, Undesirable Blood Group" and condemned "the drift towards discrimination."[36] The sharp reaction occurred despite the fact that the CNTS had taken into account such concerns and had relied upon a questionnaire focused on personal behavior, not on group membership. Donations were to be always accepted when other persons were present, even if the sample had to be later set aside.

The editors of the ministerial circular were even more cautious. Prior to publication they had submitted the circular to the Consultative Committee for Blood Transfusion, which, fearing that donors might be made to feel uncomfortable, had reluctantly approved it. In the end, the circular asked the blood centers to identify "at-risk individuals by means of a clinical examination." Only by a note given to donors was self-exclusion of those at risk to be practiced.

As was true in the case of the CNTS, caution did not preclude criticism. *Le Matin*, despite being very close to the Socialists in power, characterized the DGS's method as "indiscreet." The very serious *Le Monde* ran a headline, "Health and Private Life" and questioned whether AIDS represented such a serious threat "that for medical reasons it was necessary to inquire into the private lives of blood donors."[37]

Remarkably, the recommendations contained in the circular were seldom applied at a local level. A survey conducted in February 1984, to which only half of the centers replied, found that half of the respondents had never made any mention in their screening either of AIDS or of sexual orientation. Ninety percent of the CTS's considered their donors to be risk-free, and only nine centers stated that they systematically asked questions on "private life."[38] Only a reminder published in January 1985 pointed out the legal responsibility of the blood centers in case of transmission.

The sensitivities provoked by efforts to screen out those who might pose a risk to the blood supply are highlighted by the reluctance to move swiftly to prohibit donations by prisoners. Blood donation in prisons started in the 1950s, increased in the 1970s, and reached its peak in 1982–84. These two years corresponded to the period in which the French production of factor VIII concentrates developed rapidly. It also coincided with a period of growing repressive measures against drug addicts, resulting in an increase in the number of intravenous drug users in prison. The blood centers' main motives for collecting in prisons were of a practical nature: in a few hours they could harvest large quantities of blood. For the inmates, it was a welcome break in daily monotony and an opportunity they rarely missed. For the prison administration, blood donation was a way of enabling inmates to exercise their civil rights during detention and to participate in the duty of solidarity. Blood donation was considered an act of "social reintegration."[39] Indeed, at the Ministry of Justice, blood collection in prisons was administratively attached to the Department of Social Reintegration.

When the risk of AIDS became known, the CNTS immediately stopped its collections in prisons, in April 1983, followed by those blood centers that depended on the Parisian Public Hospital administration. Unfortunately, however, these forerunners did not make public their initiative. The Circular of June 20, 1983, on donor screening did not even mention the necessity of avoiding risky collection venues. Indeed, in 1984 the authorized number of blood collections in each prison was increased.

It was only in the spring of 1985 that the full dimensions of the dangers inherent in prison blood collection were clarified. A prison physician reported that 54% of inmate donors belonged to various risk groups.[40] Efforts on the part of the Director General for Health to formally prohibit blood collection in prisons met with resistance within the Health Minister's cabinet because of strong commitments to the ideology of social reintegration. It was only in the latter part of 1985 that prison blood collection dropped to a tenth of its former level following a joint warning issued by the DGS and the prison administration. The ban was not, however, officially declared: the two central administrations simply warned local officials by telephone. The Prime Minister's office and the chancellery preferred not to be involved in decisions on the matter because establishing a link between inmates and AIDS was considered politically undesirable, a potential cause for "social stigmatization."[41] Blood collection was continued in several prisons until 1989 and only stopped completely in 1991. Blood from prisons accounted for less than half of one percent of the total national supply until 1985, but those donors were responsible for as much as 25% of the cases of contamination through blood.[42]

Testing Blood

The advent of testing for blood contamination was made possible by the development of the HIV antibody test, and mandatory screening of donated blood became an urgent demand from transfusion leaders and others concerned with the blood supply at the beginning of 1985. The urgency of the situation was underscored by a profoundly troubling epidemiological memorandum prepared by Dr. Jean-Baptiste Brunet from the DGS. On the basis of AIDS prevalence found in the donors of two Parisian blood centers, Brunet demonstrated that "It is probable that all the products prepared from pools of Parisian donors are currently contaminated."[43] The official decision to introduce mandatory screening was announced in Parliament by the prime minister, and became applicable on August 1, 1985. France was thus one of the first European countries to institute mandatory screening of blood, yet it is clear that such screening could have been instituted three months earlier. Documents now available as a result of official inquiries reveal the play of interests and concerns that delayed such testing.

First, the French authorities sought to protect the French market from an invasion by American HIV antibody test kits produced by Abbott. The latter had filed an application, on February 11, 1985, for authorization from the National Health Laboratory (LNS) to market the test, at a time when the French firm Diagnostics-Pasteur was not yet ready to face international competition in its own domestic market. Its initial price was almost twice as high as Abbott's. Abbott's marketing license was therefore delayed. The second problem concerned the financing of blood screening, which necessitated lengthy negotiations with the Social Security Department before the latter would agree to the integration of such costs into the official prices for blood products, for which health insurance would have to foot the bill. Third, a small group of AIDS specialists, notably Dr. Brunet, stressed the necessity of providing free and anonymous testing facilities *before* blood screening was introduced, to avoid a situation in which at-risk persons might donate in order to determine their own antibody status. Finally, there were ethical concerns about what precisely would be told to those who tested positive, given the uncertainty of the clinical significance of this finding.[44] Indeed, some argued that given the risk of discrimination and the psychological burden of being informed about a potentially inaccurate or uninterpretable test result, individuals should not be notified of the results of donor testing.

These issues were discussed at an inter-ministerial meeting called by the prime minister's main adviser on May 9, 1985. The decision was taken to postpone approval of the American Abbott test in order to provide Diagnostics-Pasteur with time to enhance its own prospects. Central to that decision was the influence of those who sought to give priority to financial and industrial considerations over those that touched on matters of public health. After the meeting, the prime minister's and the health minister's chief advisers agreed that despite the importance of protecting French industrial interests, the early introduction of screening could be politically advantageous in a pre-electoral period. France's image abroad would be enhanced; the press and physicians would be satisfied.[45] Thus, just two days after the prime minister's announcement in Parliament that France would require testing of blood donations, on August 1, 1985, the Pasteur test was given its marketing license. A month later, the Abbott test was licensed.

Remarkably, the prime minister himself made the formal determination[46] —based on the advice of both ethical and medical authorities—that those who tested positive would have to be informed of their antibody status. Finally, on the question of whether testing of blood donations could commence in the absence of venues where those who wanted to know if they carried antibody to HIV could be tested, the advice of AIDS experts was ignored. Such anonymous and free test sites did not open in France until 1987, although health insurance coverage for antibody tests ordered by physicians was available in February 1987.

Viral Inactivation of Factor Concentrate

When the blood scandal broke in France, a central element of the controversy was the question of when viral inactivation of clotting factor could have been instituted. Like so much else surrounding blood, involved was a mix of scientific uncertainty, dogma regarding the risk-free nature of volunteered blood, and national industrial policy.

Although the CNTS had begun to explore the possibility of viral inactivation in 1983, the leadership of the fractionation center at Lille only came to appreciate the urgency of the matter in mid-July 1984. But even in late 1984, the president of the French Hemophilia Foundation still expressed uncertainty about the benefits of heat treatment. Writing in *Hémophile*, he stated that although the data on such processing were "interesting" it was crucial to "wait for the results of experiments being conducted by French experts."[47] In the interim, hemophiliacs should "trust their experts and doctors and the products they prescrib[ed] to us." When Jean-Baptiste Brunet informed a November 1984 meeting of the Consultative Committee that both French and international studies were conclusive regarding the efficacy of heat treatment, an eminent expert on the treatment of hemophilia replied that this "still needed to be proved."[48] As late as March 1985, a specialist writing in *Hémophile* could assert that it was only a matter of "intellectual deduction" that heat treatment could inactivate HIV, for the process had been designed to confront the challenge of hepatitis B. Other, *French*, studies were needed. As the Lucas report[49] was later to show, treatment specialists were doubtful about the reliability of foreign studies.

By the spring of 1985, doubts began to vanish and pressure from hemophiliacs for large-scale importation of heated products began to mount. Brunet had prepared a memorandum stating that "all batches of [concentrate] produced by the CNTS were probably contaminated" with HIV. But with such alarming epidemiological data at hand, France was utterly unprepared to provide inactivated concentrate. In April, Lille was just testing its heating process. In June the CNTS attempt at heat treatment failed for technical reasons.

Given the urgency of the matter, the CNTS could have undertaken the massive importation of inactivated concentrate. That, however, would have meant the failure of national industrial policy entrusted to it by the public authorities. As a consequence the CNTS chose to embrace an ultimately disastrous "transition period" during which untreated concentrates would still be distributed. In the absence of a clear understanding of the potentially dire implications of a delay, the Hemophilia Association declared that only as of October 1 should the distribution of untreated factor concentrate to be prohibited, even if that necessitated massive importation.[50]

Despite the fact that officials responsible for the distribution of factor concentrate knew that "the probability of not having contaminated batches is very slight,"[51] they continued to press for the use of remaining stocks. In June 1985 Dr. Michel Garretta, director of the CNTS, wrote a memorandum urging that the use of untreated factor should remain "standard procedure except for specific requests."[52] A CNTS memorandum of August 1985 was sent to two Parisian hospitals asking them to "try to distribute untreated products to seropositive hemophiliacs."[53]

The decision to introduce the transition period provoked no more than a single written protest, addressed on July 5 to the president of the National Blood Transfusion Society. The concerned physician referred to his professional conscience in asking for the immediate prohibition of unheated products. The letter was circulated throughout the many national commissions and organizations until the end of November, when officials concerned with hemophilia treatment policy stated that it was no longer relevant.

Two DGS decrees, both issued on July 23, 1985, closed the affair. One instituted mandatory screening of all blood donations on August 1; the other declared that unheated products would no longer be paid for by the health insurance as of October 1, amounting to a prohibition. The CNTS started heated production in mid-September 1985. At the same time, a circular from the DGS made viral inactivation compulsory for all production centers.

But even then untreated stocks in patients' homes, in hospitals, and CTS's were not recalled. Only the treatment center in the city of Rouen recalled products from its individual patients.[54] An inquiry carried out in 112 blood centers concluded that significant unused stocks still existed on September 1, amounting to a total of 30 million IU, only part of which were returned to the CNTS for destruction.[55]

The policy that covered the transition period was formulated by transfusion leaders, legitimized by advisory bodies, and then endorsed by the DGS. The health minister never intervened. It was during the transition that unsafe concentrate was provided to trusting hemophiliac patients. When illness and death crept up on the close-knit community of hemophiliacs in the following years, notably during 1988–90, they argued that they had agreed to the delays and the transition period only because they had never been made privy to the data made available to officials by Jean-Baptiste Brunet in March 1985.

The Epidemiological Aftermath[56]

Epidemiological factors, clinical practices, and the process of policy making contributed to the iatrogenic disaster of blood-borne AIDS in France. As of December 1996, 1743 cases of AIDS, including 89 pediatric cases, were reported as a result of transfusions. Two thirds of the patients have died. Five hundred and forty-three hemophiliacs, including 51 children, of a total hemophiliac population of 5000 had developed AIDS because of contaminated clotting factor. One hundred and eighty-seven heterosexual cases of AIDS were linked to the blood-borne HIV infection of sexual partners.

HIV infection is, of course, more widespread. It is estimated that between four and six thousand cases of infection occurred because of transfusions or the use of blood products. More than 1200 hemophiliacs—40% of the 3000 people with severe hemophilia—were infected.

Nevertheless, a comparison of regional data clearly shows that the general prevalence of AIDS is the basic factor behind blood-related AIDS prevalence—regions with the highest prevalence of AIDS have the highest number of transfusion-related AIDS. Thus the Parisian region (Ile-de-France), the Marseilles and Cote-d'Azur region, and the French West Indies (Antilles-Guyane) with the highest rate of AIDS cases per million population (1,801.8) had an AIDS case rate from blood transfusion and products of 69.4 per million population. In the regions with the lowest AIDS prevalence, blood-related contamination is also far lower (Franche-Comté, l'Alsace, Nord Pas de Calais). In Franche-Comté, with an overall case rate of 210.1 per million, the case rate from blood was 12.8.

While geography was destiny for blood transfusion recipients, the picture was more complex for hemophiliacs, whose rates of infection varied according to the policies of the transfusion centers and the prescribing practices of doctors. The relative protection afforded by a low AIDS prevalence or by donor screening—when effectively implemented—was neutralized by the technique of pooling thousands of

donations. Thus the sad case of Aquitaine, which holds the record for AIDS prevalence related to the blood system with 74.4 cases per million population. The Bor-
deaux blood transfusion center—the supplier of drugs to hemophiliacs in the region—
had relied on the largest prison in the region for blood. At the other extreme we find
the Nord-Pas de Calais region (case rate 9.1), which combines the lowest AIDS prevalence in the country with the fact that the regional transfusion center at Lille was the
first in France to introduce a heating technique, in the spring of 1985.

Mobilization, Public Action, and Litigation

One night in 1989, Dr. Michel Garretta, who was then engaged in negotiations with
the European Community concerning the forthcoming open market for blood products, discovered that his car was burned in protest. The following year he was deco-
rated with the *Ordre National du Mérite*, on the request of the president of the Republic, despite the reservations of the health minister, who was already involved in
ongoing negotiations over the question of compensating hemophiliacs infected with
HIV. The turn of the decade marked a watershed; what demands had been made in
prior years because of HIV in the blood supply would pale when compared to the
explosion of outrage that would ensue. The number of recorded cases of full-blown
AIDS related to blood treatment had shot up in 1988–89, and the perception of the
problem changed. Victims of blood-borne AIDS transformed themselves into a vital
political force.

Victims without Voice

The emergence of effective, organized protest on the part of hemophiliacs had to
overcome a number of obstacles rooted in the nature of the blood collection system,
the relationship of hemophiliacs to their physicians, and the legal regime surrounding blood. But as protest emerged it met with opposition from vested interests. Voluntary blood donors tolerated no criticism on blood issues and acted as powerful
spokespersons for the blood centers. When in a May 1986 television interview several hemophiliacs expressed doubt regarding French products, the president of the
Blood Donors' Association wrote to the AFH president to protest. "The CTS cannot
accept unwarranted attacks on the quality of their blood. Voluntary blood donors
have never asked for the slightest thanks from those who benefit fully from their generosity. There is no reason why they should stand for insults from them. Hemophiliacs' total dependence on the donors' voluntary, free gesture make their attitudes unjust
and almost odious."[57]

The AFH had no allies. In part, this isolation was self-imposed. Hemophiliacs refused contact with the newly created associations for the defense of people with AIDS, which they considered responsible for the blood contamination. The opposition by gay men and professionals caring for drug addicts to the screening of blood donors and even of blood samples reinforced this argument. Furthermore, the AFH wanted to remain outside the social mobilization around AIDS in order to avoid any association between hemophilia and the stigmatized epidemic. "We invited the editors-in-chief of the newspapers to explain our situation and ask them not to talk about us. You see, hemophiliacs are always boys. We didn't want to be linked to homosexuality. It's not so long ago that we were a stigmatized people." (interview) The newspapers complied with the request until 1990.

Initially, hemophiliacs hid their seropositivity for fear of losing their jobs or, in the case of children, not being accepted in school. It was in the struggle for compensation that hemophiliacs shed their accommodationist political strategy.

Legal and political dispute erupted when a minority of dissenters, who criticized the Hemophilia Association's low-profile strategy focused on behind-the-scenes negotiations, broke with the AFH. Jean Garvanoff, an atypical hemophiliac who had not been part of the "community" of patients and caregivers, sought to make the hemophiliac problem public, to mobilize the press and political parties, including the National Front, which seized the case as an opportunity to criticize the political establishment.

From 1986, when the non-socialist parties returned to power, the AFH had tried to obtain aid from the Minister of Health, who refused "to pay for the socialists' mistakes." (interview) If there was governmental or medical responsibility, hemophiliacs would have to take the matter to court. The minister, however, set up a commission to study medical and social benefits for hemophiliacs with AIDS. Following recommendations put forward in May 1988, the Minister subsidized the Hemophilia Association so that it could pay a social worker to assist families with financial difficulties. Despite growing internal contentiousness, the Association was to adhere to its choice for a collective, united approach: "There was terrible internal friction with those who wanted legal action, even violent action, including against the AFH leaders—I personally received written threats—but we thought that in legal action only a part of the hemophiliacs would be able to supply proof—proof of dates, of the doctor's fault, etc.—and obtain compensation. We opted for solidarity between all of us, so that *everyone* might obtain something." (interview)

Several activists broke away from the AFH and filed claims in the courts. The first such moves occurred in March 1988 against the CNTS for the misdemeanor of merchandising fraud. A second series followed in April, broadening the affair to include the National Health Laboratory, the National Ethics Council, and even the AFH, all on the grounds of manslaughter and non-assistance to persons in danger.

In April 1989, Jean Garvanoff, together with his brother—also a hemophiliac—and the other dissidents, founded a second association, the *Association des Polytransfusés*, as an alternative to the AFH. The new association filed a third series of claims against both the CNTS and the AFH for fraud and non-assistance to those in danger.

1991: The Year Things Fell Apart

The flames of discontent were fanned by the media. Anne-Marie Casteret, a journalist at the weekly *L'Evénement du Jeudi*, undertook her own inquiry, which in 1992 would appear as a book, *L'affaire du Sang*. In April 1991 her magazine published the minutes of the internal CNTS meeting at which the continued distribution of factor VIII concentrates, known to be contaminated, was planned. This news sparked off a vehement press campaign that was to so define the French experience. Other newspapers started their own investigations and, day by day, the public, astounded and avid for further revelations, discovered new documents stamped "confidential."

The blood scandal that emerged in 1991 was shaped by a veritable press war that provided the foundations for a new kind of medical journalism.[58] *Le Monde*, with its long-standing tradition of medical journalism, was locked in conflict with less established journalists trying to assert themselves. While the former adopted a posture emphasizing the "medical disaster" and collective errors, the insurgent journalists pinpointed the decisions made by individuals underscoring both their mistakes and malicious acts. The press grasped the opportunity to modify its relations with politicians, the medical profession, and the legal world—three areas of society in which the French press had relatively little autonomy. The affair provided an opportunity for young journalists to assert themselves in a highly competitive professional sphere, as medical journalism shifted from the hands of doctors to those of journalists wanting to specialize in medical issues. The blood affair also encouraged investigative journalism, a relatively undeveloped field in France.

While the Minister of Health remained silent, transfusion officials and journalists confronted one another on TV and in the medical press. The former argued that without the distribution of at-risk concentrates, hemophiliacs would have died from loss of blood. They claimed that there had not been enough heated products at the time on the world market, and that the problem had been similar in other countries. Based on new documents, which they discovered, journalists denounced "the monopoly" that prohibited doctors from prescribing inactivated drugs produced abroad.[59] A cabal among the state, doctors, and Dr. Garretta had betrayed the interests of hemophiliacs.

Dr. Garretta resigned on June 3, 1991, considering himself the victim of "an aggressive and partial press campaign of orchestrated disinformation."[60] In the ensuing months the press made public what seemed to be a picture of sordid financial relations within the blood sector. For the press, the contaminated blood affair had become a question of dirty money.

In September 1991 the report by the General Inspectorate for Social Affairs was issued. Known as the Lucas Report, it established an official chronology of events and decisions and pointed out the incoherence within the decision making system. The Lucas Report also provided an important document that journalists had sought in vain, the minutes of the inter-ministerial meeting in May 1985 in which it was decided to delay introducing the AIDS blood test in order to give Pasteur-Diagnostics a better chance in the marketplace. The press was henceforth to turn its attention to those "responsible in the ministries."[61] The scandal turned political. It was in this context that criminal charges were brought against four leaders in the field of blood transfusion and public health. It was also in this context that Françoise Mitterand, president of the Republic, entered the fray.

On November 10, 1991, the president of the Republic announced during a televised speech that "we need a law, we need Parliament as a whole to be involved in the measures that have to be taken to compensate [for] damages which can never be entirely compensated." Legislation—the law of December 31, 1991—establishing a public indemnification plan was unanimously approved by Parliament.

Whatever its shortcomings, such as the tendency to mischaracterize technical issues raised by the blood scandal, the press had effectively drawn attention to the victims of tainted blood and had mobilized public opinion. In so doing it had forced the government to act.

The Long Road to Compensation

The political system of the Fifth Republic, which provides wide autonomy to the executive, affords limited capacity for initiative in the French parliament. Unlike the National Assembly, however, the Senate can define its own agenda. The struggle for compensation began in 1987, when the Social Commission, in a conservative Assembly, drew up a report proposing a compensation scheme for HIV blood victims that was never put on the agenda.[62] Transfusion recipients, who were not at all organized, later found a highly effective spokesman in a senator who had a family member infected by a blood transfusion. He mobilized interest in transfusion-associated AIDS within the Senate and helped to found an association to defend the interests of transfusion recipient victims, the *Association de Défense des Transfusés*. The Senate tabled a bill in 1990 and suggested public compensation for all victims contaminated before December 31, 1986.

The return of the Socialists to power in 1988 opened the way to a collective compensation scheme, albeit under pressure. Negotiations for the first compensation scheme were held together with the insurance companies, without consulting the AFH. "The Health Minister's cabinet telephoned us, saying they were preparing a plan for us and asking a few technical details. We were never asked to give our views on it. Afterwards we were simply informed of the result, the mixed fund, and the amount of money given to it." (interview)

This first compensation scheme was limited to hemophiliacs. It was presented by the government as an exceptional case and as an act of "solidarity," as opposed to a "reparation for injury" in the legal sense of the term. In July 1989 a protocol agreement, known as the "Éven Agreement" after the Minister of Health, was signed by four parties: the insurance companies, the AFH, the transfusion institutions, and the state. It provided for payment by the insurance companies of a fixed sum of 100,000 FF (US$ 20,000) to each seropositive hemophiliac. The state was to indemnify acute AIDS cases, with payments depending on age and family situation but not exceeding 620,000 FF (US$ 120,000). A widow would receive 170,000 FF with 40,000 FF for each child (US$ 34,000 and US$ 8,000, respectively). The insurance companies, following convention, demanded that each beneficiary give up the right to institute further legal proceedings. The minister's advisers, on the other hand, insisted that the state's compensation fund should not be bound to the renunciation of further legal proceedings. While most hemophiliacs accepted the plan, the wealthier did not. Once again, the cohesion of the hemophiliac community was threatened. The *Association des Polytransfusés* sharply criticized the scheme. So too did the press and the opposition parties. Public opinion was also unfavorable. At the center of the criticism was the antagonism to the reliance, at least in part, on private financing.

Implementation of the controversial compensation scheme was lengthy. As a result, in 1990 the AFH embarked on a strategy of political mobilization for a new compensation law. Thus a scheme designed to diffuse the conflict became the occasion for further protest. The regional and local sections of the AFH actively lobbied with letters and petitions addressed to all deputies, senators, and local politicians. At the same time, the senate and the new association of transfusion recipients pushed for a general compensation law for *all* victims. The law for victims of terrorism, which had been passed in 1990, became the common reference for all parties concerned.

For both medical and legal experts, a central concern raised by the issue of compensation entailed the problem of who should bear the burden of proof and how such determinations would effect the concept of responsibility for medical errors. If the onus remained on victims to prove the precise nature of the medical fault, most would find the path to compensation all but foreclosed. However, if no showing of fault was necessary, doctors and medical institutions would be permitted to escape professional liability.[63] Neither seemed acceptable. And so, ultimately, a consensus was reached that sought to preserve the advantages of a no-fault system with those of a liability-based approach. Victims were to be freed from the burden of legal proof, but in cases where evidence existed of specific acts leading to infection with HIV, legal procedures would permit plaintiffs to seek compensation from those who were responsible.

Once the principle of compensation had been accepted, it was necessary to determine the class of eligible beneficiaries. Should only hemophiliacs be covered, or should transfusion recipients be covered as well? And if transfusion recipients were covered, why not transplant recipients and those who had become infected through artificial insemination? If those who had suffered from such medical accidents deserved compensation, why not individuals infected through occupational injury? In the end, all such individuals were deemed eligible. Gay leaders and some allied Parisian intellectuals who opposed the "blood and medically oriented" compensation policy as unjust, asked why the medically infected should be treated differently from others infected with HIV. They found no political support for their argument, though, except from the National AIDS Council (*Conseil National du Sida*). The *Conseil* criticized the "moral distinction" between the "good," "innocent" AIDS victims and the "bad," "guilty" ones. Like the earlier government report,[64] the National AIDS Council's perspective derived from a commitment to oppose all forms of discrimination, even the creation of special programs *for* those with AIDS. The government responded to such criticism by emphasizing that it was not AIDS itself which was a national calamity justifying compensation and national solidarity but the spread of HIV through the national transfusion system.

The Compensation Fund, established by the 1991 Act, provides compensation for all people infected with HIV through medical treatment or actions, including transfusion patients, their infected partners (for unmarried partners, the question remains open, but these cases are generally accepted), their children, and their heirs. Five years later, in 1996, health care workers infected occupationally would be added to those entitled to the Fund's benefits under the same conditions. The new Fund was state-financed. It received a single endowment of US$ 220 million from insurance companies, the result of negotiations on the previous compensation plan, and a state subsidy renewed annually in accordance with the Fund's needs. The Fund guarantees applicants a swift decision on their cases without legal procedures (three months for acceptance of the case, and three months further for calculating the compensation sum fixed by the Fund).

Under the new law, victims have two available paths: they may seek compensation from the Fund without having to present proof of culpability—the presence of HIV infection and of previous blood-related treatment is sufficient; or they may, through litigation, seek to obtain higher compensation—if, for instance they believe a particular act of medical malpractice can be proved. Those who pursue the path of litigation are not barred from seeking compensation from the Fund if they fail in the courts.

The level of compensation from the new Fund is much higher than previously established sums and takes into account damages in the way they would be assessed by a court of law. Emotional distress due to infection, handicap from the illness, loss of years of life, and economic losses for the victims and their heirs are all considered. For a diagnosed AIDS case in an adult man with an average income, compensation may range from the equivalent of US$ 150,000 to US$ 400,000. Compensation for emotional distress and damage to health are calculated according to age, with young people entitled to far more than older people. According to the 1992 and 1993 annual reports of the Compensation Fund, indemnities paid out for economic loss may vary considerably. In that two-year period they ranged from $3,000 to $500,000 per case. Between March 1993 and February 1994, the Fund handled 11,000 cases (4000 involved victims and 7000 family members).[65] Experts estimate the total amount that France will pay out to its HIV blood victims at around 6 to 7 billion French francs (US$ 1.2 to 1.4 billion).[66]

The broad scope of the HIV compensation scheme and its generosity provoked demands for extension of its underlying principle to others. Mounting social pressure for compensation came from victims of other transfused pathologies, notably hepatitis. The AFH strongly supported hepatitis C compensation because many hemophiliacs were affected. Liver specialists also supported the proposal. The underlying question was whether compensation should be extended to *all* medical accidents. As these are often linked to transmissible disease or to scientific and technological innovations, it was argued that victims should be freed from the onus of legally proving "medical mistakes." An initial proposal for such broadly based compensation was, in fact, first put forward two years before the passage of the 1991 act, supported by the numerous small associations of medical victims and the last Socialist Health Minister Bernard Kouchner. The latter commissioned a social scientist to examine the question. The resulting Ewald Report, published in October 1992,[67] strongly supported the idea of compensation for all victims of iatrogenic injury as a logical step forward for the welfare state. However, the medical profession and the opposition raised strong objections, arguing that it would mean the end of individual responsibility and would be too costly. In an obviously political maneuver the government, however, tabled the bill at the end of 1992, and it had no chance of surviving the spring 1993 elections.

Turning to the Courts: Civil Litigation and Criminal Prosecution

Nearly 2000 cases involving transfusion recipients and hemophiliacs have been brought before the courts. The central question posed by these cases is whether the legal standards that govern medical practice or product liability will apply.[68] Doctors and hospitals have an *obligation de moyens* (a legal obligation to provide all available care). They can be held liable by patients if they fail to provide treatment that is technically available, or if they are negligent. Producers and suppliers, on the other hand, have an *obligation de résultats*, an obligation to produce expected results. The *Cour de Cassation* relied on a notion of product liability in cases involving medical institutions covered by civil jurisdiction. By contrast, the judgments of the administrative courts dealing with public entities varied.[69] Several of them, as well as the appeals courts, maintained the *obligation de moyens* and demanded proof of negligence. From 1991, administrative courts adopted the notion of product liability. In June of that year the Administrative Court of Marseilles ordered two hospitals to pay a total of FF 600,000 (US$ 120,000) to a transfusion recipient on the basis of hospitals' *obligation de résultats*.

Finally, at the end of 1991, the Administrative Court in Paris ordered the State to pay FF 2 million (US$ 400,000) in damages to a hemophiliac because it had not prohibited the distribution of unheated products after it had been warned by Jean-Baptiste Brunet that virtually all factor concentrate was contaminated with HIV. The court stated that "once information on a public health disaster had been made available, it was the responsibility of the State to withdraw the contaminated or risky products." It also found that mandatory screening of blood donations could have been instituted three months earlier than it was. This judgment, establishing public responsibility, was confirmed twice, by the Administrative Court of Appeal in 1992 and by the *Conseil d'État* (March 9, 1993).

Lawsuits brought by hemophiliacs and those infected through blood transfusions thus began to establish the contours of the responsibility of physicians and medical institutions to those who were in their clinical care. But such suits paled in terms of the high drama associated with the laying of criminal charges against officials responsible for the French blood system. It was the trial of those individuals that would rivet the attention of the French public and that would mark the experience of France as unique among other nations that confronted the iatrogenic tragedy of AIDS and blood.

The criminal inquiry under the investigating judge in Paris lasted for two years and led to charges against four individuals: Dr. Michel Garretta, director of the CNTS; Dr. Jean-Pierre Allain, scientific director of the CNTS and adviser to the Hemophilia Foundation; Professor Jacques Roux, director general of health; and Dr. Robert Netter. The process of coming to an agreement over the precise nature of the charges to be leveled was characterized by extended controversy that occupied legal specialists and filled the press. In the end, two options remained: fraud regarding the quality of blood products sold, classified as an "offense" (*délit*); and poisoning, defined as the administration of a harmful substance *known* to lead to death, and classified as a "crime." The implications of a finding of guilt for an offense, as contrasted with a crime, were stark. In the case of fraud, the maximum penalty was four years imprisonment. Poisoning could incur a life sentence.

Jurists and especially the victims' lawyers were divided over the appropriate charges to be brought. Involved was not just the question of the potential severity of the punishment but the pragmatic matter of which charges would be most likely to elicit a guilty verdict. Each camp wrote a book defending its standpoint.[70] Both parties solicited the opinions of eminent professors of law, which led to a stormy academic debate on the legal meaning of "poisoning." The urgency of coming to a resolution of this conflict compelled the parties to reach some practical agreement. The investigating judge, the public prosecutor, most of the victim's lawyers, and the government agreed to limit the charges to "offenses": fraud and non-assistance to persons in danger. Although criticized for being no more than a *délit d'épicier* (a minor misdemeanor), fraud was chosen in order to satisfy both the victims and public opinion. The choice of a "minor offense" ensured that the trial would indeed take place and that guilty verdicts with punishments would follow. Had the indictment been for poisoning, there was concern that a popular jury would balk at finding doctors guilty.[71]

The public prosecutor thus charged the defendants with having failed to take steps that might have protected hemophiliacs and blood transfusion recipients.[72] Dr. Garretta was accused of having "lied and manipulated" in order to protect the industrial interests of the CNTS. Dr. Allain was said to be guilty of duplicity in defending Dr. Garretta's decisions on heat treatment even though he privately found them mistaken. The director general of health, Professor Roux was allegedly accountable for having failed to stop the distribution of unheated clotting concentrates, although he could have done so by ministerial decree. Dr. Netter, asserted the prosecutor, could have authorized the marketing of the Abbott HIV antibody test kit but had yielded to those who insisted that the French-produced Pasteur kits be given priority. Finally, both Drs. Roux and Netter had been guilty, charged the prosecutor, of a dereliction of duty in not having warned the minister of health of the gravity of the situation. It was the failure of Netter and Roux—two senior civil servants— that implicated the state in this catastrophe.

The trial opened on June 22, 1992, in a tense, tiny courtroom.[73] Pressure from hemophiliacs wanting to attend was so great that the trial was moved to a larger venue. Public authorities, fearing an attack against the accused—by means of a syringe containing a victim's contaminated blood—decided that the public would have to be searched at the entrance. On the first day of the trial, such searches did occur. But Dr. Allain opposed such measures and threatened not to participate in his own trial if the searches continued. Allain prevailed, and these security measures were halted. In the courtroom one could hear members of ACT-UP chanting slogans against the state and doctors. The trial was headline news for four months.

Testimony by the prime minister, the minister of social affairs, and the minister of health was heard on July 24, one month into the trial.[74] Each of them— and notably the prime minister—bowed before the pain of the victims. This gesture caused murmurs and protests among the hemophiliacs, while the ACT-UP slogan, "AIDS—The politicians knew—They murdered" could be heard from the street. The eagerly awaited hearing was disappointing. All three former ministers claimed not to have been informed that the failure to heat-treat products could result in contamination.

The judgment of the court was handed down on October 23, 1992.[75] Dr. Garretta was found guilty and was sentenced to four years in prison and a fine of FF 500,000 (US $100,000). Allain was sentenced to four years in prison, of which two years were suspended. Director General Roux received a suspended sentence of four years' imprisonment. Dr. Netter was acquitted. The judgment also stipulated that the National Blood Transfusion Foundation, the parent organization of the CNTS's, bore civil responsibility and was ordered to pay FF 9.2 million (US $1.8 million).

The spectacular criminal trial turned out to be a Pandora's box from which a seemingly never-ending legal dynamic emerged. The *délit d'épicier* was not enough to shake off death, so omnipresent in the affair[76]; hence the victims' disappointment and anger and the attraction of the indictment for poisoning. A public opinion poll found that 85% of those surveyed found the trial to be "unsatisfactory"; 75% demanded that the "politicians stand trial."[77]

The legal process was driven forward by the process of appeal. Convinced of his own innocence, Dr. Allain sought a rehearing and, as a consequence, compelled the appeals court to retry the cases of all four defendants. On July 17, 1993, the court of appeal confirmed the previous judgment, making only minor adjustments in the sentences. The court did, however, increase the plaintiffs' award from 9 to 15 million French francs.

Dr. Allain turned to the *Cour de Cassation*, the highest and last level of judicial appeal. But this appeal led to a remarkable turn of events. In June 1994 the reporting magistrate submitted a report to the criminal chamber of the court not only rejecting Dr. Allain's appeal but arguing that the facts of the case made clear that what was involved was not the offense of fraud but the crime of poisoning. Lawyers for Allain and Garretta declared that any move to retry their clients would produce an appeal to the European Court of Human Rights on the grounds that individuals may not be tried twice for the same offense, and an international group of scientific and medical notables, including several Nobel prize recipients, supported the embittered defendants. Nonetheless, the effort to press the president of the Republic to grant a pardon to the two blood officials was unsuccessful.

Nothing more tellingly underscores the continued search for guilty parties deserving of punishment in the *scandale du sang* than the investigation opened by the Paris prosecutor's office in 1995, leading to the investigation of 13 people by early 1996 and 11 more by April 1997. This new criminal case caused much surprise when it was learned that even Jean-Baptiste Brunet, the AIDS epidemiologist who sounded the first and most persistent warnings concerning HIV contamination, was being investigated. Unlike the earlier investigation, this effort was clearly aimed at extending the net of culpability.

The effort to bring to justice those responsible for the contamination of the blood supply is not restricted to functionaries but has reached the highest levels of the state. The first trial highlighted the role of the prime minister and the ministers of social affairs and health as well as the "pre-eminent role of their advisors."[78] But how was one to organize a trial of three high-ranking government officials?[79] This question has engaged the parliament since mid-1992.

The blood victims, the press, and public opinion pressed for the trial of the "politicians," whereas the opposition parties saw an opportunity to discredit the Socialists. One of the accused, former prime minister Laurent Fabius, believed that a hearing of the charges would be desirable, although not before the *Haute Cour de Justice*, associated with trials for high treason. Believing he would be acquitted, he asked to be judged by a Court of Honor. Despite his effort to confront the issue directly, the political career of this top young socialist politician suffered.

Parliament encountered problems comparable to those of the courts but of even greater complexity in its attempt to institute legal proceedings. The process was characterized by missteps and was caught up in a more general constitutional reform, changes to the *Haute Cour de Justice* and the reform of the entire code of criminal law. Finally, four years after it first considered the matter, agreement was reached to commence an investigation under the charge of "complicity in poisoning." The entire process came to an unexpected conclusion when in March 1997 the public prosecutor, politically close to the conservative party in power (the RPR) since 1993 and known for his opposition to the "criminalization of public life,"[80] declared that there were no grounds for prosecution. In his voluminous 400–page report, he argued that "complicity" implied the *active* participation in or intervention by the accused.[81] Although he held the prime minister ultimately responsible for his government and severely criticized the "apathetic" attitude of the health minister and the low level of involvement of the social affairs minister, he declared that such failings did not add up to complicity in poisoning. The ministers were *politically* responsible, and that was a matter to be dealt with by the electorate, not by the criminal courts. Although subject to extensive press commentary, the issue failed to provoke the passionate exchange that might well have occurred when the *scandale du sang* was still fresh.

What seemed a final decision in March 1997 was soon revealed as yet another twist in a complex legal path. In June 1998, the public prosecutor formally requested that the *Cour de Justice de la République*'s investigation commission drop the charges of complicity in poisoning (*Complicité d'empoisonnement*) that were pending against former Prime Minister Laurent Fabius, former Minister of Social Affairs Georgina Dufoix, and former Minister of Health Edmond Hervé. In his request, the prosecutor stated that there was insufficient evidence that the decisions of those officials in the 1980s were motivated by industrial policy rather than public health, and reasonable grounds to believe that institutional pathologies of the French medical system caused the three individuals to be insufficiently informed about the danger of HIV-tainted blood.

The Prosecutor's request was reinforced by a July 1998 decision of the *Cour de Cassation*, France's highest court. According to the judgment, which came in a case involving HIV transmission through heterosexual contact, the crime of poisoning (*empoisonnement*) requires that those charged *intended* to kill. In raising the bar on poisoning charges by requiring the element of intent, the court settled a long-festering legal dispute over the definition of poisoning and struck a potentially fatal blow to the continuing investigation of physicians and other experts for their involvement in the blood scandal.

Advocates lost little time in responding to this legal setback. Within days of the decision, the association of transfusion recipients presented a new criminal complaint, arguing that health officials should be prosecuted on charges of "failure to assist people in danger" (*non-assistance à personne en danger*) and "failure to denounce a crime" (*non-dénonciation de crime*). On July 17, 1998, the Investigation Commission of the *Cour de Justice de la République* decided that it would, despite the request of the prosecutor, move ahead with the trial of the three former ministers. Rather than relying on the charge of complicity in poisoning, however, the commission will try them for involuntary manslaughter (*homicide involontaire*) and involuntary bodily injury (*atteintes involontaires à l'intégrité physique*), crimes with penalties of up to three years imprisonment and a $100,000 fine. It is possible that the former ministers will fight the court's decision, and the prosecutor may also appeal. Whatever their actions, it is clear that the conflict over HIV and blood continues to inspire legal innovation, and has been a vehicle for organized groups of patients to become a force in contemporary health politics.

Reforming the National Blood System

The protracted legal struggles and the search for culprits overshadowed, in some ways, the more mundane, but ultimately more significant, reform of the blood system designed to preclude future catastrophes. Reform had been on the agenda since the mid-1980s, given the need to make French policy compatible with that of the European Community. Finally, in the midst of the scandal, legislation reforming the blood system was passed on January 4, 1993. The previous institutions and decision-making structures—the National Blood Center, National Health Laboratory, the Pharmaceutical Department of the Ministry of Health, and the national expert commissions—were all abolished. The supervisory authority of the DGS was reinforced and the functions of the former blood institutions redistributed to newly created bodies with independent expert authority.

Safety control procedures and market agreements for all pharmaceuticals, including blood and blood products, were placed under the responsibility of the new National Agency for Pharmaceuticals, a public body. The French Agency for Blood, a public administrative body, was given the responsibility of defining national blood policy and of monitoring its implementation. It was also given authority to grant official authorization to the CTS's and to control their activities. An independent expert committee was established, the Committee for Blood Transfusion Security, to inform and advise the minister of health. A system of blood surveillance and monitoring with precise obligations regarding case traceability was also established. Blood centers were to be obliged by law to keep records enabling them to trace and identify each individual donation, donor, batch of blood and drug distributed, as well as each recipient. The law also required them to reinforce donor screening. Hospitals and clinics were obligated to inform every patient of a blood transfusion. Finally, efforts were made to contact all previous patients who had received transfusions during the period 1980–92 so that they might undergo HIV testing and receive compensation in the event of infection.

Autologous transfusion for non-urgent surgery was finally officially recognized and fully reimbursed by the national health insurance fund, overcoming the resistance to both autologous and directed donations, which had been viewed as violating the formerly sacrosanct principle of anonymous donation on a nationwide basis. The catastrophe of AIDS had shaken the ideology that had placed at its center the "good donor" as a guarantor of national solidarity.

The new organization of the blood sector was completed by a reform of university training. The Ruffie report of February 1993 provided new standards for the training of physicians who would serve as blood center doctors.[82] The transfusion field, which was formerly attached to hematology, became an autonomous medical and scientific specialty within medical faculties. No longer was the management of blood to be seen as a subdiscipline of hemopathology. It was, rather, to be viewed as entailing the provision of healthy blood, as part of public health. The training reform put an end to the "intellectual isolation"[83] of transfusion professionals.

Conclusions

The *scandale du sang contaminé* was unquestionably the most costly way, financially and politically, of reforming the blood transfusion system. The compensation law, the criminal case, and the personal intervention of President Mitterand were not enough to spare the Socialists from having to pay for the collapse of a national myth.

Many unsolved problems crystallized in the blood scandal. HIV arrived in a system with no helm, governed by a postwar ideology of national independence and solidarity. In the aftermath of the blood scandal, profound changes in the organization of the blood system and in the politics of those dependent on that system occurred. The major shift in the policy network also amounts to a *redefinition of the symbolic value of blood*. The hemophiliac association now advocates a system of "selected, regular, seronegative plasma donors and, when possible, genetic production [of concentrates] without donation."(interview) Thus the blood sector is no longer viewed as the noble medical expression of social solidarity but rather as a technical, consumer-oriented domain. Blood has lost its special status as a "part of the human body." It has descended into the category of normal drugs.

The consequences of the HIV/blood accident are numerous and far reaching. The criminal case as well as the fall of the war-born celebration of blood donors has marked the end of the position that French physicians have held in society since the Third Republic. The entire transfusion sector has been modernized by profound reform, as has the organ transplantation system. Public health structures and institutions have been reinforced. A Higher Committee for Public Health has been created and entrusted with regular reporting to the government on public health issues.

The significant mobilization of the legal system also had far-reaching consequences. The relationship between medicine, science, and law has been adjusted. The ensemble of legal proceedings condemned an obsolete conception of science that demands irrefutable evidence before action can be taken by officials responsible for public health.[84] Out of the blood controversy emerged a new notion of the place of risk in administrative law. The need to act in the face of *potential* risk was established.

The changes and reforms were not, of course, solely the result of the HIV/blood catastrophe; the need for change had been recognized long before. The blood scandal, with its important media mobilization did, however, help to remove the obstacles to reform at many levels, most notably within the political system. Precisely because the tragedy of blood in France could not be traced to international factors, precisely because it was "home-grown," did the *scandale du sang* have such profound ramifications.

NOTES

1. On March 31, 1995, France accounted for 56.2% of the recorded cases in the European Union. Data from the European Center for the Epidemiological Monitoring of AIDS, Paris.

2. TV interview TF 1, November 3, 1991; *Le Monde*, November 5, 1991.

3. Declaration by the conservative UDF, *Le Monde*, November 5, 1991.

4. *Quarterly Report*, No. 36, December 1992, European Center for the Epidemiological Monitoring of AIDS, Paris.

5. Marie-Angèle Hermitte, *Le sang et le droit. Essai sur la transfusion sanguine*, (Paris: Éditions du Seuil, 1996). In this excellent historical and legal analysis of the French blood transfusion system, Hermitte highlights the amazing, virtually total ignorance of those run-

ning the French blood transfusion system as to foreign cases and the debates and solutions in other countries.

6. Doris Marie Provine, "Courts and the Political Process in France," *Courts, Law and Politics in Comparative Perspective*, ed. Jacob, Blankenburg, Kritzer, Provine, Sanders (New Haven: Yale University Press, 1996), pp. 177–248.

7. "La mise en examen des cabinets ministériels," *Pouvoir*, 68, Seuil, 1994.

8. The standpoints of the National Front are presented in the book by its medical adviser, Dr. F. Bachelot. See François Bachelot and Pierre Lorane, *Une société au risque du Sida*, (Paris: Éditions Albatros, 1988).

9. Pierre Favre, *Sida et Politique, les premiers affrontements (1981–1987)* (Paris: Éditions l'Harmattan, 1992).

10. Aquilino Morelle, *La défaite de la santé publique*, (Paris: Éditions Flammarion, 1996).

11. Alain Ehrenberg, *L'individu incertain* (Paris: Éditions Calmann-Lévy, 1995).

12. Jean Baptiste Brunet, "Comportement français," *Les Temps modernes*, 567 (October 1993), pp. 52–56.

13. Bruno Jobert, and Monika Steffen, *Les politiques de santé en France et en Allemagne*, Observatoire européen de la protection sociale (Espace Social Européen) (Paris, 1994).

14. Marie-Angèle Hermitte, *Le sang et le droit. Essai sur la transfusion sanguine* (Paris: Éditions du Seuil, 1996).

15. Hearing of Professor J. Ruffié, Inquiry Commission of the Senat. SÉNAT, 1992. *Rapport de la Commission d'enquête sur le système transfusionnel français en vue de son éventuelle réforme, créée en vertu d'une résolution adoptée par le Sénat le 17 décembre 1991* (rapporteur: C. Huriet), document No. 406, Paris, p. 34.

16. Hermitte, *op. cit.*, p. 96.

17. Jane Kramer, "Bad Blood," *The New Yorker* (October 11, 1993), pp. 74–95.

18. Michel Setbon, *Pouvoirs contre Sida. De la transfusion sanguine au dépistage: décisions et pratiques en France, Grande-Bretagne et Suède"* (Paris: Éditions du Seuil, 1993).

19. *Ibid.*

20. Sénat, *Rapport de la Commission d'enquête sur le système transfusionnel français en vue de son éventuelle réforme, créée en vertu d'une résolution adoptée par le Sénat le 17 décembre 1991* (rapporteur: C. Huriet), document No. 406, Paris (1992), p. 34.

21. IGASS/IGSJ, Joint report of the Inspection Générale des Affaires Sociales and the Inspection Générale des Services Judiciaires, November 1992, *Rapport d'enquête sur les collectes de sang en milieu pénitentiaire. Observations suite à la communication du rapport. Réponses de la mission et synthèse de l'enquête. Annexes.* (Report No. IGAS: SA 07 92 119, No. IGSJ: RMT 13 92), Paris.

22. *Ibid.*, p. 109.

23. Morelle, *op. cit.*, p. 211.

24. Hermitte, *op. cit.*, p. 132.

25. Jean Pierre Soulier, *Transfusion et Sida, le droit à la vérité* (Paris: Éditions Frison-Roche, 1992): p. 90.

26. Setbon, *op. cit.*, p. 88.

27. *Ibid.*, p. 85.

28. Soulier, *op. cit.*, p. 107.

29. Monika Steffen, and Martine Bungener, "Les politiques médico-sociales en France," *Les politiques de santé en France et en Allemagne*, ed. Bruno Jobert, and Monika Steffen, *op. cit.*

30. See Annexes in Soulier, *op. cit.*

31. Minutes of the AFH (French Hemophiliac Association) General Assembly, June 1983.

32. *Hémophilie*, February 1983.

33. Soulier, Annexes 7–1, 7–2, and 8, pp. 184–188.

34. Danièle Carricaburu, 1993, L'Association Française des Hémophiles face au danger de contamination par le virus du Sida: stratégie de normalisation de la maladie et définition collective du risque," *Sciences Sociales et Santé*, No. 3–4, October, vol. IX, pp. 55–61.

35. Internal documents, European Center for the Epidemiological Monitoring of AIDS, Paris.

36. *Libération*, June 16, 1983.

37. *Le Monde*, June 16, 1983.

38. Joint report IGASS/IGSJ, *op. cit.*, pp. 106–107.

39. *Ibid.*, p. 18, Annex 83.

40. *Ibid.*, p. 164, Annex 133, Report of Dr. Espinoza.

41. *Ibid.*, p. 176.

42. *Ibid.*, pp. 62–63.

43. Dr. Jean-Baptiste Brunet, Mémorandum of March 12, 1985, DGS, Health Ministry.

44. Comité Consultatif National d'Éthique pour les Sciences de la Vie et de la Santé, *Rapport concernant les problèmes éthiques posés par l'appréciation des risques du Sida par la recherche d'anticorps spécifiques chez les donneurs de sang*, Paris, May 13, 1985.

45. Morelle, *op. cit.*, pp. 80–81.

46. Michel Lucas, 1991, *Transfusion sanguine et Sida en 1985. Chronologie des faits et des décisions pour ce qui concerne les hémophiles*, Report by the head of the IGASS inspection board (Inspection Générale des Affaires Sociales) (Paris, September, 1991), p. 42.

47. *Hémophilie*, Editorial, October, 1984.

48. Professor Duclos, quoted by Morelle, *op. cit.*, p. 311.

49. Lucas, *op. cit.*, pp. 22–24.

50. *Hémophilie* 102, September 1985.

51. Lucas, *op. cit.*, Annex 23.

52. *Ibid.*, Annex 28.

53. *Ibid.*, Annex 29.

54. *Ibid.*, p. 53.

55. Soulier, Annex 27, pp. 66, 213.

56. Data from the Réseau National de Santé Public, Paris.

57. Letter and further documents reproduced by Anne-Marie Casteret, *L'affaire du sang* (Paris: Éditions La Découverte, 1992), pp. 196–209.

58. Patrick Champagne, in collaboration with Dominique Marchetti, "L'information médicale sous sontrainte. A propos du 'scandale du sang contaminé,'" *Actes de la recherche en sciences sociales* 101–102 (March 1994): 40–62.

59. Anne-Marie Casteret, *L'affaire du sang* (Paris: Éditions La Découverte, 1992), pp. 196–209.

60. *Ibid.*, p. 233.

61. *Ibid.*, p. 237.

62. Monika Steffen, *The fight against AIDS. An international public policy comparison between four European countries (France, Great Britain, Germany, Italy)*. (Grenoble: Presses Universitaires de Grenoble, 1996).

63. Laurence Engel, "Vers une nouvelle approche de la responsabilité. Le droit français face à la dérive américaine," *Esprit*, 6 (June 1993), pp. 5–31.

64. Claude Got, *Rapport sur le Sida. Rapport au Ministre de la Santé* (Paris: Éditions Flammarion, 1988).

65. Fond d'Indemnisation, annual reports, 1992, 1993, *Rapport annuel sur le dispositif d'indemnisation des hémophiles et transfusés: mars 1992–février 1993; Rapport annuel sur le dispositif d'indemnisation des hémophiles et transfusés: mars 1993–février 1994*, internal reports to the parliament and to the government, Paris.

66. *Le Monde*, November 5, 1994.

67. François Ewald, *Le problème français des accidents thérapeutiques: enjeux et solutions*, Report to the Minister of Health and Humanitarian Action (September-October 1992) Paris.

68. Hermitte, *op. cit.*

69. *Ibid.*, p. 275.

70. For the two points of view, see Sabine Paugam, *Un sang impur. L'affaire des hémophiles contaminés* (Paris: Éditions JC Lattès, 1992); Caroline Bettati, *Responsables et coupables. Une affaire de sang* (Paris: Éditions du Seuil, 1993).

71. Paugam, *op. cit.*, p. 89.

72. Laurent Greilsamer, *Le procès du sang contaminé*, (Paris: Éditions Le Monde-Documents, 1992). This book published the main documents of the trial: the prosecutor's nearly 70–page charge, the judgment of nearly a hundred pages, and an account of the court hearings. Except where otherwise indicated, the following citations are from these court documents.

73. Paugam, *op. cit.*, pp. 67–92.

74. Greilsamer, *op. cit.*, pp. 159–172.

75. *Ibid.*, pp. 215–305.

76. J. P. Delmas Saint-Hilaire, "La mort: la grande absente de la decision rendue dans l'affaire du sang contaminé par le tribunal correctionnel de Paris," *La Gazette du Palais* (March 9, 1993).

77. BVA Opinion Poll—Prévention Santé, *Revue Française des Sondages*, 82 (December 1992), pp. 3–8.

78. "La mise en examen des cabinets ministériels," *Pouvoir* [quarterly journal], 68 (Paris: Seuil, 1994).

79. "Who is responsible? Who is guilty?" *Esprits* [monthly journal], 6 (1993).

80. *Le Monde*, March 13, 1997.

81. Jean-François Burgelin, Procureur général à la Cour de Justice de la République, *Réquisitoire* of March 11, 1997.

82. Jacques Ruffié, *Rapport sur l'enseignement, la formation et le recrutement en transfusion sanguine*, Report to the Minister of Health and Humanitarian Action, and to the Minister of National Education and Culture (Paris, 1993).

83. Hermitte, *op. cit.*, p. 18.

84. *Ibid.*, pp. 286–350.

4

From Trust
to Tragedy
HIV/AIDS and the
Canadian Blood
System

Norbert Gilmore and
Margaret A. Somerville

In May 1993, after six months of hearings into the disastrous impact of the AIDS epidemic on hemophiliacs and blood transfusion recipients in Canada, a House of Commons Committee called for a formal inquiry. The Committee recognized that it was essential to undertake an in-depth examination of the events leading to the contamination of the blood supply in the 1980s, in particular with HIV, and to recommend policies to secure the safety and enhance the efficiency of the blood collection and distribution system. Characteristic of the fractious politics surrounding the Canadian blood system, amplified by federal-provincial jurisdictional issues, it took another six months for the Privy Council to order a formal inquiry.

The Commission of Inquiry into the Blood System in Canada—known as the Krever Commission after the judge who chaired it—began hearings in October 1993. Dramatic testimony, especially from those who were infected by blood treatment, received, often daily, front-page coverage. By the time of its final hearings in November 1995, the Commission had cost over $14 million, had collected 50,000 pages of testimony from hundreds of witnesses, and had assembled more than half a million pages of submissions and documentary evidence.

Public attention given to the Krever Commission reflected and contributed to a widespread sense of dismay regarding the blood system. The sense of trust and pride it had evoked was shattered by revelations of incompetence and apparent indifference on the part of those responsible for its operation. Where safety should have been the central concern, internecine politics had prevailed. Canadians had been failed by their blood system, and as a consequence HIV had become, in the early 1980s, a silent predator. As death, disease, and suffering increased in the late 1980s and early 1990s, so too did the anger and distrust of the public, especially the hemophilia community. A 1996 public opinion survey made clear the depths of distrust that had emerged in the wake of the "AIDS–blood system" disaster. When asked what frightened them most about surgery, 22% of respondents replied "fear of blood transfusion," whereas only 16% reported they feared dying during surgery.[1]

Background to Disaster

Canada's blood system appeared to be both secure and successful in the 1970s. Screening for hepatitis B (HBV) was in place, making treatment with blood and blood products safer than ever before. Major advances in cardiac surgery, transplantation, dialysis, and chemotherapy became possible with the use of blood and blood products. Much of the system's success was due to the loyalty and generosity of Canadian donors. They were a trusted and trusting resource.[2] Every year, 700,000 Canadians donated blood, with 87% of them doing so, on average, twice a year.[3] As unpaid volunteers, they were considered "lifesavers,"[4] who donated the "gift of life."[5] Over 200,000

Canadians received blood or blood products annually. The health and longevity of Canada's 2300 hemophiliacs improved dramatically because of the availability of cryoprecipitate, and improved even more when concentrated preparations of factor VIII became available in 1978.

Most hemophiliacs quickly switched to factor VIII. It was more efficacious and convenient than cryoprecipitate. It was also more stable, easily stored, and readily accessible, so that many hemophiliacs could self-administer it at home. Quantities of factor VIII concentrate distributed by the Canadian Red Cross Society (CRCS) skyrocketed from less than 3 million units in 1978 to more than 30 million units two years later; in the same period, cryoprecipitate use dropped from about 30 to 15 million units and remained more or less stable thereafter. By 1984, the CRCS was distributing more than 43 million units of factor VIII annually. As a result of advances in therapy, life expectancy more than doubled, and morbidity such as crippling joint disease plummeted.[6] In 1983–1984, warnings about a risk of HIV infection from using concentrate, and recommendations that cryoprecipitate should be used instead had little impact.[7] Few people wanted to switch, especially when, at the time, so few hemophiliacs had developed AIDS. Much later, and by then far too late, the warnings and recommendations would be found to have been far from sufficiently cautionary.[8]

Compounding the failure to replace concentrate with cryoprecipitate was the institutional inability to establish the efficient manufacture of blood products in Canada. The CRCS was committed to a self-sufficient blood supply, with blood collected from Canadian donors and blood products manufactured in Canada from that blood. The system was self-sufficient in whole blood, erythrocytes, platelets, leukocytes, plasma, and cryoprecipitate, but it lacked the capacity to manufacture blood products. Instead, it relied on American fractionators to manufacture them from plasma that originated in Canada, increasing the cost of blood products.

Starting in 1976, the CRCS pressed federal and provincial governments to develop a national plasma fractionation capacity. Finally, in 1980, federal and provincial ministers of health responded. They elected to expand their existing domestic plasma fractionation capacity rather than choosing to build a state-of-the-art plasma fractionation plant.[9] One year later, the CRCS was instructed to ship its plasma to a Canadian fractionator, rather than to U.S. fractionators. That effort to make Canada self-sufficient in factor VIII concentrate was, however, unsuccessful. Factor VIII production failed to meet Canadian needs; inefficient, outdated manufacturing methods wasted more than 50,000 liters of plasma,[10] and non-Canadian-origin plasma and products had to be imported to supplement the shortfall.[11] As a consequence, almost 50% of Canadian factor VIII concentrate had to be made from American plasma, at a time when that plasma was probably the world's most HIV-infected. As the editor of the *Canadian Medical Association Journal* noted in 1993,

Spain . . . imported 90% of its blood-clotting products from the U.S., and 82% of its 2700 hemophiliacs were infected with HIV. Belgium, on the other hand, imported no concentrates, and only 4% of its 800 hemophiliacs were infected with HIV. Canada depended on imports for 45% of its concentrates, and about 43% of its hemophiliac population was infected.[12]

The Canadian blood system was a world unto itself, involving federal and provincial ministries of health, the CRCS, federal and U.S. regulators, plasma fractionators in Canada and the United States, hospitals across the country where blood and blood products were administered, and health care professionals who prescribed them. The CRCS is the system's most prominent component.[13] It was founded in 1896 as a humanitarian organization to provide domestic disaster relief and health care in war zones. Its first Canadian volunteer blood donor clinic was held in January 1940. That same year, a research team in Toronto revolutionized medical care when it developed a method to dry plasma, allowing it to be easily stored, shipped, and reconstituted. It became a staple for treating injured soldiers in World War II. The first peacetime donor clinic in Canada opened in 1947, and the Blood Transfusion Service (BTS) developed over the next few years to provide nationwide availability of treatment with blood and blood components. Beginning in the 1980s, it included 17 quasi-autonomous centers where over a million donations were collected each year, which were then processed into 1.5 million units of blood and blood components.[14] A national headquarters coordinated, set standards, oversaw the budget, and provided reference laboratory services. Most of the operations were funded by the provincial governments and "overseen" by them.

The Federal government makes transfer payments to the provinces for health care under the *Canada Health Act*.[15] Under the Canadian constitution, health care is a provincial responsibility, and provincial governments supplement the federal funds and provide health care services. Treatment with blood and blood products is made available through the health care system of each province, and provincial governments pay for most of the operating costs of the blood system. As is true for health care in general, the Federal government has direct authority over the blood system in only two ways. First, it can tie certain conditions to the acceptance of its funds; for instance, it requires the provinces to prohibit "private billing" by physicians. Second, it has constitutional power to legislate to ensure the purity and safety of food and drugs, and it can regulate the production and quality of biologicals, including blood and blood products. It exercises this authority through the *Food and Drugs Act*. This Act gives Health Canada the power to license and inspect CRCS operations with regard to the manufacture of blood products, and recall defective or unsafe products, but it it did not exercise legal control over whole blood and its components (as opposed to blood products) until 1989.[16] The political reality was, however, that the federal government could inform, plead with, and cajole the provinces but could not "tell" them directly to respond to threats facing the blood system.

The Canadian Blood Committee (CBC) was established in 1981 to direct, coordinate, and finance the blood system. This can be viewed as an institutional expression of the complex of provincial and federal relations on matters involving the blood supply. Its members were the federal and provincial ministers of health. The CBC's work was strongly influenced by an advisory subcommittee that included members appointed by Health Canada, the CRCS, as well as members representing three Canadian plasma fractionators, and members representing the Canadian medical, hospital, pathology, hematology, anesthesia, and cancer associations.

At the time HIV infiltrated the blood supply, federal regulatory intervention was being de-emphasized because of political considerations.[17] Other health concerns such as air pollution, acid rain, aboriginal health, and a backlog of new drug approvals competed for limited federal regulatory resources. Ironically, confidence in the blood system weakened its claim on what little regulatory capacity existed, or as a senior Health Canada bureaucrat testified at the Krever Commission years later, ". . . the government didn't feel compelled to regulate the Red Cross because of its reputation. . . ."[18] Similarly, a former Bureau of Biologics (BoB) director testified, "The bureau left regulating the blood system to the Red Cross. . . . It thought the blood agency could do the job, considering it had been collecting blood for about 40 years and had a good international reputation."[19]

The Canadian Hemophilia Society (CHS) was the major "consumer" voice in the blood system. Its members include about two thirds of the hemophiliacs in Canada.[20] It was founded in 1953[21] as a national, not-for-profit community organization of people with inherited clotting disorders such as hemophilia A and B. Its mission has been to "[i]mprove the quality of life for all persons with hemophilia and related conditions"[22] through education and support for hemophiliacs and their families, and to improve their treatment. There are ten provincial chapters and a national headquarters located in Montreal. It has a Medical/Scientific Advisory Committee (MSAC) that includes professionals treating people with clotting disorders. Some of the people infected with HIV by blood transfusions joined the CHS in 1988 and organized themselves as the "HIV-T Group" that now numbers about 100 members. CHS input into the blood system has grown during the past decade, paralleling its evolution from a quiet, grassroots organization to a militant and sometimes angry guardian of the interests of those treated with blood and blood products. The transition was facilitated by a hard-fought, successful campaign to win financial assistance from government for its members infected with HIV.

The blood system was governed by committee, consensus, and liaison between federal and provincial government departments and the CRCS. In theory it could have worked well. In practice, however, subsequent enquiry has shown it operated as an "old boys" network: well-meaning, self-satisfied, homogeneous, risk-averse, and loyal to those it regarded as members of the team. No mechanism existed to assure public accountability.

On the eve of the AIDS epidemic, the Canadian blood system was cumbersome, prey to inertia and bureaucratic lethargy. Most critically, there was no clear line of authority that would have permitted the system as a whole to respond rapidly and effectively to an emerging threat like that posed by AIDS. Even a decade later, the Krever Commission concluded in its *Interim Report*:

> The respective function, authority, and accountability of each party [in the blood system] are not well defined. Nor . . . is there currently any legislation or agreement which formally establishes the roles and responsibilities of the organizations dedicated to the supply of blood and blood products.[23]

These were among the most glaring faults of the blood system, little appreciated at the time. Consequently, the system faced the necessity of a radical overhaul, which has now taken place.

Missed Warnings

In the spring of 1981, cases of AIDS began to surface in Montreal, Toronto, and Vancouver. None of them were related to blood or blood products. Indeed, the first warning about a possible threat to Canada's blood system came from the United States. In July 1982, the CDC reported that three U.S. hemophiliacs had developed AIDS.[24] One month later, the BoB warned the CRCS that "there was a theoretical risk that an unknown transmissible agent present in [blood products] may be responsible for AIDS," and suggested the CRCS inform physicians and warn them to be vigilant for manifestations of AIDS in hemophiliacs.[25] At the same time the message was reassuring; there was no "evidence," it said, that Canada's blood supply was contaminated. No mention was made of responses that might be considered to protect the blood supply or those who used it from the threat of the new disease.

In December 1982, worrisome results of a study of 34 Montreal hemophiliacs were published in *Canada Diseases Weekly Report*.[26] Many of the hemophiliacs had profound, unexplained immune defects.[27] Proof that the system had been contaminated came four months later, when a British Columbia hemophiliac died on March 31, 1983 from an AIDS-defining opportunistic infection.[28] The case went unnoticed by the public[29] until March 1984, when it was discussed by the media.[30] This first case confirmed that blood products had transmitted HIV in Canada. How frequently this could occur remained unknown. In the summer of 1984, when Health Canada obtained a small supply of HIV antibody tests, blood samples from Montreal hemophiliacs, collected in 1982, were assayed.[31] The results were catastrophic: 56% were infected.[32] The data were circulated within Health Canada in the late summer of 1984 but had little apparent impact.[33] Those responsible for the safety of the blood system took no emergency action. In December 1984, a national consensus conference was finally organized. The participants agreed to make heat-treated factor VIII concentrate available. But they agreed to do so only after a further six-month delay. Donor screening was going to be possible within a few months, necessitating responses from many of those who attended the conference. Yet donor screening and the preparations that would be required to implement it were not discussed at the conference. Incongruously, four days earlier, the data on the Montreal hemophiliacs was published as a letter to the editor of the *New England Journal of Medicine*.[34]

In November 1982, the CDC reported that three adults had developed AIDS following blood transfusions.[35] The report provoked controversy[36] and acrimonious debate in the United States,[37] but almost none in Canada. The first case of AIDS in Canada attributable to a blood transfusion was a pediatric patient reported to Health Canada in August 1983.[38] It was not a reportable case of AIDS, because there was no case definition of pediatric AIDS. As a result, its impact on the then prevailing practice in the blood system was minimal. Canada's first case of transfusion-associated AIDS in an adult was reported by Health Canada in April 1985. It, too, went almost unnoticed. By then, based on data from the United States, no one doubted that blood transfusions could transmit HIV infection.

False Hopes and Feeble Responses

What is most remarkable about the torpid pace with which those responsible for the blood supply responded to the risk of AIDS is that the lack of adequate response coexisted with fears in the general population. A 1984 national poll showed 34% of Canadians would avoid "receiving [a] blood transfusion . . . because of concern about getting AIDS."[39] It was a fear that would continue to grow, even after donor screening had radically dimished that risk. In 1987, a poll showed "[e]ight of ten respondents fear[ed] getting AIDS from a blood transfusion."[40] Such fears did not translate into effective political pressure to secure the blood supply. Instead, they elicited efforts to reassure the public that the risk from blood and blood products was minimal and should not interfere with needed treatment.

Those responsible for the blood system conceptualized the risk from blood transfusion as the incidence of reported blood-related AIDS cases. Until April 1985, there were no reported Canadian cases of transfusion-associated AIDS in Canadian adults. This meant the risk was considered zero, although it was expressed, as it was in the United States, at about one in a million. This was an easily understood and reassuring number. It was probably more reassuring than the more accurate statement that the risk was unknown. In the spring of 1985, six months before donor screening was implemented nationally, a small study of Toronto donors found 0.37% of them to be repeatedly ELISA reactive. It was a staggering number: as many as one out of every 270 donors tested may have been infected.[41] Even when those numbers were known by federal government and CRCS officials, they were not disclosed to the public until a Krever Commission hearing in 1993.

The CBC was passive in responding to the emerging threat. Individual provincial ministers did not appear to press the committee as a whole to respond; the committee, in turn, did not press individual ministers and their governments to respond. It was only in December 1984, at the request of the CRCS, that the CBC convened a consensus conference to expedite the availability of heat-treated factor VIII. Its record on screening for HIV antibodies was even less timely. The CBC never demanded from the CRCS a plan to implement donor screening. Instead, it waited until May 1985 when it received such a plan from the CRCS. In the face of this sluggishness, Health Canada bypassed the CBC and called delegates from provincial departments of health to Ottawa in July 1985 to help coordinate and expedite responses to protect the blood supply. The meeting took place three months after donor screening was implemented in the United States. The meeting addressed the need to establish a Canadian capacity for HIV antibody testing outside the context of blood banking. There is little doubt that the availability of alternative testing sites was an important issue: The concern was that people who had engaged in activities that were high risk for transmitting HIV might see donating blood as the only way to have access to an HIV antibody test. But at that juncture donor screening should have been the preeminent concern. Even at that late date, however, the urgency to implement screening was ignored. It would take years for the cumulative impact of this and other missed opportunities to be fully appreciated. As each misstep became public, the once cherished blood system was plunged deeper into disrepute.

Excluding Donors at Risk

In March 1983, after alerting the medical community to the possibility that AIDS might be transmitted by blood,[42] the U.S. Public Health Service advised all agencies collecting blood and plasma in the United States that anyone considered at risk for developing AIDS should be excluded from donating blood and plasma.[43] Those populations to be barred from blood donation included men who had sex with men, members of the Haitian community, injection drug users, and the sexual partners of any of those individuals. One week later, the CRCS asked donors belonging to those populations to refrain voluntarily from donating.[44]

The Canadian approach to donor exclusion was a "softer" one than that of the United States, shaped by the former system's ideology of trust and altruism. Questioning potential donors about whether they might be at risk for AIDS was viewed as an expression of distrust of those who had selflessly provided blood without remuneration. It represented an affront in the face of generosity.[45] There was also concern about discrimination and offense to the groups singled out. Moreover, there was a risk such questioning would dissuade individuals from donating, leading to shortages.[46] Rather than being directly interrogated, potential donors were asked to read information about AIDS and the groups who should exclude themselves from donating. They could, if they chose, discuss this information with a CRCS nurse. Such an approach, it seemed at the time, would be a "no-lose" one, or in the words of a CRCS official in June 1984:

> The Canadian Red Cross Society further considered that, as donation is entirely voluntary in Canada, donors have a particularly high sense of community responsibility and will, therefore, refrain from donating if they are properly informed and are not caused embarrassment.[47]

With time, the screening of Canadian donors became more sophisticated, and the information provided to potential donors became more pointed. From April 1984, donors were asked to read a pamphlet that specifically addressed the logic and importance of donor exclusion; in April 1985, the pamphlet included information about "high risk" activities and symptoms of AIDS.[48] Beginning in 1986, donors were interviewed to ensure that they read the information presented to them, were in good health, had no symptoms of AIDS or HIV infection, and had no reason to be excluded. But they were not asked expressly about their sexual and drug-using activities. However, in this instance, Canadian measures to deter infected donors, which lacked the directness of those adopted in some other countries, appear to have been as effective as other approaches.[49]

For some of those who were excluded, the measures adopted to protect the blood supply carried the burden of stigma. This was especially the case for members of the Haitian community in Canada. The exclusion unleashed a wave of discrimination against the community and its members.[50]

Canada's gay communities were offended by the exclusion of men having sex with men, but they did not protest the exclusion forcefully; nor were they subjected to discrimination as intense as that experienced by the Haitian community. Instead, some gay communities rallied to educate their members not to donate.[51]

In 1986, the CRCS implemented "CUE"—or confidential unit exclusion—requiring donors to complete a simple form that instructs the CRCS whether their donation could be used for treatment or should only be used for research, which meant in practice that those donations would be discarded. As its name indicated, the CUE instruction was confidential, necessitating the availability of a private space where donors could complete the self-exclusion form. Lacking such space, but using CUE nonetheless, the CRCS asked the CBC in 1987 to provide funding for this purpose. It was only in 1990 that the CRCS finally received it.[52] This delay illustrated yet again how little the system had changed from five years earlier when delays in commencing donor screening occurred. But soon calls for change would shake the system.

Antibody Screening

The CRCS began screening every blood donation for HIV antibody on November 4, 1985, seven months later than the United States, six months later than Australia, three months later than France, and a month later than Germany and the United Kingdom.[53]

Health Canada's Bureau of Medical Devices (BMD) first approved an HIV test kit in May 1985,[54] almost 10 weeks after the same test was approved for marketing in the United States,[55] but it did not fast-track its evaluation of the kits.[56] Indeed, two weeks after test kits were approved for marketing in the United States, the BMD made an unprecedented announcement that it would require premarketing evaluation of any antibody test before it could be licensed, despite the fact that the kits had been thoroughly evaluated in the United States. Why the BMD decided to subject test kits that would be used to screen blood donations (as opposed to diagnostic testing) to premarketing evaluation, why it did not accept American approval data, and why it did not utilize front-line donor screening experience from the United States was not explained. It was during this self-imposed delay that the BMD found that some test kits performed poorly, although this did not add further to the delay in the approval of kits that performed satisfactorily.

Further impeding the introduction of donor screening was the fact that the CRCS was unprepared to use the results of tests being evaluated by the BMD. It decided to undertake its own evaluation of test kits. Ultimately it selected the kit adopted by the American Red Cross months earlier. But even then, screening could not be implemented without the approval of and funding from the CBC. The CRCS planned to begin screening within three months of receiving funding. In May, the CRCS finally submitted its implementation plan to the CBC. A month later, the Committee met and approved the plan "in principle" but refused to fund it. Requests by the Chair of the National Advisory Committee on AIDS—NAC-AIDS[57]—and a former president of the CRCS failed to persuade the committee to approve funding. The CBC finally approved funding in August, which meant testing could not begin before the end of October. Committee members who represented some provinces were concerned about the cost of donor screening, and they refused to approve funding until they had obtained authority to do so from the ministers they represented. The Committee, which might have been expected to lead the system in implementing safety measures, including donor screening, had become an impediment.

In contrast to the delays in implementing donor screening, HIV testing was made available to the public across the country relatively quickly. There was widespread concern at the time that some people might donate blood as a way to be tested. Were that to occur, more rather than fewer infected donations could enter the blood supply. Therefore, "alternative testing sites" needed to be established across Canada, if possible before donor screening began. Doing so was a provincial responsibility, and neither the CRCS nor the federal government could "order" the provinces to make testing easily available. In an effort to mobilize the provinces, the CRCS threatened that it would refuse to notify donors whom it found to be HIV seropositive until alternative testing sites were operational. Second, NAC-AIDS established two task forces in order to expedite the establishment of alternative testing. One developed information that provincial governments could use to educate physicians about HIV antibody testing,[58] while the other assessed the diagnostic laboratory services that would be necessary to support public testing.[59] Third, as noted above, Health Canada invited delegates of provincial ministries of health to meet in July 1985, in order to convince them to move quickly to establish alternative testing sites. Only the CBC, mandated to oversee the blood system, remained uninvolved, even though it had been informed about the importance and urgency of establishing alternative test sites. These efforts were successful. By the time donor screening began, testing was available in almost every clinic and physician's office across the country.

The importance of implementing alternative testing sites was, however, later forgotten, a sign of the seeming inability of the Canadian blood system to learn even from those times it had "done right" and from its own successes. Fortunately, in this case, no harm ensued. In April 1996, the CRCS implemented a second HIV test to screen donors, P24 antigen screening. Its purpose was to narrow the "window period" during which infected donors without sufficient antibody to show on test results would go undetected. The test was brought into blood centers, but was not made available to the public. However, preliminary results of a 1996 survey of 6,000 potential donors, including some who were rejected, showed that P24 antigen screening did not prompt people to donate in order to be tested for HIV infection. But, unhappily, the study also showed that one in every 200 respondents were already donating blood in order to be tested for HIV. Even more worrisome was the finding that approximately 50 of them knew they were HIV seropositive when they donated.[60] Although none of their blood was used for transfusions, it emphasized the importance of maintaining a vigilant screening system.

In the face of the perceived limits of screening, pressure mounted in Canada for both autologous and directed donations. Autologous donations, in which individuals could predonate blood for their own use, were considered too costly and complicated to justify their collection and storage. But in the face of persistent public pressure, the CRCS relented and began collecting autologous donations in 1987. However, because of its financial concerns, the CBC forbade it to promote or advertise this service and refused to fund it until 1990.[61] The number of autologous donors grew from approximately 5000 in 1990–1991 to an estimated 26,000 in 1995–1996. The number is unlikely to further increase, because autologous donations are feasible for only about 10% of those who require transfusions.[62]

The CRCS was more steadfast in its refusal to collect directed donations, considering them less safe, especially because high-risk individuals might feel pressured into donating blood in order to avoid humiliation or disclosure that they were HIV-infected or had engaged in high-risk behavior.[63] The CRCS also believed that errors were more likely with directed donations because collecting, processing, and storing them is more complex. They were also more costly.[64] It was only under threat of a court action sought by the parents of a child in need of a transfusion that the CRCS yielded, at least for donations from parents to their children.[65]

Heat Treatment of Factor VIII Concentrate

Heat treatment of factor VIII concentrate reduced hepatitis B transmission,[66] suggesting to many that it might also reduce transmission of HIV. Nonetheless, as late as October 1984 the CRCS recommended the use of untreated material. It did so because of (1) ". . . inconclusive evidence that such [heat treated] products as are available to date are free of virus infectivity"; (2) "yields of factor VIII can be up to 25% lower than the untreated product"; and (3) "Canadian fractionators . . . are not yet licensed for the production of heat treated factor VIII concentrate."[67] In November 1984, when the Bureau of Biologics licensed one U.S. fractionator to manufacture heat-treated factor VIII for the Canadian market, it also informed the CRCS that all untreated factor VIII should be replaced with heat-treated product as soon as possible. Because the CRCS had done little to secure a supply of heat-treated factor VIII before the BoB's announcement, it was not until April 1995 that it secured a supply of heat-treated material. Indeed, the CRCS was fortunate to obtain a supply that quickly, for it lacked the capacity to produce heat-treated factor VIII concentrate and had to rely on American manufacturers at a time when heat-treated material was in great demand and short supply.

Blood authorities faced two dilemmas in switching to heat-treated factor VIII concentrate. First, in the face of an inadequate supply, who should be treated with the safer products? Second, how and when should untreated stock be removed from the system? The CBC responded to the first dilemma by quickly organizing a consensus conference, inviting federal and provincial officials, specialists in transfusion medicine, representatives of commercial plasma fractionators, the Canadian Hemophilia Society (CHS), and other experts to meet in December 1984.[68] Everyone participating in the meeting knew the urgency of making heat-treated concentrate available.[69] They also knew that heat-treated factor VIII concentrate was unlikely to be available for at least four months. They agreed to start distributing heat-treated factor VIII by May 1985 and to stop distributing untreated concentrate by July 1985.[70] The Conference minutes make no mention of the disposal or recall of untreated factor VIII concentrate.

The Conference mandated the Medical/Scientific Advisory Committee of the CHS to undertake the job of establishing criteria for the use of heat-treated factor

VIII until there was an adequate supply.[71] In April, the CHS board of directors approved the triage criteria proposed by its Advisory Committee. Heat-treated factor VIII concentrate would first be reserved for hemophiliacs who had never been exposed to untreated blood products; next, it would be made available to hemophiliacs who had been treated least with such products or had received only cryoprecipitate. Younger hemophiliacs would receive priority.

Lists of those eligible to receive heat-treated factor VIII concentrate in the switchover period were drawn up in some hemophilia treatment centers. As it turned out, there was little need for what some hemophiliacs called their *Schindler's List*. Stunningly, only one million of the 15 million units the CRCS received at the time were ever distributed, presumably in an effort to use stocks of untreated material that otherwise would have had to be recalled and destroyed.[72] As Andre Picard, a journalist who has written extensively on the blood system reports.

> Had the Bureau of Biologics done its job and ordered unsafe products destroyed, had the consensus conference emphasized safety, had the Red Cross resisted the temptation to use up existing stocks, heat-treated products would have been distributed to everyone months earlier, and no priority list would have been required. . . .
>
> As if that weren't enough, in several instances untreated products that were returned by one hemophiliac were redistributed to another to ensure that they were used.
>
> Products considered unsafe in Regina were returned to the Red Cross warehouse in Ottawa and were immediately sent out to Montreal. . . .[73]

There were additional problems. Untreated factor VIII, manufactured from plasma of American donors, known to be HIV-infected, was not recalled,[74] and lots of concentrate that had been manufactured from plasma collected in San Francisco, with its high AIDS prevalence, were recalled within the CRCS, but hemophilia treatment centers and hemophiliacs were not warned to return stocks they had received. As a result, only 208 of 3326 potentially contaminated vials were returned.[75] Even the recall of untreated material after July 1985, when only heat-treated factor VIII concentrate was being distributed across the country, was slipshod.[76]

Two years after the introduction of heat-treated factor VIII concentrate, in October 1987, six Canadian hemophiliacs in British Columbia and one in Alberta were diagnosed as being HIV-infected. Each had been treated with donor-screened, heat-treated factor VIII concentrate from one manufacturer, Armour Pharmaceuticals Co.[77] Armour's method of heat treatment, it turned out, failed to inactivate HIV completely. Its heat-treated concentrate was recalled in the United Kingdom in October 1986, and the FDA revoked its license to market concentrate in the United States in January 1987. The Bureau of Biologics did not revoke Armour's Canadian license,[78] and the concentrate that infected these seven Canadian hemophiliacs continued to be imported until their infection was discovered in October 1987.[79]

A decade later, as a reaction to controversy over contaminated blood products, the CRCS twice recalled blood products at the request of the Bureau of Biologics and Regulations (formerly the BoB). The recalls involved products made from the plasma of individuals, or their relatives, who developed Creutzfeldt-Jakob disease (CJD)—a disease never convincingly shown to be transmitted by blood products. Even then, the first recall was delayed until it was disclosed at the Krever Commission that a recent donor had died of CJD.[80]

Looking Back, Sometimes . . .

When the CRCS began screening donors, it announced that it would undertake trace-backs to seek out donors when a recipient of their blood or components developed HIV infection,[81] and undertake look-backs to seek out recipients of blood, components, and products from donors later found to be HIV-seropositive. Both were understood to be laborious, time-consuming, and expensive.[82] In 1986, the CRCS tried unsuccessfully to have Health Canada, through NAC-AIDS, take on the responsibility of tracing recipients of infected blood, claiming it was a public health, not a blood system, concern. Less than one quarter of such recipients have ever been notified.[83] In one highly publicized lawsuit, the CRCS was found guilty of negligence for not taking reasonable steps to ensure that a recipient who had received blood from a seropositive donor had been informed of this exposure.[84]

In 1989, NAC-AIDS took a different approach to informing recipients. Because HIV testing was easily accessible, recipients could discover if they were infected by visiting their physicians and being tested. The committee recommended that voluntary HIV antibody testing might be advisable for anyone who had received a blood transfusion between 1977 and the time donor screening began and strongly recommended testing for recipients of unscreened, pooled blood products.[85] Those recommendations had little impact at the time.

Four years later, a Toronto pediatric hospital notified almost 1800 parents that their children had received blood or blood products before donor screening was implemented.[86] The decision to notify the parents was controversial, arrived at by a committee of parents, health professionals, and experts. Six children were subsequently discovered to be infected. Only 3% of contacted parents refused to have their children tested.[87]

Several provincial governments then mounted public advertising campaigns advising people treated with blood and blood products to consult their caregivers and consider being tested for HIV infection.[88] As many as 1.5 million people received treatment between 1980 and 1985,[89] and it was estimated that almost 100 of them were infected, possibly unknowingly exposing their partners and offspring to HIV, and depriving themselves of health care and financial assistance.[90] In the six months following public announcements in Ontario, 12,500 recipients of blood and blood products were tested, of whom only six were seropositive. In Quebec, a similar number of people were tested and seven were found to be infected.[91] Thus, the quest to persuade potentially infected recipients to be tested was unsuccessful, although its importance was reiterated by the Krever Commission in its *Interim Report*.

Body Counts: The Aftermath of Policy and Organizational Ineptitude

At the end of 1985, blood safety precautions were at last in place. Although there was little appreciation for the ultimate toll that HIV would take on transfusion recipients and hemophiliacs, a grim picture was emerging. Fifty-six percent of hemophiliacs in Montreal were infected by the end of 1982; by 1988, 74% of hemophiliacs with severe disease were estimated to have been infected.[92] The number of people infected by blood transfusions would not be estimated until 1993, but data from around the time that donor screening began were ominous, showing that as many as one in every 270 donors in Toronto, in February 1985, may have been seropositive[93]; one Montreal hospital found 8 of 4000 blood units were repeatedly ELISA reactive when tested in late summer of 1985[94]; and the CRCS found 211 seropositive donors in the first year after screening began.[95] In 1993, between 900 and 1400 transfusion recipients were found to have been infected, and as many[96,97] as 100 were infected between the time donor screening began in the United States and when it began seven months later in Canada.[98] By the time these numbers were reported, the public was demanding to know why so many Canadians were infected. The personal face of death, disease, and suffering seen almost daily in newspapers, on television reports and before the Krever Commission was convincing evidence of a catastrophe.

Assembling Against Dissembling: Patients Turn Activist

Individuals who received blood transfusions in the 1980s were dispersed across the country, without an organization to represent or promote their interests. Unlike those with hemophilia, who received care in specialized centers and belonged to, or identified with, the CHS, they were not an identifiable community. Because AIDS and HIV infection were stigmatizing diseases in Canada, many of those who had been exposed through blood and blood products denied their risk, and those who were infected or who had developed AIDS often hid themselves to avoid being scapegoated, discriminated against, and mislabeled as "gay." Eventually, the fear of exposure would be cast off and transfusion recipients and members of the hemophilia community would mobilize into a group of activists not unlike the gay communities.[99]

Autumn 1985 found members of the hemophilia community shocked and angered by the increasing death and disease related to HIV. A small group decided to act. They quietly collected documents and pieced together a story of ineptitude, indifference, and alleged negligence. The *Archival Study*, as it became known, was first used in 1988 in an effort to pressure the federal government for financial assistance that would ameliorate the suffering and financial plight of HIV-infected hemophiliacs. In the spring of 1988, the drive for assistance was strengthened when the Royal Society of Canada released a comprehensive report on AIDS that recommended compensation for persons infected with HIV through transfusions or blood products.[100]

In August 1988, members of the CHS met with the Federal Minister of Health. For the first time, the depth of the failure of the Canadian blood system in the face of HIV was brought squarely to the attention of Health Canada. Supported by the *Archival Study*, the CHS claimed that the blood system had failed hemophiliacs because there was no national blood policy, and no national agency appeared willing to take emergency action. There was a substantial wastage of factor VIII from Canadian plasma, resulting in increased dependence on American blood products during the critical years of HIV transmission. There were delays in implementing measures to protect the Canadian blood supply against transmission of HIV, and there were inadequate and incomplete efforts to recall potentially harmful products from distribution.[101] A 1988 study of 1000 Canadian hemophiliacs showed just how terrible were the economic burdens of this failure. Eighty-four percent of those hemophiliacs had little or no life, disability, or supplementary health insurance; 62% had no group insurance; 50% were having difficulty at work or school; and 43% already had mounting medical costs.[102]

In December 1989, Health Canada announced it would pay $30,000 annually for four years to every Canadian infected by blood treatment. It limited assistance to four years, thinking most of those assisted would die within that period.[103] An estimate that lawsuits brought against the government by infected hemophiliacs and transfusion recipients could cost in excess of $1 billion was one reason why Health Canada was persuaded to provide assistance.[104] The assistance was popularly referred to as "compensation" but the government expressly declared that its Extraordinary Assistance Programme was not compensation, because the government was not admitting "legal liability or responsibility."[105] Consequently, recipients had to agree that accepting assistance did not imply actionable fault on the part of the government.

The assistance provided by the federal government did not meet the expectations of the CHS. Whatever additional assistance would be forthcoming, including continuation of the program beyond four years, would have to come from provincial governments, because the federal government saw them as being responsible for the blood system and, therefore, any harms that resulted from it. Provincial governments had not contributed to the Extraordinary Assistance Programme. They united in refusing to supplement the assistance or continue it beyond its four-year life span. But, in 1991, after a struggle with the CHS, provincial governments relented and agreed to contribute to an assistance program that would permit people infected by blood treatment to continue to receive assistance indefinitely.

When the federal program expired, it was replaced by one that paid each infected person a lump sum of $22,000 as well as $30,000 a year for life, with a smaller payment made to spouses and children after the death of the recipient of the infected blood product or transfusion. The new program was funded by a consortium of federal and provincial governments, the CRCS, blood product manufacturers, and insurance companies. To receive assistance, applicants had to waive their right to sue any members of the funding consortium. They also had to sign on to the program before March 15, 1995. Many eligible for assistance were angered by the closing date, for it required that they act before the Krever Commission released its final report and before a pending lawsuit brought by the infected wife of a transfusion recipient was decided. Nevertheless, 1078 people signed on for assistance, with only a handful of people refusing, preferring instead to seek compensation in the courts.[106]

The struggle of the hemophilia and transfusion-recipient communities for assistance politicized their members and strengthened those groups. In the process, the CHS evolved from a quiet, publicity-shy organization to a forceful and well-organized advocacy group. Not only did it press for blood safety, it demanded a full-scale federal investigation into the Canadian blood system.[107] That effort would bear fruit with the appointment of the Krever Commission.

Litigating the Failures of the Blood System

Courts have provided an important forum for examining Canada's contaminated blood catastrophe. There has been one criminal case resulting in the conviction of a man who donated blood knowing he was HIV infected,[108] but no criminal charges, as late as 1997, had been laid against any persons with responsibility for the blood system or decision making concerning it. This might, however, change. Depending on the facts documented in the Krever Commission report, some people could be charged with criminal offenses. Although the commission itself must not assign criminal blame, the Supreme Court of Canada has held that it may "find facts" that could potentially lead to criminal charges.[109] Individual citizens can bring criminal charges under Canadian law. The Canadian Hemophilia Society has threatened to do so against individuals whom it perceives as having acted in a criminal manner in not protecting the health of hemophiliacs and transfusion recipients. As of late 1998, no such charges have been brought.

In February 1997, the Royal Canadian Mounted Police began an investigation of an incident involving the CBC that might well lead to criminal charges.[110] In May

1989, CBC members from nine provinces approved the destruction of verbatim records of the committee's deliberations dating from 1981.[111] In 1994, the minutes of the CBC meeting at which the decision to destroy the records was taken were discovered in documents submitted to the Krever Commission. The destruction was investigated by the Federal Information Commissioner, who in January 1997 reported that the CBC had willfully destroyed the verbatim records of its deliberations to ensure that they would not become public. The documents were destroyed two weeks *after* the CBC received a formal request for copies, under the Federal *Access to Information Act*. The Information Commissioner's report states that the committee was under pressure from the CRCS "not to release documents to the public because they might be useful in lawsuits that had been filed by victims of the [tainted blood] tragedy."[112]

There has been a plethora of civil suits involving the blood system brought against the CRCS, federal and provincial governments, manufacturers of blood products, and physicians treating hemophiliacs and blood transfusion recipients. These cases involve, among other issues, matters of liability, public health reporting requirements, and the rights of parents to provide directed donations to their children. The number of civil suits would have been greater, but many HIV-infected hemophiliacs and transfusion recipients waived their right to sue as a condition of being given government assistance. Further, as late as 1997, some HIV-infected persons were waiting for the report of the Krever Commission before deciding whether to undertake legal action.

One set of civil cases raised questions about the liability of the CRCS for its failure to exclude high-risk blood donors who transmitted HIV to those who received transfusions. The cases were heard by the Ontario Court (General Division) as a group because they involved the same donors. Two of the blood recipients are now deceased; the other, a child at the time he received a transfusion, is infected but healthy. One major issue in these complex cases was whether the adults who contracted AIDS and died from infected blood and blood products did so as a result of negligence on the part of the CRCS in not screening out high-risk donors and failing to warn blood centers and physicians, and through them blood recipients, of the risk of HIV transmission through blood. The plaintiffs were given blood from the same two high-risk donors—gay men who had sex with multiple partners. Neither was an eligible donor at the time, but self-exclusion policies then in place were ineffective in dissuading them from donating. In a 170-page judgment, the court found that one of these donors would have been dissuaded from donating if the CRCS had been more direct and explicit with respect to the characteristics and symptoms of persons who should not give blood. In establishing what would have constituted a non-negligent standard of conduct for the CRCS in this respect, the court referred approvingly to the approach taken in the United States. Accordingly, the CRCS was held liable for negligence in the case of recipients injured as a result of receiving that donor's blood. Although the CRCS, likewise, breached its legal standard of reasonable care in failing to screen out the second donor, the recipient of that donor's blood did not recover in negligence against the CRCS, because the court found that even had the CRCS met the required standard of care to dissuade high-risk donors from donating, that donor would still have given blood. Therefore, the CRCS's breach of the standard of care was not the legal cause of the recipients becoming infected by receiving HIV-infected blood. The CRCS was also found negligent in failing to warn health care institutions that used its blood and blood products—especially hospital blood banks—of the risks of transfusion-associated AIDS.[113]

Another civil suit raised important questions regarding the notification of persons exposed to HIV by blood treatment. In 1990, the wife of a recipient of an HIV-tainted transfusion found that she had been infected by her husband, Mr. Pittman, through sexual intercourse. In 1985, the CRCS had found that the donor of the blood received by Mr. Pittman was HIV-seropositive. In 1986, it informed the hospital where Mr. Pittman received his treatment about the HIV-infected blood. The hospital informed Mr. Pittman's physician in 1989 of the potential exposure. The physician tested Mr. Pittman for HIV antibodies but did not inform him of the confirmed positive result, believing that he was too ill and old to pose a sexual risk to his wife and that informing him would create an undue psychological burden. The wife sued the physician, the hospital, and the CRCS. The court found each negligent for delays in the look-back program and the failure to warn Mr. Pittman that he had been exposed to HIV-tainted blood.

In a lengthy and complex judgment on negligence, the court held that the duty of the CRCS and the hospital consisted of two separate components, a timely "look-back" for recipients of blood from HIV-seropositive donors and a timely communication to those recipients or their physicians that they had received potentially infected blood. Importantly, and surprisingly, the court also held that the CRCS had an obligation to monitor hospitals' progress in tracing the recipients of such blood and the outcome of the warning given to recipients. The hospital was held negligent for failing to ensure that the recipient's physician had sufficient knowledge and information to warn the recipient of the risk of HIV infection, and for not following up to ensure that there had been no difficulties for the physician in warning the recipient.[114] This ruling means that those who notify intermediaries of a risk of HIV infection must take reasonable steps to ensure that they notify individuals who have been placed at risk for HIV infection.

Motions for certification of class action suits against the CRCS for alleged negligence in providing HIV-infected blood were brought in Quebec and Ontario in 1993.[115] Neither was permitted to go forward on the grounds that the claims did not raise common issues, because it could not be assumed that transfusion had caused the infection in all the persons who had received a blood transfusion and were infected with HIV.

An important case involving public health law concerns the notification of blood donors whose donation could not be tested for HIV when they donated because no test was available. Between December 1984 and November 1985, the CRCS collected and stored 175,000 blood samples from donors in the Toronto area for a re-search study on hepatitis transmission. Between then and the time when knowledge of the existence of the samples became public, in 1994, a handful of the samples were tested for HIV infection. They were samples from donors whose blood was trans-fused to recipients who were later found to be HIV-infected. Tracebacks had identi-fied the donors. All other samples remained frozen and untested. In May 1995, an Expert Advisory Committee with diverse membership, set up by the CRCS, informed the CRCS that the samples should be tested unless there was evidence that the do-nor had already been tested. Further, the Committee recommended that recipients of blood from donors whose samples were seropositive should be informed, but seropositive sample donors should not be compulsorily informed because at the time of donating they had not given informed consent to such testing. Indeed, at the time of donation, the donors had been informed that no test for HIV existed.[116]

The latter part of the Expert Advisory Group's recommendation conflicted with a provision of the Health Protection and Promotion Act of Ontario that requires labora-tory operators to report to public health authorities the identities of persons whom they confirm as HIV seropositive. When Toronto's Medical Officer of Health requested the names of the donors whose samples were seropositive, the CRCS did not contest the request, but the Canadian AIDS Society turned to the courts. It sought an injunction against the Medical Officer of Health and made the CRCS a codefendant in the suit seeking to prevent the disclosure of the identities of the seropositive donors. The court held that the statute was clear; the law required disclosure, and the court was bound to apply the law, regardless of the ethical concerns this raised.[117] On appeal, the judg-ment was upheld.[118] In May 1977, the Supreme Court of Canada refused to hear a further appeal by the Canadian AIDS Society, and the names of 13 seropositive donors have been turned over to Toronto public health officials. Consequently, these donors who did not seek testing will be notified that they are HIV-infected.

Finally, controversy erupted in 1996 when the parents of a child awaiting sur-gery asked to donate blood on his behalf. The CRCS, as noted above, refused to collect their directed donations. Unable to convince the CRCS to allow them to donate, the child's parents sought a court injunction to force the CRCS to provide this ser-vice. The case was settled out of court, with the CRCS permitting the parents to donate. At the same time, the CRCS announced a new policy that would permit parents to donate blood for their children.[119]

The Krever Commission Takes Center Stage

While the courts have played an important role in settling HIV/blood-related con-flict, the central forum for airing the tragedy of blood-borne HIV in Canada has been the Krever Commission, established in 1993 by the Privy Council. The Commission's final report, due in October 1994, was delayed because of the size and complexity of Canada's blood system, the controversy and legal challenges the inquiry triggered, and opposition to the Commission on the part of many of those in the blood system. An interim report was submitted to the Privy Council and released to the public in February 1995, and the final report was released in November, 1997.[120]

The final day of Commission hearings was especially eventful, underscoring the political morass within which it was mired. On November 14, 1995, two years after the Commission began and more than a year past its initial reporting deadline, the federal government refused to turn over 30 documents that the Commission had been trying to obtain for over a year. These were Cabinet documents related to 1984 draft legislation that would have extended the federal government's regulatory control over the blood system. The legislation was not enacted until 1989.[121] The Privy Council, which established the Inquiry, refused to release the documents, because they were protected by cabinet secrecy.[122] This triggered a political storm over access to government documents, especially those considered subject to cabinet secrecy.[123]

The Commission was required by law to give advance notification, with an opportunity to reply and rebut the allegations, to individuals whom it might cite for misconduct in its final report, or who might be seen as having been involved in misconduct as a result of facts found by the Commission. On December 21, 1995, a month after its final public hearing, the Commission sent confidential notices to 90 individuals and institutions, among whom were 34 former ministers of health and 20 institutions, including Health Canada, the CRCS, the CHS, and five pharmaceutical companies. Many of the notified individuals and institutions retaliated by seeking an injunction to have the notices quashed. They argued that their rights to "natural justice" had been infringed because they had not been given a fair hearing, had not been warned they could incriminate themselves by giving evidence, and had not been accorded other due process rights. The plaintiffs also claimed that some allegations in the notices amounted to findings of civil or criminal fault.

At the hearing on the injunction, the Commission surprised the Court by announcing that only 17 individuals might be named in its report. All others who had received notices would go unnamed. The 17 individuals included 14 CRCS employees, four of whom worked in the CRCS national office, and 10 of whom were physicians working in regional CRCS centers. The other three individuals were a former director of the BoB, a former Executive Director of the CBC, and a former chair of NAC-AIDS (N. Gilmore, an author of this chapter). Although the decision to narrow the scope of persons named relieved many, it provoked protest by the CHS and others who claimed that many government officials were being shielded from blame.

The plaintiffs' suit for an injunction to prevent the Commission naming names was dismissed on June 27, 1996.[124] The Court held that an inquiry, unlike a court, "does not determine guilt or liability. Rather it aims to discover facts to explain to the public the harmful events which occurred, and on the basis of fact to recommend ways to avoid similar events in the future." This finding was upheld by the Supreme Court of Canada on September 27, 1997. In its ruling, the court held that the Commission is free to assign blame to individuals and to institutions for any "moral, legal, scientific, social or political" failures found during the inquiry process.[125] The court praised the Commission for offering procedural protection that was "extensive and exemplary" but warned the Commission that it must be careful in wording its findings not to impute any criminal culpability or civil liability to those it might name in its report.

Truth or Consequences

The Krever Commission's notices of potential misconduct to institutions responsible for the blood supply were broad in scope and suggested failure at every conceivable level.[126] Health Canada received notices of 153 potential findings of misconduct that included "failure to 'respond in an effective and timely manner' to the threats posed by . . . AIDS to Canada's blood supply and a failure of health ministers to provide leadership in responding to the AIDS crisis, notably through a lack of funding and absence of a strategy to deal with the epidemic."

The Bureau of Biologics, which the Commission found "inadequately staffed and funded because politicians did not take blood-borne diseases seriously," had failed to actively and properly exercise its regulatory authority. The Laboratory Center for Disease Control had "failed to conduct timely and effective disease surveillance . . . in a manner consistent with its mandate," in particular by failing to inform public health officials, physicians, blood donors, and users of blood products about AIDS.

The National Advisory Committee on AIDS had failed to fulfill its mandate. It had disseminated "public health information to physicians and the public that was inaccurate and insufficient," and had delayed donor screening. The CBC was "called on to answer some of the most serious allegations of wrongdoing." These included allocating money and plasma to fractionation operations that were incapable of manufacturing quality products, "based, at least in part, on political considerations such as regional economic development at the expense of the health and well-being of Canadians in general and specifically the hemophiliac community. It was also criticized for failing to create a national blood policy; failing to regulate blood donations; failing to provide hemophiliacs with blood products of sufficient quantity or quality; and directly or implicitly authorizing the CRCS to exhaust its inventory of untreated factor VIII concentrate, while knowing that such material could transmit HIV.

The CRCS, notified of 71 potential findings of misconduct, was said to have failed to adequately oversee, direct, and provide resources for the operation of Canada's blood system. It had failed to recognize that HIV could be transmitted by blood from 1982 through 1985; had not implemented adequate donor screening; had continually and persistently underestimated the risk of HIV transmission by blood and blood products; had failed to label factor VIII concentrate with a warning about the risk of HIV infection; had bought and distributed factor VIII concentrate from Armour Pharmaceuticals Inc. after its concentrate was implicated in the transmission of HIV; and had failed, until 1987, to develop a look-back procedure to locate recipients of blood and blood products from donors with HIV infection or AIDS.

Pharmaceutical companies had failed "to take adequate steps to notify consumers and physicians of the risks associated with the use of [blood] products and advise that they consider alternative therapies"; had not provided the BoB with evidence of the efficacy of viral inactivation methods in a timely manner; had made concentrate from plasma collected in places of "high AIDS prevalence" including jails and the San Francisco area; and had failed to withdraw concentrate on discovering the plasma from which it was made had come from donors with AIDS.

Finally, the CHS was cited for being slow to respond to the threat of AIDS, exposing Canadian hemophiliacs to high risk before mid-1985. The CHS had been an ineffective advocate for Canadian hemophiliacs before 1988 because it failed to provide them with complete and candid information about AIDS and the risk of AIDS. It had failed to recommend the use of heat-treated blood products because it "placed concerns about the cost of [the blood products] . . . above the immediate safety of Canadian hemophiliacs."

Reflecting the prevailing sense of dismay fueled by the scope of the Commission's potential findings, federal and provincial ministers of health decided in early 1996 to undertake a major reorganization of the blood system.[127] The ministers recognized that "a systematic failure [of the blood system] was at the root of the public health disaster," and agreed that federal and provincial governments "have to ensure that the blood system is safe, secure, publicly-funded and one that restores confidence."[128] A planning process was established that addressed accountability, management structure, and processes controlling the supply, use, and safety of blood and blood products.[129] In September 1996, ministers were presented with two options. One would strip the CRCS of its monopoly, forcing it to compete with other nonprofit blood banks for funding from the Canadian Blood Agency, the successor agency to the CBC. The other would replace both the CRCS and the Canadian Blood Agency with a single agency, the Canadian Blood Service. They opted for the latter. The new system would be guided by three principles: accountability to Federal and provincial legislatures; transparency of internal operations; and integration of the management and funding of the system. In addition, recipients of blood and blood products were to be provided with an institutional mechanism for making known their views.[130]

This dramatic effort to act decisively was quickly derailed. Public opinion was lukewarm about the proposed changes. A public opinion poll conducted by the federal government found that 45% of Canadians rejected the idea that a "totally new agency should administer blood collection in Canada"; 55% expressed continuing confidence in the CRCS.[131] Furthermore, the planned reorganization provoked the anger of Justice Krever, whose commission had as a central mission recommendations regarding the blood system's overhaul.[132] The Quebec government, which at one juncture had attempted to thwart the Krever Commission's efforts by challenging the authority of the federal government to oversee or investigate blood, broke ranks with the other provinces, by announcing that it would develop its own independent blood system.[133]

In the midst of conflict and turmoil, a decision was made to delay the restructuring of the blood system until after the Krever Commission issued its final report. When it became clear that the Commission would fail to meet its new April 1997 deadline, ministers once again took up the matter. A fragile coalition of federal and nine provincial ministers of health determined that a new Canadian Blood Service would be operational by June 1998, if possible, and no later than September.[134] To achieve that goal would entail a formidable effort. Yet it was felt that there was little time to lose. Reflective of the state of disarray that confronted the ministers was the precipitous decline in blood donations nationwide. In Quebec, for instance, the stock of blood had dropped to less than 30% of normal levels in August 1997, causing the CRCS to declare a province-wide state of alert.[135] Donations in other parts of Canada had fallen by as much as 40%.[136]

In shaping the new system, the architects of the Canadian Blood Service sought to avoid the pitfalls that had bedeviled the discredited blood system. Central to that endeavor was an attempt to keep it at arm's length from governments and free of political interference. Hence politicians and bureaucrats were to be excluded from the governing board of the Canadian Blood Service.[137] Nonetheless, even at the moment of its creation, the new system could not be insulated from the political divide in Canada. Quebec made clear its determination to establish an independent blood system. In so doing it posed the most serious challenge to building a strong, responsive, integrated blood system in Canada. Almost one quarter of the blood collected and distributed in Canada comes from Quebec.

To effectuate its own plans, Quebec called upon the CRCS to be the purveyor of blood and blood products in the province.[138] That request came at a moment when the Canadian Red Cross Society had decided to withdraw from the new Canadian Blood System rather than serve only in the capacity of a recruiter of donors—the sole function it was to have under proposals of the federal and provincial health ministers.[139] Furthermore, the request on the part of Quebec came just as the CRCS had announced that it was, because of the huge debts and large liability incurred during the past 15 years, in danger of bankruptcy.[140]

Refusing to wait for the Krever Commission to report, federal and provincial governments moved ahead.[141] To some the haste suggested a political maneuver on the part of those who bore responsibility for the system's past failures.

Writing to the *Globe and Mail*, one critic declared:

> Health bureaucrats have been trying to get their hands on the blood system for decades. . . . Now, in the wake of the tragedy they helped to create, they are using the tragedy to complete their takeover, moving as quickly as they can before the incriminating Krever inquiry lands.[142]

The report of the Krever Commission was released on November 26, 1997. A searching examination of Canada's blood system, the report has become a critical tool in the reshaping of the system at a moment when many Canadians are fearful of having to be treated with blood and blood products and are increasingly unwilling to give blood to a system they do not trust. How long will it be before Canadians once again view blood as the "gift of life?" That question is the bitter legacy of the AIDS years. We hope that the system now being established will allow a shift from tragedy to trust.

NOTES

1. M. Quinn. "Poll Suggests Canadians Don't Trust Blood Supply," *Family Practice* (Toronto) (May 13, 1996), p. 6.

2. *Canadian Red Cross 1990 Blood Donors' Consultative Opinion Forum* prepared and administered by Delphi Consultative Surveys & Research (International) Ltd., Winnipeg MN. Over 3000 donors considered the CRCS to be a highly esteemed, trustworthy institution when they were surveyed.

3. Division of HIV/AIDS Epidemiology, *Proceedings of National Forum on the Findings of the Report on HIV Infection in Transfusion Recipients in Canada, 1978–1985, Ottawa, 6 September 1994.* Ottawa, Division of HIV/AIDS Epidemiology, Bureau of Communicable Disease Epidemiology, Laboratory Centre for Disease Control, Health Protection Branch, Health Canada, 1994, Appendix B, p. 6.

4. Commission of Inquiry on the Blood System in Canada: *Interim Report.* Ottawa, Ministry of Supply and Services Canada (Canada Communication Group—Publishing), 1995, p. 82 [Catalogue No. CP32–62/1-1995].

5. A. Picard. "Distrust of Blood System Outweighs Inherent Safety," *The Globe and Mail* (Toronto) (April 24, 1996), p. A5.

6. T. L. Chorba, R. C. Holman, T. W. Strine et al., "Changes in Longevity and Causes of Death among Persons with Hemophilia A," *Am J Hematol,* 45 (1994), pp. 112–121; I. M. E. Berntorp, T. Löfqvist, H. Petterson, "Twenty-five Years' Experience of Prophylactic Treatment in Severe Hemophilia A and B," *J Int Med,* 232 (1992), pp 25–32. F. R. Rosendaal, C. Smit, E. Briët, "Hemophilia Treatment in Historical Perspective: a Review of Medical and Social Developments," *Ann Hematol,* 62 (1991), pp. 5–15.

7. In February 1983, the Medical and Scientific Advisory Committee of the Canadian Hemophilia Society recommended hemophiliacs switch from factor VIII concentrate to cryoprecipitate whenever that would be feasible. Despite its publication in *Canada Diseases Weekly Report* (Canadian Hemophilia Society Medical and Scientific Advisory Committee, "Reduction of AIDS Risk: Recommendations for Physicians Treating Hemophiliac Patients," *Can Dis Weekly Rep,* 26 (9) [March 1983] pp. 49–50), the recommendation appeared to have had little impact at the time (A. Picard, *The Gift of Death. Confronting Canada's Tainted Blood Tragedy* (Toronto: Harper Collins, 1996), pp. 92–96). The Bureau

of Biologics warned the CRCS in 1983 about the possibility of HIV transmission by blood products, requesting they ask physicians prescribing blood products to be vigilant about this possible risk, but it did not require them to inform those treated with blood products. (K. Dunn, "HIV and Canada's Hemophiliacs: Looking Back at a Tragedy," *Can Med Assoc J*, 148 (1993) pp. 609–612.) Until October 1984, the CRCS recommended hemophiliacs continue to use non-heat-treated factor VIII concentrate (D. H. Naylor, J. B. Derrick, "Heat Treated Coagulation Factor Products," *Hemophilia Ontario*, 16(3) (1984) pp. 2–3) but was unable to make heat-treated material available before late in the spring of 1985.

8. M. Kennedy, "Hemophiliac Group Told It's On Spot in Blood Scandal," *The Gazette* (Montreal) (May 4, 1996), p. A13.

9. Canadian Press, "Politicians Share Guilt, Blood Inquiry Told," *The Globe and Mail* (Toronto) (May 10, 1995), p. A5.

10. K. Dunn, "HIV and Canada's Hemophiliacs: Looking Back at a Tragedy," *Can Med Assoc J*, 148 (1993), pp. 609–612.

11. A. Picard, "U.S. Blood Blamed for Cases of AIDS," *The Globe and Mail* (Toronto) (November 17, 1992), p. A4.

12. K. Dunn, "HIV and Canada's Hemophiliacs: Looking Back at a Tragedy," *Can Med Assoc J*, 148 (1993), pp. 609–612, at p. 612.

13. The most up-to-date, authoritative description of the Canadian Blood System is in Commission of Inquiry on the Blood System in Canada, *Interim Report*. Ottawa, Ministry of Supply and Services Canada (Canada Communication Group–Publishing), 1995, pp. 5–15 [Catalogue No. CP32-62/1-1995]. Other sources include J. McDuff, *Le Sang qui tue. L'affaire du Sang Contaminé au Canada.* [Lethal Blood: Canada's Contaminated Blood Scandal] (Montreal, QC: Editions Libre Expression, 1995); V. Parsons, *Bad Blood. The Tragedy of the Canadian Tainted Blood Scandal* (Toronto: Lester Publishing Ltd., 1995); A. Picard *The Gift of Death. Confronting Canada's Tainted-Blood Tragedy* (Toronto: Harper Collins Publishers Ltd., 1995).

14. Division of HIV/AIDS Epidemiology, *Proceedings, op. cit.*

15. *Canada Health Act.* S.C. 1984, c.6.

16. Pursuant to the *Food and Drugs Act*, the federal department of health (Health Canada) through its Bureau of Biologics and Regulations is responsible for regulating all biological drugs, including blood, blood components and blood products that are listed in Schedule D of the *Food and Drugs Act* (W. Kondro, "Canada: Blood Transfusion Inquiry," *Lancet*, 341 [1993] pp. 1465–1466).

Division 4 of the Act deals with all biological drugs, including plasma collection by plasmapheresis. Division 8 deals with all drugs, including biologicals, and includes requirements for investigational and new drug submissions. There are guidelines but no regulations specific to the collection and processing of blood and blood components. The five sets of guidelines emphasize good manufacturing practices and have resulted in the development of standard operating procedures, center audits, and standardization of operations.

Manufactured blood products became subject to regulation when the first commercial production license for their manufacture and sale was issued in 1968. Plasmapheresis was added to Schedule D in 1978. (SOR/78/545, Canada Gazette Part II, p. 2895) Beginning in 1983, the CRCS asked Health Canada to make the collection, processing and distribution of blood and blood components subject to regulation by adding them to Schedule D. But it was not until 1989 that this occurred. (SOR/89-177), Canada Gazette Part II, Vol. 123, No. 8, p. 1. A public explanation has never been given for the six-year delay that occurred at a critical time when donor screening was being implemented.

Blood is now included in Schedule D, but it is regulated differently from commercial, manufactured products such as albumin, immunoglobulin preparations, and coagulation factor concentrates. Blood and its components are not considered "products," rather they are defined as components of a health care service. (A. Robinson, "What Happens to Donated Blood?" *Can Med Assoc J*, 152 [1995] pp. 521–524)

17. Canadian Press, "Torries Blamed for Lack of Regulations for Blood," *The Gazette* (Montreal) (November 4, 1995), p. A9.

18. Canadian Press, "Torries Blamed for Lack of Regulations for Blood," *The Gazette* (Montreal) (November 4, 1995), p. A9.

19. Canadian Press, "Blood Safety Not Priority for Agency, Inquiry Hears," *The Globe and Mail* (Toronto) (October 26, 1995), p. A2B.

20. Canadian Hemophilia Society, *The Canadian Hemophilia Society Fact Sheet* (Montreal: Canadian Hemophilia Society, 1992).

21. *Ibid.*

22. *Ibid.*

23. Commission of Inquiry on the Blood System in Canada: *Interim Report*. Ottawa, Ministry of Supply and Services Canada (Canada Communication Group–Publishing), 1995, p. 9 [Catalogue No. CP32-62/1-1995].

24. Centers for Disease Control, "Pneumocystis carinii Pneumonia among Persons with Hemophilia A," *Morbidity and Mortality Weekly Report*, 31 (July 16, 1982) pp. 365–367.

25. K. Dunn, "HIV and Canada's hemophiliacs: looking back at a tragedy," *Can Med Assoc J*, 148 (1993) pp. 609–612, at p. 610.

26. C. Tsoukas, H. Strawczynski, A. Fuks et al, "Decreased Cell-mediated Immunity in a Symptomatic Hemophiliac with the Immunologic Status of Asymptomatic Hemophilia Patients—Quebec." *Can Dis Weekly Rep*, 8–50 (December 11, 1982) pp. 249–250.

27. C. Tsoukas, F. Gervais, A. Fuks et al, "Immunologic Dysfunction in Patients with Classic Hemophilia Receiving Lyophilized Factor VIII Concentrates and Cryoprecipitate," *Can Med Assoc J*, 129 (1983) pp. 713–717.

28. A. Picard, "Paying the Price of Tainted Blood," *The Globe and Mail* (Toronto) (November 18, 1992), p. A1.

29. Laboratory Centre for Disease Control, "A Hemophilia Patient with AIDS—British Columbia," *Can Dis Weekly Rep*, 9 (1983) p. 90.

30. Anonymous, "AIDS Inquest Delayed in B.C. over Legal Bill," *The Globe and Mail* (Toronto) (March 16, 1984), p. 5.

31. J. McDuff, *Le sang qui tue. L'affaire du sang contamine au Canada* [Lethal Blood: Canada's Contaminated Blood Scandal] (Montreal: Editions Libre Expression, 1995), pp. 105–116.

32. A. Picard, "Ottawa Knew Blood Tainted: AIDS Specialist Warned of Contamination a Year before Action," *The Globe and Mail* (Toronto) (July 20, 1993) p. A1.

33. D. McDougall, "Red Cross Played Down AIDS Risk: Scientist," *The Gazette* (Montreal) (October 25, 1995), p. A14.

34. C. Tsoukas, F. Gervais, J. Shuster et al., "Association of HTLV-III antibodies and cellular immune status of hemophiliacs," *N Engl J Med* 311 (1984) pp. 1514–1515.

35. The first case of AIDS attributable to a blood transfusion was reported to the CDC in January 1982; subsequently, two additional cases were discovered, in June 1982, when records requesting authorization from the CDC to use pentamidine to treat *Pneumocystis carinii* pneumonia were reviewed at the CDC; in July 1982, the CDC alerted the medical community about the possibility of transmission of AIDS by blood transfusions (Centers for

Disease Control, "Possible Transfusion-associated Acquired Immune Deficiency Syndrome (AIDS)—California," *Morbidity and Mortality Weekly Report* 31 [1982] pp. 652–654). The first report in a medical journal of this possiblity was not published until November 1983 (J. Jett, M. D. Kuritsky, J. A. Katzmann et al., "Acquired Immunodeficiency Syndrome Associated with Blood-Product Transfusions," *Ann Intern Med*, 99 [1983], pp. 621–624). This publication had an explosive impact on understanding the association between exposure to blood or blood products and transmission of AIDS. Numerous cases were recognized and reported soon thereafter (see M. D. Grmek, *History of AIDS. Emergence and Origin of a Modern Epidemic*. Trans. R. C. Maulitz and J. Duffin [Princeton NJ: Princeton University Press, 1989], pp. 37–39.)

36. W. A. Check, "Preventing AIDS Transmission: Should Blood Donors Be Screened?" *JAMA*, 249 (1983) pp. 567–570.

37. J. Marx, "New Disease Baffles Medical Community," *Science*, 217 (1982) pp. 618–622, and discussion in M. D. Grmek, *History of AIDS: Emergence and Origins of a Modern Pandemic* (Princeton, NJ: Princeton University Press, 1990), pp. 161–163. Attempts to publish a report of this syndrome attributable to transfused blood were unsuccessful until 1984, when the report, refused by the *New England Journal of Medicine*, was finally published in the *Journal of Infectious Disease* (S. M. Gordon, F. T. Valentine, R. S. Holzman et al., "Acquired Immunodeficiency Syndrome Possibly Related to Transfusion in an Adult without Known Disease-Risk Factors," *J Infect Dis*, 149 [1984] pp. 1030–1032).

38. N. Lapointe, Z. Chad, G. Delage et al., "Malnutrition and Concomitant Herpesvirus Infection as a Possible Cause of Immunodeficiency in Haitian Infants," [letter] *N Engl J Med*, 309 [1983] pp. 554–555.

39. Gallup poll commissioned by Health and Welfare Canada, September 1984, as reported in National Advisory Committee on AIDS: *AIDS in Canada. Annual Review 1984–1985*. Ottawa, Health and Welfare Canada, Appendix 4.

40. R. Ludlow, "Fear and Loathing in Canada: Poll Shows Widespread Ignorance," *The Gazette* (Montreal) (December 13, 1987) p. A4.

41. B. Buchner, Clinical Evaluation of Abbott HTLV III EIA for the Detection of Antibody to Human T-cell Lymphotropic Retrovirus Type III (Toronto: Canadian Red Cross National Hepatitis Reference Laboratory, undated). Testing was carried out between February 5 and 19, 1985, as indicated by an attached memorandum to this document, addressed to B. Buchner from C. Archibald. It is not clear if the ELISA results were adequately confirmed by Western Blotting. [Personal communication from Dr. M. Davey, former Assistant Director, CRCS Blood Transfusion Service, September 8, 1997.]

42. Centers for Disease Control, "Possible Transfusion-associated Acquired Immune Deficiency Syndrome (AIDS)—California," *Morbidity and Mortality Weekly Report*, 31 (1982) pp. 652–654.

43. Centers for Disease Control, "Prevention of Acquired Immune Deficiency Syndrome (AIDS): Report of Inter-agency Recommendations," *Morbidity and Mortality Weekly Report*, 32 (1983) pp. 101–103 [March 4, 1983].

44. Press release, "AIDS," (Ottawa: Canadian Red Cross Society, March 10, 1983).

45. D. McDougall, "Canadian Red Cross Balked at Screening Blood Donors for Fear of Offending Them," *The Gazette* (Montreal), (May 24, 1995), p. A10.

46. A. Picard, "Red Cross Officials Feared Scaring Donors, Inquiry Told," *The Globe and Mail* (May 18, 1995), p. A7.

47. J. B. Derrick, "AIDS and the Use of Blood Components and Derivatives: the Canadian Perspective," *Can Med Assoc J*, 131 (1984) pp. 20–22, at p. 20.

48. A. Picard, "Red Cross Slow in Screening, Panel Told," *The Globe and Mail* (Toronto) (September 20, 1994), p. A4.

49. R. Remis, A. Vandal, *An International Comparison of Transfusion-associated HIV Infection: How Well Did Canada Do?* A report prepared for the Krever Commission (Exhibit X1279).

50. A. Picard, "Labelling of Haitians as Blood-Donor Risks Called Devastating," *The Globe and Mail* (Toronto) (September 27, 1994), p. A6.

51. The problem of gay exclusion resurfaced a decade later when, in 1995, University of Victoria students complained to the British Columbia Human Rights Commission, claiming that excluding male donors who have sex with men was discriminatory. (D. Bueckert, "Gays File Complaints Because They Can't Donate Blood," *The Gazette* [Montreal] (February 20, 1995), p. A5). The Commission ruled such exclusion discriminatory but justifiable in view of the need to ensure blood safety (Anonymous, "Red Cross Makes the Right Move," editorial from the *Vancouver Sun* [February 21, 1995] printed in *The Gazette* [Montreal], [February 22, 1995], p. B3). In some universities the issue became prominent; blood drawings were cancelled at three universities when male students who had sex with men threatened to donate. (E. Lamarre, "UQAM and Carleton Cancel CRC Blood Drives," *McGill Tribune* [Montreal] [February 11, 1997], p. 1).

52. Testimony by the CRCS at the Krever Commission, Ex 867, Vol. 199, Table 5, p. 2, and Table 6, p. 7.

53. M. Trebilcock, R. Howse, R. J. Daniels "Do Institutions Matter? A Comparative Pathology of the HIV-Infected Blood Tragedy," *Virginia L. Rev.* 82 (1996) pp. 1407–1492.

54. Krever Commission, Exhibit 635, Vol 32, Tab 33. This date is seven weeks later than the widely reported but erroneous April 1985 date when BMD approved a test kit for the first time (see, for example, The Standing Committee on Health and Welfare, Social Affairs, Seniors and the Status of Women of the House of Commons reported that a first test was approved for marketing on April 1, 1985, and a second one approved on April 18 (Standing Committee on Health and Welfare, Social Affairs, Seniors and the Status of Women, *Tragedy and Challenge: Canada's Blood System and HIV*. Ottawa, House of Commons, Minutes of the Standing Committee on Health and Welfare, Social Affairs, Seniors and the Status of Women, Issue No. 19, May 1993, p. 40, and Picard in his exhaustive report of the tainted blood tragedy, states that a testing kit was first approved on April 1, 1985 (A. Picard, *The Gift of Death* [Toronto: Harper Collins Publishers Ltd., 1995], p. 130).

55. The U.S. Public Health Service required that, as of January 11, 1985, all blood should be screened for HIV antibodies, but this was contingent upon approval of screening tests for this purpose by the government (Centers for Disease Control, "Provisional Public Health Service Interagency Recommendations for Screening Donated Blood and Plasma for Antibody to the Virus Causing the Acquired Immunodeficiency Syndrome," *Morbidity and Mortality Weekly Report* 34 [1985] pp. 1–5). The first test was approved on March 2, 1985.

56. Testimony by Dr. P. Gill at the Krever Commission, Vol. 201, October 25, 1997, p. 42432.

57. This consensus conference of federal and provincial government authorities, the Canadian Blood Committee, and interested parties took place in Ottawa on December 10, 1987.

58. The Task Force on Preparation of Guidelines on the Management of Persons with Positive AIDS Screening Tests met on June 17, 1985, in Ottawa.

59. The Task Force on the AIDS-Virus Testing Service for HTLV-III/LAV Antibody met on July 17, 1985, in Ottawa.

60. J. A. Chiavetta, A. Glulivi, F. Tam, P. Gill, " Evaluation of Blood Donor Test Seek-

ing and Possible Magnet Effect of HIV p24 Antigen Testing," *Canadian Journal of Infectious Diseases,* 8 (Suppl A) (1997), p. 42A.

61. Canadian Press, "Public Not Told about Blood Storing Service," *The Globe and Mail* (Toronto) (June 13, 1995), p. A15.

62. N. Robb, "Concerns of Patients, MDs are Transforming Transfusion Medicine," *Can Med Assoc J* 154 (1996), pp. 391–396.

63. Canadian Press, "Hemophiliacs Not Warned about Blood from San Francisco," *The Globe and Mail* (Toronto) (May 17, 1995), p. A19.

64. A. Picard, "Red Cross Urged to Quit Blood Business," *The Globe and Mail* (Toronto) (September 21, 1994), p. A2.

65. D. McDougall, "Blood Boss Defends Lack of Action," *The Gazette* (Montreal) (November 1, 1995), p. A7.

66. J. A. Levy, G. A. Mitra, M. F. Wong, M. Mozen, "Inactivation by Wet and Dry Heat of AIDS-associated Retroviruses during Factor VIII Purification from Plasma," *Lancet,* 1 (1985) pp. 1456–1457.

67. D. H. Naylor, J. B. Derrick, "Heat Treated Coagulation Factor Products," *Hemophilia Ontario,* 16(3) (1984), pp. 2–3. [newsletter of the Canadian Hemophilia Society/Ontario chapter]

68. One of the authors (N.G.) was chair of NAC-AIDS from 1983 until 1989.

69. Standing Committee on Health and Welfare, Social Affairs, Seniors and the Status of Women, *Tragedy and Challenge: Canada's Blood System and HIV. Report of the Standing Committee on Health and Welfare, Social Affairs, Seniors and the Status of Women,* Ottawa, House of Commons, Government of Canada, May 1993, p. 19.

70. Annex 2. Recommendations of the Consensus Conference on Heat-Treated Factor VIII, Ottawa, December 10, 1984, from Record of the Consensus Conference on Heat-Treated Factor VIII. Ottawa's Capital Congress Centre, Ottawa, Ontario, December 12, 1984. Ottawa, Canadian Blood Committee, December 24, 1984.

71. Record of the Consensus Conference on Heat-Treated Factor VIII. Ottawa's Capital Congress Centre, Ottawa, Ontario, December 12, 1984. Ottawa, Canadian Blood Committee, December 24, 1984.

72. A. Picard, *The Gift of Death. Confronting Canada's Tainted-Blood Tragedy* (Toronto: Harper Collins Publishers Ltd., 1995), pp. 119–120.

73. *Ibid.,* at pp. 119–120.

74. D. McDougall, "Warning Ignored: Red Cross Figured Bad Blood Was Already Used Up, Inquiry Told," *The Gazette* (Montreal) (April 11, 1995), p. A10.

75. Canadian Press, "Hemophiliacs Not Warned about Blood from San Francisco," *The Globe and Mail* (Toronto) (May 17, 1995), p. A19.

76. A. Picard, "Red Cross Urged to Quit Blood Business," *The Globe and Mail* (Toronto) (September 21, 1994), p. A2.

77. R. S. Remis, M. V. O'Shaughnessy, C. Tsoukas et al., "HIV Transmission to Patients with Hemophilia by Heat-Treated, Donor-screened Factor Concentrate," *Can Med Assoc J* 142 (1990), pp. 1247–1254.

78. D. McDougall, "Blood Boss Defends Lack of Action," *The Gazette* (Montreal) (November 1, 1995), p. A7.

79. J. Coutts, "U. S. Firm Sold Suspect Blood Factor," *The Globe and Mail* (Toronto) (October 6, 1995), p. A1.

80. A. Picard, "Blood Agencies Disorganized," *The Globe and Mail* (Toronto) (November 29, 1995), p. A2.

81. V. Hogan, S. Mankikar, A. Adatia, N. B. Whittemore, Anti-HIV lookback programme of the Canadian Red Cross Society. Abstract (T.B.P. 359) presented at Vth International Conference on AIDS, Montreal, June 4–9, 1989.

82. G. Wanamaker, "Scandal Resurfaces over HIV-tainted Blood," *Family Practice* (Montreal) (December 7, 1992), p. 25.

83. V. Parsons, *Bad Blood: The Tragedy of the Canadian Tainted Blood Scandal* (Toronto: Lester Publishing, 1995), p. 178.

84. *Pittman Estate v. Bain et al* *1994) 112 DLR(4th) 257; 19CCLT (2d) Ont Ct Gen Div, as reported in A. Picard, "Blood Liability Put at $1 Billion," *Globe and Mail* (Toronto) (January 29, 1996), p. A1.

85. Health and Welfare Canada, "Human Immunodeficiency Virus Antibody Testing in Canada," *Can Dis Weekly Rep* 15(8) (1989) pp. 37–43.

86. A. Picard, "Thousands Need Tests, HIV Experts Say," *The Globe and Mail* (Toronto) (May 19, 1993), p. A5.

87. S. M. King, M. Fearon, C. Major, D. Cook, "Results of the HIV Information Project for Transfusion Recipients at the Hospital for Sick Children—Toronto, Ontario," *Can Communicable Dis Rep* 20(10) (1994), pp. 77–79.

88. R. Mackie, A. Fuller, "Ontario Expands Testing for HIV: Transfusion Patients At Risk," *The Globe and Mail* (Toronto) (July 22, 1993), p. A1.

89. A. Picard, "Thousands Need Tests, HIV Experts Say," *The Globe and Mail* (Toronto) (May 19, 1993), p. A5.

90. Division of HIV/AIDS Epidemiology, *Proceedings of National Forum on the Findings of the Report on HIV Infection in Transfusion Recipients in Canada, 1978–1985, Ottawa, 6 September 1994.* Ottawa, Division of HIV/AIDS Epidemiology, Bureau of Communicable Disease Epidemiology, Laboratory Centre for Disease Control, Health Protection Branch, Health Canada, 1994.

91. Quebec AIDS Coordination Centre: Operation Transfusion: 1978–1985. Press release. Montreal, Quebec AIDS Coordination Centre, October 1994.

92. K. Dunn, "HIV and Canada's Hemophiliacs: Looking Back at a Tragedy," *Can Med Assoc J*, 148 (1993), pp. 609–612.

93. Report from Dr. M. Davey of the CRCS to Dr. A. K. Das Gupta of the BMD, dated April 24, 1985, entitled "Re: *Abbott anti-HTLV III Test Kits*." The report was prepared by Ms. C. Archer of the CRCS for Dr. B. K. Buchner of the CRCS, dated February 21, 1985.

94. A. Picard, *The Gift of Death: Confronting Canada's Tainted Blood Tragedy* (Toronto: Harper Collins Publishers Ltd., 1995), p. 134; J. McDuff, *Le Sang qui tue: L'affaire du Sang Contamine au Canada* [Lethal Blood: Canada's Contaminated Blood Scandal] (Montreal: Editions Libre Expression, 1995), p. 199.

95. M. Davey, Demographic and Donor Profile, Anti-HIV Screening for Period November 1, 1985 to October 31, 1986, National Summary. Ottawa, Canadian Red Cross Society Blood Transfusion Service, November 24, 1986.

96. M. Davey, Demographic and Donor Profile, Anti-HIV Screening for Period November 1, 1985 to October 31, 1986, Province of Quebec. Ottawa, Canadian Red Cross Society Blood Transfusion Service, November 24, 1986.

97. A. Picard, "Montreal Clinic Had High HIV Rates," *The Globe and Mail* (Toronto) (September 26, 1994).

98. Division of HIV/AIDS Epidemiology: *Proceedings of National Forum on the Findings of the Report on HIV Infection in Transfusion Recipients in Canada, 1978–1985, Ottawa, 6 September 1994.* Ottawa, Division of HIV/AIDS Epidemiology, Bureau of Communicable

Disease Epidemiology, Laboratory Center for Disease Control, Health Protection Branch, Health Canada, 1994

99. R. Mickleburgh, "Group Admits Role in Scandal," *The Globe and Mail* (Toronto) (April 22, 1994), p. A5.

100. Royal Society of Canada, "AIDS: A Perspective for Canadians," background papers. (Ottawa: The Royal Society of Canada, 1988), p. 6.

101. A. Picard, *The Gift of Death. Confronting Canada's Tainted-Blood Tragedy* (Toronto: Harper Collins Publishers Ltd., 1995), pp. 163–164.

102. V. Parsons, *Bad Blood. The Tragedy of the Canadian Tainted-Blood Scandal* (Toronto: Lester Publishing, 1995), p. 214.

103. A. Picard, *The Gift of Death. Confronting Canada's Tainted-Blood Tragedy* (Toronto: Harper Collins Publishers Ltd., 1995), p. 167.

104. A. Picard, "Blood Liability Put At $1 Billion," *The Globe and Mail* (Toronto) (January 29, 1996), p. A1.

105. C. Gray, "Health-related Compensation Claims: the Line Forms on the Right," *Can Med Assoc J*, 142 (1990) pp. 1360–1361.

106. W. Kondro, "Curtailed Canadian HIV Compensation," *Lancet*, 343 (1994) pp. 783–784.

107. D. Page, "Hemophilia and HIV Infection," *Can Med Assoc J* 148 (1993) pp. 1870–1871.

108. *R v. Thornton* (1991) O.J. No. 25 (Ontario Court of Appeal); (1993) 2.S.C.R. 445.

109. A. Picard, "Krever Allowed to Lay Blame," *The Globe and Mail* (Toronto) (September 27, 1997).

110. A. McIllroy, "RCMP to Probe Loss of Blood Files," *The Globe and Mail* (Toronto) (February 6, 1997), p. A1.

111. A. Picard, "Blood Panel Destroyed Records," *The Globe and Mail* (Toronto) (August 31, 1995), p. A1.

112. A. McIlroy, "Key Blood Documents Destroyed," *The Globe and Mail* (Toronto) (January 23, 1997), p. A1.

113. T. Claridge, "Ontario Judge Finds Red Cross Negligent," *The Globe and Mail* (Toronto) (October 9, 1997), p. A1.

114. *Pittman Estate v. Bain et al.* (1994) 112 DLF(4th)257; 19 CCLT(2d) Ont Ct Gen Div, as reported in A. Picard, "Blood Liability Put At $1 Billion," *Globe and Mail* (Toronto) (January 29, 1996), p. A1.

115. *Sutherland et al. v. Canadian Red Cross Society and Her Majesty The Queen in Right of Ontario.* Ontario Court (General Division) No. 16523/93, Feb. 15, 1994 and *Godin v. The Canadian Red Cross Society and the Attorney General of Quebec* (August 10, 1992) per J. Belanger; Court of Appeal of Quebec No. 500-09-001564-921, May 10, 1993.

116. Expert Advisory Committee to the Canadian Red Cross Society: Report of the Expert Advisory Committee to the Canadian Red Cross Society on Stored Serum Samples. Ottawa, The Canadian Red Cross Society, August 4, 1994.

117. *Canadian AIDS Society v. Ontario* (1996) 25 O.R. (3d) 388 [Ont. Ct. Gen. Div.].

118. *Canadian AIDS Society v. Ontario* (1996) 31 O.R. (3d) 798 [Ont. Ct. Gen. Div.].

119. A. Picard, "Red Cross Eases Donation Ban," *The Globe and Mail* (Toronto) (March 28, 1996), p. A1.

120. Commission of Inquiry on the Blood System in Canada: *Interim Report.* Ottawa, Ministry of Supply and Services Canada (Canada Communication Group–Publishing), 1995 [Catalogue No. CP32–62/1-1995].

121. M. Grange, "Ottawa Denies Krever Key Data," *The Globe and Mail* (Toronto) (November 15, 1996), p. A2

122. Canadian Press, "Rock, Privy Council Differ Over Blood Documents,"*The Globe and Mail* (Toronto) (November 27, 1996), p. A10.

123. H. Winsor, "Krever Releases Letters on Document Request,"*The Globe and Mail* (Toronto) (June 28, 1996), p. A1.

124. A. Picard, "Court Lets Krever Probe Proceed," *The Globe and Mail* (Toronto) (June 28, 1996), p. A1.

125. A. Picard, "Krever Allowed to Lay Blame," *The Globe and Mail* (Toronto) (September 27, 1997), p. A1.

126. References to the allegations of potential misconduct discussed here can be found in A. Picard, "Krever Allegation Revealed," *The Globe and Mail* (Toronto) (February 12, 1996), p. A1; M. Kennedy, "Hemophiliac Group Told It's On Spot in Blood Scandal," *The Gazette* (Montreal) (May 4, 1996), p. A13; and T. Claridge, "Allegations Against Firms Revealed in Court Filings," *The Globe and Mail* (Toronto) (April 12, 1996), p. A6.

127. A. McIlroy, "Red Cross Switches Gears with Firing,"*The Globe and Mail* (Toronto) (March 25, 1997), p. A1.

128. R. Brennan, "Quebec Will Go It Alone on Blood: Rochon,"*The Gazette* (Montreal) (September 10, 1996), p. A8.

129. J. Coutts, "Blood System Eclipses Medicare on Agenda," *The Globe and Mail* (Toronto) (September 9, 1996), p. A6.

130. M. Kennedy, "Bureaucrats Urge Private Blood Agency Replace Red Cross," *The Gazette* (Montreal) (September 9, 1996), p. A4.

131. M. Kennedy, "Most Believe Red Cross Should Run Blood Supply," *The Gazette* (Montreal) (August 20, 1996), p. A7.

132. Canadian Press, "Task Force to Go Ahead with Report Despite Krever," *The Gazette* (Montreal) (August 8, 1996), p. A10.

133. J. Coutts, "Quebec to Set Up Own Blood System,"*The Globe and Mail* (Toronto) (September 10, 1996), p. A1.

134. M. Borsellino, "New Blood Authority Promised by Next Year," *The Medical Post* (Toronto) (September 23, 1997), p. 93.

135. Anonymous, "Red Cross Issues State of Alert," *The Gazette* (Montreal) (August 1, 1997), p. A7.

136. R. Mackie, "New Blood Agency a Must, Wilson Says,"*The Globe and Mail* (Toronto) (July 24, 1997), p. A3.

137. R. Mackie, "New Blood Agency a Must, Wilson Says,"*The Globe and Mail* (Toronto) (July 24, 1997), p. A3.

138. E. Thompson, "Red Cross Might Stay," *The Gazette* (Montreal) (October 23, 1994), p. A1.

139. G. Abbate, "Red Cross to Stop Collecting Blood," *The Globe and Mail* (Toronto) (July 31, 1997), p. A5.

140. A. McIlroy, "Stakes Raised as Red Cross Hints at Collapse," *The Globe and Mail* (Toronto) (September 15, 1997), p. A3.

141. M. Borsellino, "New Blood Authority Promised by Next Year," The Medical Post (Toronto) (September 23, 1997), p. 9

142. T. Corcoran, "Blood on Their Hands," *The Globe and Mail* (Toronto) (September 27, 1997), p. A7.

5

The
Never-Ending
Story?

The Political and
Legal Controversies
over HIV and
the Blood Supply
in Denmark

Erik Albæk

On October 3, 1996, the Danish Supreme Court pronounced its judgment in a case brought by three Danish hemophiliacs against the Ministry of Health, the National Board of Health, and a Danish pharmaceutical company. The court's judgment was the conclusion of what had become a never-ending story about the struggle of Danish hemophiliacs to protect themselves from HIV and to place the responsibility for their becoming infected. It was a struggle that became publicly known as the blood scandal.

This scandal had the most extensive and protracted judicial sequel in Danish political-administrative history. Although the many judicial tribunals that reviewed claims of the aggrieved found grounds for criticizing Danish blood policy and its implementation, they did not sustain the hemophiliacs' central charge. Politicians, civil servants, and blood product manufacturers had not endangered lives by acting negligently when they had postponed the introduction of heat treatment of blood products and HIV antibody testing of blood donations. Indeed, the conclusion to be drawn from the many judicial interpretations of the Danish hemophiliac case is that despite the widespread perception in the Danish population, there was in legal terms never a "blood scandal."

But as the Danish case reveals, such findings may be irrelevant in politics: For although hemophiliacs were unsuccessful in their efforts to place legal responsibility, their *political* struggle against the Danish health system was remarkably successful. The Danish Hemophiliac Society (DHS) was successful in demanding heat treatment of factor concentrate and screening for the HIV antibody in all donor blood despite the advice of the country's top medical authority, the National Board of Health (NBH). And by exploiting the common perception in Denmark that the health authorities were guilty of gross negligence and to a large extent responsible for the HIV infection of Danish hemophiliacs, the DHS obtained the largest compensation ever granted to a patient group in the history of the Danish health system.

The extraordinary success of the hemophilia society's political effort was not due to its potential for mass mobilization. When HIV appeared, there were approximately 350 hemophiliacs in Denmark. Rather, hemophiliacs had seized upon a very efficient, alternative channel for political influence: the media. In a public health care system, it is difficult for the responsible authorities and politicians not to capitulate to patients' demands when their problems are structured and defined skillfully in the media and when they know how to exploit institutional and political conflicts in the policy system.[1]

Blood and Hemophiliacs: The Ironies of Therapeutic Progress

In the 1970s the safety of the blood supply became a concern for health authorities, not only in Denmark but also internationally. Extraordinary developments in transfusion medicine and especially in hemophilia treatment had dramatically increased the need for plasma, which could not be easily met. Therefore, several private pharmaceutical companies had established large-scale programs for commercially based blood collection in the developing countries, which among other things meant an increased risk of infection.[2] The risks were exacerbated by the technology of factor concentrate production. Derived from pooled plasma from thousands of units, the new therapeutic agents vastly increased the probabilities of contamination for hemophiliacs.

In 1977, these developments caused the Ministry of the Interior to form a blood products committee to examine collection and distribution of blood as well as the production of fractionated blood products. In its 1980 report, the committee listed recommendations from WHO, the European Council, and International Red Cross that national blood transfusion service not be run commercially; that voluntary, unpaid donors be used; and that countries strive for national self-sufficiency in blood and plasma.[3] Denmark had a noncommercial blood transfusion service that relied on unpaid volunteer donors. It was, however, not self-sufficient.

The goal of Danish self-sufficiency could possibly have been reached in a few years, had it not been for yet another advance in hemophilia treatment. Approximately 10% of treated hemophiliacs developed inhibitor—antibodies against factor concentrate. In Bonn, Germany, a hematologist had experimented with inhibitor treatment in which he injected megadoses of factor. The treatment was controversial, among other reasons because the hematologist had not conducted research and accounted for his results in a scientifically conventional way. In the beginning, the Danish NBH was skeptical because it believed that the treatment's efficacy had not been sufficiently documented. Furthermore, the treatment was extraordinarily expensive. Needless to say, Danish patients felt differently. Unless they had access to the "Bonn protocol," they would have to resort to more traditional and much less efficient treatment methods. Ultimately, a Danish hematologist negotiated with an international blood products manufacturer to donate a sufficient amount of factor concentrate so that a single patient could go to Bonn, start the treatment, and thus help bury the international skepticism that the treatment had engendered.[4]

The Danish hemophiliac underwent a successful Bonn protocol in 1977/1978. Thus, the NBH lost its argument for not approving the treatment method. Because of the expense of the Bonn treatment, an obvious solution was to carry out the therapy at Danish hospitals. Eventually all Danish inhibitor patients underwent the Bonn protocol.

In November 1983, one hemophiliac underwent the Bonn protocol to the tune of US$ 3.7 million[5] and for the first time, the expenses in connection with hemophilia treatment created a political stir. The press had a field day. Initially, the hemophiliac's home county, the financially responsible authority, did not want to help pay for his treatment. However, after several years of feel-good stories in the media about dramatically increased life expectancy and improved quality of life, hemophiliacs had gained a great deal of sympathy among Danes. And when some newspapers presented this specific case as a question of cold, calculating politicians who were passing a death sentence, the politicians had to yield to the demand for treatment.

In this instance, the hemophiliac's home county managed to turn the treatment into a national political issue, so that Interior Minister Britta Schall Holberg became responsible for hemophilia treatment. Thus, one headline read, "Iron-Britta barters with life and death."[6] Later, the minister would be called much worse names. The furor surrounding this case underscored the fact that discussions of priorities within the health sector are taboo in Danish culture and politics. In connection with an article with the headline "Should money decide if hemophiliacs will live,"[7] prominent Danes said, for example, "We have to pay what it costs" and "Who should die?" The Interior Minister's predecessor and political adversary didn't mind fishing in troubled waters and stated, "No doubt—we must treat."

But cost was not the only challenge posed by the Bonn protocol. Danish self-sufficiency policy was never intended to cover the consumption of the extraordinary amounts of factor concentrate needed for inhibitor treatment. For example, in the course of one year, one third of the total Danish factor consumption was used to treat a single hemophiliac. Because it was impossible to get factor produced in Denmark in the quantities required in the inhibitor treatment, it became necessary to import factor produced in other countries.[8] During this period, imported factor was prescribed not only to inhibitor patients but also to many other hemophiliacs as well.[9] In this context, the centrality of self-sufficiency to the goal of limiting blood-borne infections was utterly lost sight of by hemophiliacs, practicing hematologists, the DHS, and the NBH. It would turn out that these imported factor products were contaminated with HIV.[10]

Policy Responses

First Lessons

As early as 1982, Danish doctors became aware of U.S. information that blood could be a medium for AIDS transmission. Even before the discovery of HIV and the possibility of antibody screening, there were initiatives to reduce the risk of AIDS transmission through blood. First, there was a series of measures to exclude at-risk persons from the donor pool. In May 1983, the NBH recommended in an AIDS memorandum that homosexual men refrain from donating blood.[11] That recommendation was formalized in July 1983 when, in accordance with emerging international practice, the NBH officially requested that homosexual males refrain from donating blood. It was a request that was strongly resented by the the National Danish Organization for Gays and Lesbians.[12]

In September 1983, this July initiative was supplemented by general blood donor information about AIDS requesting that people in high-risk groups and their sexual partners exclude themselves as donors.[13] Two years later, an NBH letter dated August 27, 1985, to the Danish blood banks required blood donors to sign a statement at each drawing stating that they had read an AIDS information pamphlet and that they did not belong to one of the risk groups mentioned in the pamphlet.

In addition to donor exclusion, screening of donor blood for hepatitis B was fully implemented by June 1, 1983, and from then on functioned as a surrogate marker for AIDS. Finally, Danish self-sufficiency of blood and blood products was made a priority. In letters to the county authorities dated September 11, 1984, and March 19, 1985, the Ministry of the Interior outlined a plan that could contribute to a higher degree of Danish self-sufficiency of blood and blood products. The plan called for increased plasma delivery to producers by, among other things, increasing the price of plasma.

Close relations between Danish AIDS researchers and the Pasteur Institute in France made it possible to test 22 patients with severe hemophilia in the spring of 1984, only a few months after HIV had been isolated and the first test for HIV antibody became available.[14] The study revealed how rapidly the infection of hemophiliacs had taken place and the role that the market in blood had played in that tragedy: 64% of the examined Danish hemophiliacs were infected with HIV. Part of a Danish-Scottish mapping of the prevalence of HIV among hemophiliacs, the study also showed that seropositivity was directly correlated with the consumption of commercial factor concentrate obtained from the United States.[15]

Encounters over Heat Treatment

Exclusion of gay donors had sparked some conflict, yet there was little dispute regarding most of the initial measures to secure the blood supply. Only when heat treatment of blood products and, later, screening for HIV antibody emerged as possibilities did controversy take hold. In the fall of 1984, the first scientific evidence appeared that heat treatment of blood products markedly reduced the risk of HIV transmission. On December 22, 1984, the full Danish-Scottish hemophilia investigation was published in the *Lancet*. The authors recommended treating newly diagnosed hemophiliacs with concentrates from donors from low-risk areas.[16] An accompanying editorial recommended heat treatment of factor concentrate. West Germany implemented virus inactivation on January 1, and Sweden on February 22, 1985.

Gradually, hemophiliacs learned of these developments, although the news traveled slowly. The message at the 1983 and 1984 World Federation of Hemophilia congresses was that hemophiliacs were at greater risk of dying from inadequate treatment of their bleeding disorders than from infection with HIV. At the end of 1984, foreign sources as well as Danish hematologists informed the Danish Hemophilia

Society of the introduction of heat treatment in other countries. Still, it was not until the beginning of 1985 that a hemophiliac medical student happened to come upon the study published in the *Lancet* that showed that 64% of the Danish hemophiliacs were infected.[17] The authors had sent the results to the chairman of the NBH expert committee on AIDS and the head of the NBH division responsible for epidemic diseases, thinking that the information would be passed on to the relevant authorities and other concerned parties.[18] However, this did not happen. "I was probably too busy with the big epidemic" (i.e., HIV infection among homosexuals), as the expert committee chairman later explained.[19]

But the hemophiliacs' physicians had begun to worry. As early as December 1984, NBH received the first application for permission to use a foreign, heat-treated factor preparation, and in the spring of 1985, the number of applications increased. At that time, no Danish or foreign heat treated clotting factor preparations were registered with the NBH—a requirement for the sale and distribution of drugs in Denmark. In special cases the board can grant an exemption from the registration rule and permit sale or distribution of limited amounts of a medicine that is not marketed in Denmark. But in the early 1980s, the use of exemptions had gradually become so widespread that the NBH moved in the spring of 1985 to reimpose tighter control so that the standards of safety that accompanied NBH registration would not be circumvented.

The replies to the exemption applications for heat-treated factor concentrate were long under consideration. And hemophiliacs, increasingly aware that the only known effective approach to preventing HIV transmission involved access to such treatment, were becoming worried as more and more were informed that they were already infected. On March 9, 1985, the Hemophiliac Society held its general meeting. The mood was close to resignation. A young board member made the unusual proposal to write directly to the interior minister to explain the hemophiliacs' situation to her. Not only did he get support for his proposal, he was also elected chairman of the Society. On March 13, he sent his polite two-page letter to Minister Britta Schall Holberg. The Society requested that all hemophiliacs immediately be switched to heat-treated factor concentrate, and that all Danish clotting factor manufacturers immediately introduce heat treatment as a permanent element of the manufacturing process. Moreover, the Society proposed introduction of HIV-antibody screening in all donor blood as soon as possible. West Germany, it was noted, had already introduced or decided to introduce similar measures.[20]

The Society's letter to the minister was a dramatic break with its normal way of dealing with the health authorities. It entailed the possibility of damaging the Society's relationship with important individuals and institutions. Clearly the appeal would create political problems with the minister of the interior who was committed to self-sufficiency in blood and with Danish manufacturers.[21] It also revealed an important fissure within the Hemophilia Society.

While the DHS medical committee agreed with the proposal to introduce HIV-antibody screening in all blood as soon as possible, it was split on the possible benefits of demanding an immediate introduction of heat treatment and a complete switch-over to exclusive use of heat-treated factor preparations. Although a hemophilia physician from Copenhagen University Hospital argued in favor of immediate heat treatment, the majority believed it would be a death blow to the Danish self-sufficiency policy, because no Danish manufacturer could deliver heat-treated preparations. Production of factor concentrate would come to a halt and might well never resume.[22]

In an April 9, 1985, letter to the NBH, the DHS medical committee pointed out that the effects of heat treatment had not yet been scientifically proven. Because the risk associated with the use of untreated Danish factor still seemed small, the committee recommended continued use for the time being. However, it did recommend using heat-treated factor concentrates for children under four years of age and for all other hemophiliacs who had no detectable HIV antibody.[23] The DHS was not pleased with the chairman of the medical committee, who worked at Aarhus University Hospital, one of the three Danish blood preparation manufacturers.[24] When he stepped down a year later — for reasons having nothing to do with AIDS — he was replaced by the Copenhagen University Hospital physician who had supported the DHS' heat treatment request.[25]

The DHS did not immediately receive an answer from the Ministry of the Interior. Even after the World Health Organization issued a global recommendation of heat treatment on April 26, 1985, there was silence. Professional disagreements, institutional confusion, and problems of coordination were responsible for the delays in responding to the requests for exemption to the rules regarding registration and for the pace with which the hemophilia society's appeal was considered.

The NBH drug division responsible for blood products presented several reasons for not recommending heat treatment immediately. Some of these reasons were medical, some technical, some financial, yet others involved consideration for the interests of Danish manufacturers. It remains unclear which factors were overriding, but from the perspective of the hemophilia society it was the interests of the manufacturers that had come to dominate NBH deliberations.[26]

The drug division believed that untreated Danish concentrate was safer than heat-treated foreign products that relied on plasma of unknown quality. Skepticism about the efficacy of various approaches to heat treatment and uncertainty about whether such treatment might cause changes in the antigen properties of clotting factor added to the concerns. Thus the Division refused to recommend the general distribution of nonregistered heat-treated factor preparations.[27]

It is clear that concerns about the well-being of Danish manufacturers of blood products as well as the price of factor concentrate militated against meeting the demand for heat treatment in the spring of 1985. General permission to use foreign heat-treated factor concentrate would mean that no hemophiliacs would be willing to use clotting factor preparations manufactured in Denmark. Danish producers were just then testing heat treatment methods, so it would be some time before their products could be marketed.[28] Thus Danish products, including stocks, could not be used. Furthermore, even were Danish producers to begin the use of heat-treated factor, virus inactivation would mean considerable loss of factor during processing. This would not only mean a reduction in the availability of Danish blood products, but also necessitate the importation of large amounts of virus-inactivated blood products. Such a course would represent an obvious defeat for the policy of self-sufficiency. Even were a decision made to attempt to import treated factor, it was not clear that it would be possible to procure enough heat-treated factor to cover Danish demand. In all, either because of the need to import concentrate or the increased costs associated with the heightened demand for the product thought by some to be safer, the result would be additional expense for the Danish state.

On May 6, a routine meeting was held of the NBH's advisory Blood Products Committee at which, among other things, the DHS request was discussed. The next day, the Ministry of the Interior answered the DHS' March 13 request with a brief statement concluding that "we shall return to the matter when the NBH's evaluation is ready."[29] After further internal considerations and discussions at meetings on May 8 and 9, the NBH itself decided on May 17 that permission to distribute heat-treated factor concentrate would not be granted, when the application "was motivated exclusively by fear [of contracting] AIDS with a non-heat treated preparation."[30] The same terms were used by way of justification in the response to the appeals of individual applicants. The Hemophilia Society reacted sharply to this decision. In a letter of protest on June 15 to the minister of the interior, the Hemophila Society claimed that the NBH was working directly against the hematologists' attempt to introduce prophylactic measures and had apparently put the interests of Danish manufacturers above those of patients.[31] Protests from hemophilia treatment centers also occurred.

Further evaluation by the NBH of the hemophiliacs' plea for heat treatment came in connection with a 28–page general memorandum on AIDS sent to the Ministry of the Interior on June 24.[32] Until then, public AIDS initiatives had been few and scattered. As the highest medical authority in the country, the NBH now found it necessary to evaluate the AIDS situation. At the same time, the NBH had received clear political signals from the interior minister and her permanent secretary that the Board could not spend more on health care.[33] Unhappy with the savings-minded minister, the NBH chose to ignore her political signals. Instead, the NBH memorandum presented an unprioritized list of possible AIDS efforts, which might cost an estimated US$ 4.2 million in 1985 and $15.3 in 1986. In a cover letter, the NBH urged the Ministry to find the resources necessary to reduce the spread of AIDS and to track the epidemiology of the new disease.[34]

Despite its commitment to an enhanced effort on AIDS, the memorandum made clear that screening of blood and heat treatment of factor concentrate were not high on the list of concerns. Even though the NBH memorandum in principle was an unprioritized list of efforts, it concluded that at present it would "be more appropriate" to spend resources on AIDS for information directed to the general public and for targeted campaigns directed at those most at risk than on screening blood. The memo's justification for recommending a postponement of the introduction of donor blood screening echoed the Board's earlier view that such an effort would not be cost beneficial, because it would prevent but one case of transfusion-associated AIDS per year *if* no other prevention measures were introduced. It was estimated that a general screening of donor blood would mean extra costs of between US$ 3.2 and $6.4 million per year, and the extra costs related to a transition to heat-treated factor concentrate were estimated to be US$ 0.8 million.

The memorandum did state, however, that over the next few months the NBH would require that all registered factor preparations be virus inactivated. Furthermore, it said that the Board would issue permission to hospitals to distribute virus-inactivated factor preparations if they applied for permission to do so. In a June 18 letter, the board notified Aarhus University Hospital that the NBH would now be able to grant applications for general distribution of heat-treated factor preparations to hospitals.[35] A copy of the letter was sent to the responsible hemophilia physician at Copenhagen University Hospital.

If relations between the NBH and the minister had been chilly, they reached subzero temperatures when the minister received the NBH June 24 memorandum. And if the communication mode between Board and Ministry had sometimes been odd, it now became absurd. The NBH memorandum made the minister furious: in part, because the press received it just as she did, and, in part, because it failed to indicate where the resources to fund the AIDS effort would come from. In the minister's opinion, to present such seemingly "medically founded" proposals involved "no cost to the NBH."[36] But it confronted the Ministry with the politically difficult task of identifying the required resources.

The minister was painfully aware of the information asymmetry that necessarily exists when decision-making power is conferred on professional groups. Did the memorandum reflect a medical assessment or was it an expression of professional group interest? The minister believed that the memorandum "stank of pressure" to obtain larger appropriations. Like many of her predecessors, she wanted to reduce the NBH's independence, to bring it under her political direction, and she noted in the margin of her copy of the memorandum that it was "another death blow to the NBH's future."[37] She demonstrated her anger over the memorandum in a handwritten, "private" letter to the NBH director, and wrote among other things "that the NBH will be asked to indicate where in the health care sector, including the NBH's own area, the money will be found."[38] Of course, her anger toward the NBH did not diminish when she read the private letter in the press.

Hemophiliacs were frustrated and angry with the NBH memorandum as well as with the interior minister's assessment of it. Despite the apparent recognition of the importance of viral inactivation, the NBH was in no hurry to act. And on the all-important issue of screening, a decision to move forward had yet to be made. Hemophiliacs simply did not believe that they were being heard, whereas the producers' interests were apparently being given serious consideration. In a letter dated July 29 to the Parliamentary Committee on Municipal Affairs,[39] the DHS asserted that whereas producers had direct access to the relevant authorities, were even represented on the NBH Blood Products Committee that advised it on matters involving the blood supply, neither hemophiliacs nor hematologists were so represented. In fact, in 1984, the interior minister had rejected representation on the grounds that hemophiliacs were not the only patient group with an interest in blood and blood products.[40]

Confronting what they took to be intransigence, the DHS attempted to bypass the NBH by arranging a meeting with Interior Minister Schall Holberg in order to present their case directly to her. The meeting took place on August 15. After the meeting there was confusion as to what the minister had actually said and agreed to.[41] The DHS representatives clearly understood her to have promised that hemophilia centers would be told to distribute heat-treated factor concentrate to hemophiliacs upon request. The DHS chairman immediately wrote to all members that "the Interior Minister [has] approve[d] a switch to heat-treated (AIDS safe) preparation." Within days, when a hematologist called the Ministry of the Interior to confirm the new policy, he was unable to do so. In fact, because he had mistakenly turned to the Ministry rather than the NBH, which alone had the sound authority to grant permission to modify treatment, his request to use heat-treated preparation with a patient was turned down. Resistance to change comes in many guises.[42]

Deciding to Screen Blood, Mandating Heat Treatment

Once again hemophiliacs were deeply frustrated and angry. They had tried to influence the appropriate decision makers through conventional political means and, in their opinion, factual arguments. Now they decided to exploit a totally different and occasionally extremely efficient channel of influence: the mass media. As a patient group, hemophiliacs and their demands for virus-inactivated factor concentrate possessed all the characteristics that were destined to give them massive media attention: Their interaction with the public authorities could be presented in a dramatic serial story as an intense, critical, specific, simplified, polarized, and personified conflict.[43] For the media, this was a good story, one that would sell newspapers. For hemophiliacs, who as a patient group would normally be portrayed as a weak party in conflict with a cold "system," media attention could create public awareness of their demands in a way that the authorities can rarely afford politically to overlook.

But hemophiliacs were not yet in a strong position to obtain the media attention they needed. So far, HIV infection had not shown up in Danish blood or in factor concentrate prepared in Denmark. Their case lacked a dramatic touch. The low salience of the hemophiliacs' concern was demonstrated when on July 24, the chairman of the DHS published a long comment in *Politiken*, a major national newspaper,[44] about the problems facing hemophiliacs. Even after the publication of his essay, the media seemed uninterested.[45] However, the dramatic touch that was to spark attention was not far off, and hemophiliacs soon proved that they had mastered the art of timing.

The final decision to introduce screening and heat treatment in Denmark was taken after a chaotic and dramatic sequence of events that made it difficult to tell the political and medical arguments apart. The occasion was a September 2, 1985, meeting of a county hospital committee, which discussed an account of a homosexual man who had been diagnosed with AIDS and who had given blood on three occasions between June 1983 and May 1984. Those who had received his blood, however, had all died of their primary diseases.[46] Although the account was treated at a confidential meeting, it was leaked to the press and was mentioned that same evening on the news on Denmark's only TV channel.

The minister felt misinformed and betrayed when her secretary called and informed her that evening that the case had received media attention. All along, she had been told that there had been no cases of transfusion-transmitted AIDS in Denmark. Three days earlier she had written in a newspaper comment that Danish donor blood had still not been shown to contain virus and that her political decisions had been based on these scientific realities.[47] Within hours, the interior minister issued a press release asserting that the case of transfusion-associated AIDS was completely new to her, and that she would start an exhaustive investigation. The next day, the NBH was told to carry out such an investigation and deliver a report to the minister that very day. The press rolled out big dramatic headlines. "AIDS in donor blood: We may all become infected," read one.[48] Another shouted: "Doctors injected dying patients with AIDS."[49]

Despite these banner headlines, the interior minister might well have weathered the storm if not for the fact that the DHS saw the information about the AIDS-diagnosed blood as a "policy window,"[50] through which the Society could push its own demands on the health authorities. The chairman of the DHS prepared a press release describing the plight of hemophiliacs and personally delivered it to the most important editorial newspaper staffs in the Copenhagen region. That night, he was interviewed as part of the lead story for the evening news in Denmark. By skillfully linking the hemophiliacs' demands for virus-inactivated factor concentrate to transfusion-transmitted infection, the DHS chairman used a well-known strategy in political

agenda setting[51]: He expanded the DHS conflict with the health authorities to include not only other social groups, but the entire population. Hemophiliacs became
living proof of how dangerous it was for the entire population to receive blood. Before the news program was over, the anchorperson announced that the minister had
called to inform the public that hemophiliacs would be able to receive foreign, heat-
treated factor preparations until they could be delivered by Danish producers.

The minister was justifiably angry. The NBH had actually known about the
AIDS-diagnosed donor for more than a year, but had chosen to keep this knowledge
within a tight circle in order to avoid alarming the population. The minister, on the
other hand, felt ridiculed because on several occasions—based on inaccurate information supplied to her by the NBH—she had falsely assured the population that there
were no cases of transfusion-transmitted infection in Denmark.

The minister expressed her political dilemma in unambiguous terms in a TV
interview: "For me as a politician, there is a significant difference between something that's a hypothesis on a piece of paper and something that's an established fact.
As soon as one single instance has been recorded, then it's an entirely different reality for the citizens."[52] The NBH was concerned with statistical probabilities. But the
population's tolerance for risk created the universe within which the minister had to
respond as a politician. And the population's tolerance changed dramatically when
the statistical probability became a reality.

Press coverage not only of the blood conflict but also of AIDS in general now
exploded,[53] and the press was almost unanimously arrayed against the minister. The
gay community and AIDS doctors who demanded more resources for the fight against
AIDS were against her. So were hemophiliacs who demanded heat treatment and
screening. Her own Board of Health did not like the economy-conscious minister
and could only agree with these groups. It was, however, unable to find savings elsewhere in the health care budget so that their demands could be met. The Social
Democratic chairman of the Parliamentary Committee on Municipal Affairs, whose
political motives were almost indistinguishable from his professional interest in the
case, saw an opportunity to punish a prominent minister.

The press both reflected and fed popular discontent. It "smelled blood," was
merciless in its criticism, and was not above using a sexist angle. The minister was
no longer portrayed as "Iron Britta." In what was an unusually personal campaign
for Denmark, she became the insensitive "Blood Britta," who thought only of money
and "wanted dead bodies" before she would take action.[54] The cost-conscious minister was caught in a classic political dilemma: it is far easier to win approval by supporting expansive demands on the public sector when responding to the claims of
children, the elderly, and patients, than by attempting to save taxpayers' resources by
pressing for budgetary restraint when it affects the interests of such vulnerable groups.[55]

The minister knew that she might pay a high political price for the uproar over
AIDS-diagnosed blood. Therefore, on September 3, she decided to contact the min-

ister of finance and was granted US$ 6.4 million for screening of donor blood. The decision was made in the Ministry of the Interior without consulting the NBH, and as a consequence of the inflamed atmosphere between the Ministry and the Board, the absurd communication mode continued. The minister called the NBH director at 11:15 p.m. to tell him that he would "see something unpleasant in the newspaper" the next day. At 11:55 pm, she issued a press release announcing the decision to initiate blood donor screening. Adding insult to injury, the NBH was only told of the decision in a letter dated September 4.[56]

On September 5 and 6, the interior minister met with the three Danish factor producers, and on September 10, she requested the NBH to introduce, as soon as possible, a general requirement to subject Danish as well as foreign blood products to heat treatment. This was no longer a major problem for the health authorities. On July 31, Nordisk Gentofte, a Danish blood products manufacturer, applied for approval of its first heat-treated factor preparation. Approval was announced on August 30, 1985. Shortly thereafter, the National Serum Institute, the other major manufacturer, also had a heat-treated factor preparation registered. On September 13, importers and producers of clotting factor concentrate were notified that the cut-off date for the distribution of untreated factor was October 1. At the same time, producers and importers were requested to recall factor concentrate that had not been subject to viral inactivation.[57]

In early October, the National Serum Institute informed the NBH that starting 1986, routine screening of Danish donor blood would be possible through "Western blot" analysis. In its circular dated November 1, 1985, to all Danish hospitals, the NBH stated that screening for HIV-virus antibody in all donor blood would be mandatory starting January 1.[58] Most counties started blood screening earlier.

The seeds of the Danish AIDS scandal were sown during those dramatic and chaotic September days in 1985. The press and public opinion shared the impression that a heartless minister had played Russian roulette with the health and lives of hemophiliacs and the general public. Another common impression was that weak civil servants had let themselves be bullied by a minister into considering economic instead of medical interests. Even their failure to fully inform the minister was seen through eyes critical of Britta Schall Holberg. Failure to notify the minister was understood as partly linked to the perception that given her economic views she did not want to be confronted with such information. Failure to inform the public of the presence of infected blood stemmed from a desire to shield the population from fear, when resources for screening of donor blood were not forthcoming.

But all this would probably have been forgotten—especially after the minister was transferred to the Ministry of Agriculture in March 1986 and later left Danish politics in May 1988—if not for the fact that a transition scheme had been introduced. It was that scheme that both the parliamentary opposition and hemophiliacs knew how to exploit.

Risks, Burdens, and Politics during the Transition to Safer Blood

With the introduction of heat treatment of clotting factor concentrate and screening of donor blood, everything should have been in order. And apparently it was. Things turned out quite differently, however, two years later.

Once again, the media succeeded in forcing the issue onto the political agenda. On December 8, 1987, a TV feature announced that at least one hemophiliac had been infected with AIDS after being treated with heat-treated blood products that, despite guarantees to the contrary, had not been produced from screened donor blood. Huge headlines announced the disaster the very next day.

The case seemed tangled. In early 1987, a physician discovered that her hemophilia patient was infected with HIV. It took several months before the physician was able to conclude that the infection might have occurred in a transition period before blood intended for factor production was subject to antibody screening. After the chaotic and quick but clear decision to introduce heat treatment and screening, a transition scheme permitting the use of non-screened blood in factor production until July 1, 1986, had been established. Neither the minister, *Folketinget*, nor the public, including hemophiliacs and hemophilia centers, knew about this decision. Something seemed "really wrong" here. The media immediately smelled a scandal—and a continuation to the serial story about life and death among hemophiliacs and the insensitive health system.

On December 9, 1987, the Parliamentary Health Committee announced that it expected a memorandum about and a discussion of the case in a parliamentary consultation the next day with the minister of health, Agnete Laustsen, who had recently been appointed minister of the newly created Ministry of Health. On December 14, the chairman of the Social Democratic Party wrote the prime minister and requested a judicial inquiry. Although there were an increasing number of such investigations of apparently illegal or criticizable conditions in the Danish central administration, they were still rare. And it was very rare that a judicial inquiry would be initiated immediately and without a battle. But that is precisely what occurred in this instance. On December 15, a high court judge was appointed to conduct the inquiry.

Just one day later, the recently appointed minister of health panicked. Like all the other responsible officials, she saw the issue of the blood supply as extremely volatile and had no desire to become the new "Blood Britta." On December 16, without consulting the NBH, she demanded a recall of all non-screened albumin and gamma globulin preparations. It was, she said, necessary to remove any doubts consumers might have about the risk of HIV. Denmark became the first country to take such action. The safety of these preparations had never been questioned. On the next day, the minister realized that politically inspired panic had produced a decision that, in the words of the NBH director, had "gone too far." The recall was

modified on December 17. But political considerations precluded a complete rever-
sal despite the absence of a medical justification for such action.[59]

Blood Politics and Legal Responses

The transition scheme triggered the largest and most protracted judicial sequel in
Danish political administrative history. In the *judicial* inquiry ordered by the prime
minister, the judge's mandate was to examine "if there were mistakes in the administrative procedure" regarding the use of nonscreened blood after January 1, 1986,
"and if *Folketinget* and the public had been misinformed or had gotten insufficient
information on the matter."[60]

The report of the judicial inquiry was presented on June 13, 1988, and it was an
unambiguous acquittal of the two politically responsible ministers, Britta Schall
Holberg and Knud Enggaard. More importantly, there were no grounds to fault the
decision to introduce the transition scheme or its duration. It was clear, noted the
report, that a decision was taken that all blood products distributed after October 1,
1985, must be heat treated. It was also clear that all donor blood had to be tested
after January 1, 1986. But it had never been politically decided that blood products
distributed after January 1, 1986, had to be screened *and* heat treated. The NBH
had decided that ultimately blood intended for fractionation would be screened. But
that necessitated a transition scheme so that the producers could exhaust stocks of
blood plasma drawn at the end of 1985. The transitional period was set to end July 1,
1986.

All medical knowledge at the time, noted the report of the judicial inquiry, indicated that heat treatment was sufficient to ensure virus inactivation. It was not until
the spring of 1986 that it emerged that heat treatment had its limits. Furthermore,
the judge found no reason to criticize the NBH failure to notify the Ministry about the
transition scheme, because it was not inconsistent with the political decisions that
had been taken. The scheme was a reasonable measure designed to give effect to
those decisions. However, in the implementation of the scheme and their failure to
fully inform the minister, authorities and producers had acted in ways that warranted
"serious criticism." The report did not evaluate whether the pharmaceutical firm
Nordisk Gentofte had committed punishable acts or whether civil servants had violated the statute governing their official conduct. In a political climate where the
public and the media shared the impression that hemophiliacs had been treated
scandalously and that someone had to be held accountable, the prosecution and the
responsible minister had to react to the criticism.

Consequently, a *criminal case* against Nordisk Gentofte was started in August
1988. A verdict was handed down on November 29, 1989.[61] The company was ac-

quitted of having reprocessed factor preparations against NBH guidelines and of neglect in connection with recall of factor preparations. However, the company was found guilty of ignoring NBH guidelines by letting non-screened plasma enter the production of immunglobulin and by letting plasma from HIV-positive donors enter the production of albumin, even though the risk of infection through the use of these preparations is extremely small. Likewise, the company was found guilty of mislabeling factor preparations. All such products in 1986 carried the label, "All plasma used in this product has been screened and tested negative for [HIV] antibodies." This was not always the case during the transition period. Nordisk Gentofte was fined US$4,000. Given the popular perception of scandal, this was nothing more than a slap on the wrist. The case was not appealed to the High Court.

Attuned to popular concerns, Minister of Health Elsebeth Kock-Petersen told the press that she believed that "there [was] basis for disciplinary proceedings" against the named civil servants, given the criticisms made by the judicial inquiry. On July 1, 1988, she issued a press release stating that a *disciplinary inquiry* had been initiated to determine whether there were grounds for sanctions. Only in one case did the Supreme Court judge who was in charge of the inquiry find sufficient evidence of misconduct. This one instance involved the head of the National Serum Institute's fractionation department, who had ignored NBH rules for screening and shelf life.[62] The doctor was reprimanded and was transferred to another job at the Institute.

In the *compensation case*, the DHS sued the Ministry of Health, Nordisk Gentofte, and the National Serum Institute for damages on December 14, 1987. Interestingly enough, the DHS decided not to sue international manufacturers, although the Society knew that it was precisely their products that had been contaminated. At the first sitting in the case, the defendants requested the High Court to dismiss the case on the grounds that the DHS could not act on behalf of its members. As a consequence, it became necessary for the DHS to identify HIV-contaminated members for whom specific claims for damages could be made and for whom the DHS could act as representative. In the end, nine hemophiliacs—or their relatives— participated in the case.

The High Court's judgment was pronounced on January 14, 1995, seven years after the suit was initiated. The court judged that the relevant authorities had not acted negligently by not demanding heat treatment and screening earlier. Like the judicial inquiry, the Court did not challenge the introduction of the transition scheme. However, it found that it had been too protracted. Therefore, the public authorities had incurred a responsibility to the single plaintiff, assumed to have been infected at a time when factor concentrate should have been both screened and heat treated. The court ordered the public authorities to contribute to his funeral expenses.

On April 5, 1995, three of the plaintiffs appealed the High Court's judgment to the Supreme Court. The court pronounced its judgment on October 3, 1996. The Supreme Court acquitted Nordisk Gentofte and also concurred with the High

Court's judgment that the authorities had not acted negligently in connection with the introduction of heat treatment of factor and screening of donor blood. The Supreme Court likewise found that the authorities had not acted negligently by introducing the transition scheme. However, the Supreme Court significantly departed from the High Court in its evaluation of the transition scheme. Unlike the lower court, it did not find a basis for leveling criticism. Thus those who saw in the transition the heart of the "blood scandal" had been rebuffed by Denmark's highest judicial tribunal.

The Supreme Court departed from the High Court on one other point. In a four to three decision, the majority found that because there was by mid-April 1986 sufficient knowledge about the risk of infection from foreign, non-heat-treated factor products, the NBH had been negligent in failing to grant applications for permission to use foreign, heat-treated factor preparations. Furthermore, the NBH had acted negligently in failing to call on doctors to stop the use of foreign, non-heat-treated preparations. The majority held the NBH and the Ministry of Health liable to one plaintiff, who between July 9 and August 12, 1985, had treated himself with a foreign, non-heat-treated preparation he had received in February of that year. Had his physician been contacted by the NBH, the contaminated preparation might have been returned, thus protecting the now-infected individual.[63]

Interestingly, the severest judgment of the response of the Danish system to the plight of hemophiliacs came from the *European Court of Human Rights*. In that instance, the issue entailed not the substance of the claims against the medical authorities, but the duration of the legal proceedings.

The Danish Hemophilia Society had initiated its proceedings in December 1987 in the High Court of Eastern Denmark. When almost five years later — in August 1992 — the case had not yet been decided by the High Court, the plaintiffs turned to the European Commission of Human Rights claiming a breach of Article 6§1 of the Convention for the Protection of Human Rights and Freedoms, which entitles everyone to a "hearing within a reasonable time by [a] tribunal. . . ." The case was referred to the European Court of Justice in July 1995, which in February 1996 held that the Danish state had indeed violated the plaintiffs' human rights in prolonging the compensation case for seven years and two months before reaching a judgment.[64] Given the nature of the case, the stakes involved, and the reduced life expectancy of the plaintiffs, there was, said the court, a duty of exceptional diligence. Seven plaintiffs were each awarded $16,000. In the case of two, the court held that no duty of exceptional diligence was due to the relatives of hemophiliacs who had died before the court proceeding had begun in 1987.

The Danish press presented the judgment as — finally — a great victory for hemophiliacs[65] and "A Bloody Nose for the System."[66] At the same time, the press noted that, ironically, the European Commission and the European Court themselves had taken three years and six months to try the hemophiliacs' case.[67]

In sum, careful evaluation of the many judicial interpretations of the Danish hemophiliac case must lead to the conclusion that in contrast to a widespread conception in the Danish population, there never was a blood scandal in Denmark in legal terms. Clearly, the conduct of public authorities, civil servants, producers, and importers have been subject to criticism, but it is only with the vantage of hindsight that it now appears that it would have been reasonable to introduce heat treatment of Danish factor and donor blood screening a few months earlier and to have shortened the transitional period.

The true tragedy of hemophilia and AIDS in Denmark is very different from what common perceptions had held. Hemophiliacs were infected long before the HIV virus was known and identified and before heat treatment and screening of donor blood became technically possible. Indeed, the AIDS researcher who first documented that the vast majority of the HIV-infected Danish hemophiliacs had become infected in the early 1980s told the High Court that even if heat treatment and screening of donor blood had been introduced on January 1, 1985, few, if any, hemophiliacs would have been saved from HIV infection.[68]

Paying for Injury: The Politics of Compensation

Although the efforts of hemophiliacs to place legal responsibility failed, their political struggle to obtain economic compensation and to make the health policy system more receptive to their interests and demands have been remarkably successful.

The hemophiliacs' chances of placing the legal responsibility with the health authorities or the blood products manufacturers in order to obtain economic compensation were small. At the time the hemophiliacs were infected, common compensation rules applied to injuries caused by treatments and by medicine. The so-called culpa principle informed compensation law. Injured persons had to prove that (1) the tort feasor has acted culpably, (2) the injured person has suffered a loss, and (3) there was a causal relation between act and loss. If the injured person could not satisfy each of these elements, the injury was deemed accidental and no damages were awarded.

The Hemophilia Society realized early on that this principle would make it almost impossible for hemophiliacs to meet the burden of proof. In an April 1987 memorandum, the DHS encouraged the Parliamentary Committee on Municipal Affairs to award an *ex gratie* compensation through special legislation, not only to infected hemophiliacs but also to those infected through blood transfusion, whose case the DHS chose to speak for from that moment. The memorandum evaluated the scope of the damages and arrived at the conclusion that the damages would have to be at least US$ 68,000 per person.[69]

Despite the requirements of Danish compensation law, there were a number of factors that bolstered the DHS claim for an *ex gratie* compensation. Since the 1950s, a reform of the physicians' professional responsibility had been considered,[70] and in December 1984 the interior minister established a work group to examine the possibility of introducing medical injury insurance in Denmark. Technological development as well as changes in popular attitudes meant that it was no longer considered fair that patients alone should bear the risks associated with therapeutic developments. Given the limitations of the prevailing restrictive conceptions of compensation, the working group had been given two tasks: to examine the possibility of a broader coverage of patient injuries than provided by the common compensation principles, and to find a quick and efficient way to award compensation—for example, without the involvement of the courts. It is within this context that the DHS made its claims for compensation. The DHS's second argument was that *Folketinget* had, although rarely, awarded *ex gratie* compensation. Most recently, it had done so in 1986 when under media scrutiny it had provided funds to patients who in the 1960s had been subjected to medical experiments with LSD.

The intensive media coverage of the LSD compensation case eased the way to an award. It took the Parliamentary Finance Committee only until June 3, 1987, to approve the Interior Ministry's decision to award an *ex gratie* compensation of US$ 16,000 to HIV-infected hemophiliacs. At no time did the government use "erstatning," the Danish term for compensation. Instead "godtgørelse" (making good) was used to indicate that the *ex gratie* compensation was extraordinary assistance and that the government took no responsibility for HIV infection among Danish hemophiliacs.

The DHS was far from satisfied with the compensation when its details were published in connection with the Interior Ministry's order on September 2, 1987.[71] In an October 15, 1987, letter to the Parliamentary Health Committee, the DHS pointed out, among other things, that the size of the compensation was not proportionate with the deterioration in the quality and prospect of life of those who had been infected, and that the group of recipients was too narrow because it excluded survivors of infected hemophiliacs who died before the compensation had been enacted; spouses or girlfriends who had been infected before the hemophiliacs had been informed of their infection and the risk of infection; and non-hemophiliacs infected through blood transfusion.

Just as the Hemophilia Society sent its October 1987 letter to the Parliamentary Health Committee, the media again took on the decisive role that enabled the DHS to pressure the health policy system to accommodate its demands. It started in the October issue of *PRESS*, a monthly critical Danish magazine, which published a long documentary article on the hemophiliacs' 1985 fight to introduce heat treatment of blood products and screening of donor blood; the front page headline was "Britta Schall sent 350 Danes into AIDS Hell."[72] The article rekindled public attention. Two months later the transition scheme was made public, and the DHS simultaneously decided to sue for damages in the High Court. From this moment, the widespread impression developed that the health authorities and especially the former interior minister, Britta Schall Holberg, had subjected the hemophiliacs to scandalous treatment and that they were responsible for the plight not only for the few hemophiliacs who might have been infected after January 1, 1985—the cut-off date the DHS used in the compensation case—but for all infected hemophiliacs. This misperception turned out to be decisive for the DHS' chances of broadening and increasing the compensation.

On April 6, 1988, one month before the judicial inquiry issued its final report, *Folketinget* decided to increase the *ex gratie* compensation to US$ 40,000 and ordered that the awards could also be made to patients infected through transfusion at Danish hospitals[73] and to certain relatives.[74] However, the DHS still was not satisfied. Infected sexual partners of hemophiliacs were still not eligible for damages, and the amount was not even close to fair in the Hemophilia Society's view. It therefore continued to work on increasing the sum of the compensation.

In October 1991, the DHS received support from a televised documentary "The Human Factor." The program focused on the 1985 decisions to introduce heat treatment and screening and later the transition scheme. The two reporters described the background of the documentary: "We feel that the responsibility has never really been placed. The government has compensated hemophiliacs who were infected via their factor preparations. But nobody has explained who was responsible. The amount of [US$ 40,000] for each infected hemophiliac is totally ridiculous."[75] Through comments and cross-cuts it was strongly suggested that it was not only the two interviewed hemophiliacs who had been infected—because the authorities had hesitated to introduce heat treatment and screening and because of the decision to introduce a transition scheme—but that all 89 infected hemophiliacs had been infected for the same reasons. Both allegations were wrong. Likewise, an interview with a dead hemophiliac's girlfriend left the impression that arrogant doctors had inexcusably pursued their own research interests at the expense of the woman's right to proper treatment. None of the doctors were interviewed for the program, nor was their version of the events related. Although the TV documentary generated considerable media attention, it did not result in an immediate increase of the compensation. However, the claims of the two women who had been sexually infected by hemophiliacs and who had so far been turned down for compensation were now accepted.

In August 1992, the DHS board and its lawyer decided to file their complaint before the European Court of Human Rights. On Sunday, October 4, one of the large Danish newspapers published an extensive portrait of a young hemophiliac. In prime time the following Friday, HIV contamination among hemophiliacs was the top story in one of the then most popular Danish TV programs. In the discussion, a Social Democratic member of the Parliamentary Health Committee demonstrated that he obviously had only limited or incorrect knowledge of the development of HIV infection among Danish hemophiliacs. An HIV-contaminated Hemophilia Society board member and its attorney had an easy time, and the viewers could only get the impression that the authorities were hiding something. During the following days, the Health Minister was bombarded with questions from journalists but refused to increase the compensation. "We have already discussed that matter, and it will not be re-opened."

But the minister was wrong on that count. Two weeks later, on October 23, the French hemophilia case was decided, and the leader of the French blood transfusion system was sentenced to four years in prison. Three days later, the Hemophilia Society held a press conference with, among others, a lawyer who had represented French hemophiliacs before the European Court of Human Rights in Strasbourg. It was obvious that the DHS wanted to use the press conference as leverage in its fight against the health policy system. The Society was very dissatisfied that the Danish health authorities were not willing to take responsibility for the HIV infection of Danish hemophiliacs—something health authorities in other countries had done. In addition, the DHS found it reprehensible that the Danish *ex gratie* compensations had not been raised to the level of other countries.

The strategy paid off. The press conference resulted in huge headlines and pictures in the newspapers the next day, not least because the DHS attorney at the meeting stated that there were many parallels between the French and the Danish hemophilia case; and that he would ask the police to initiate a criminal investigation against the former interior minister and two NBH top civil servants.

The press coverage made clear the profound sympathy for the hemophiliacs' demand. It demonstrated a striking lack of fundamental knowledge of the development of the hemophiliacs' HIV contamination, and an absence of any critical perspective on the DHS attorney's arguments and motives. For instance, an editorial in *Jyllands-Posten*, one of the large national papers, demanded "Names of those responsible" and stated in that connection that "more than 1000 French hemophiliacs became HIV-positive between 1984 and 1985" and that "in Denmark there were 89 infected hemophiliacs in the same period."[76] The tabloids knew how to exploit the situation. *Ekstra Bladet*, which through the years had run a systematic and, in Denmark, completely unheard of personal campaign against the former interior minister, Schall Holberg, asked the DHS chairman to participate in a telephone session on October 29, where readers could call in and comment on the case. There was a deluge of calls. The next day, an unflattering photo of the former minister covered the entire front page of the newspaper along with the text, "Danes in uproar over the hemophiliac scandal: She must be punished." Excerpts of the readers' comments filled several pages.[77]

Politicians immediately sensed the public sentiment and almost ran each other down in the rush to express their disgust over the failure to place responsibility for the HIV infection of the Danish hemophiliacs. The Social Democratic opposition party had had no part in government power during the Danish AIDS epidemic and quickly exploited public opinion, demanding that the Parliamentary Health Committee deal with the case. After an October 29 parliamentary consultation with the health and justice ministers, a member of the Radical Liberal opposition party said: "At this time, it is indecent to talk about money. However, it is important to place the responsibility for the infection of so many hemophiliacs through their vital factor medicine."[78] Adding to the furor, the Danish Broadcasting Corporation scheduled a rerun of the documentary "The Human Factor."

A day later, *Folketinget* increased the compensation to US$ 120,000 for each infected hemophiliac. In five years the sum to be paid had thus risen almost eightfold. The new compensation package granted about twice the amount initially requested by the Hemophilia Society.

However, the DHS' plans to report the former interior minister and two of her civil servants to the police created a stir in the legal community, and a few journalists started to smell the politics in the legal maneuvers.[79] A prominent law professor described the report to the police as frivolous. In his opinion, the report had no legal basis but was so full of politics that it would create a witch hunt against the former minister. He encouraged the General Council of the Bar to evaluate whether the DHS attorney had acted within the code of professional conduct.[80] The law professor was supported by a colleague when he pointed out that DHS' plans to report the former interior minister to the police was primarily part of a political game, for only the Danish Parliament can impeach a (former) minister, which, of course, the DHS attorney knew perfectly well.[81] The attorney filed his report with the minister of justice on October 3, 1992.[82] One year later the public prosecutor determined that there was no basis for bringing charges.[83]

When at last the hemophiliacs' compensation claims became the subject of a High Court decision, on February 14, 1995, the public reaction was predictable. Danes were shocked when the authorities and the blood products manufacturers were virtually exonerated. That the High Court could acquit the health authorities of their obvious responsibility could mean only one thing: the courts and the authorities were accomplices. Ordinary Danes had a "rat's chance" against the "system."

Politicians joined the public indignation. Said one, "In my 25 years in politics, I have never experienced anything worse."[84] The minister issued a press release on February 22 declaring that the parliamentary parties and the government sympathized with the HIV-infected hemophiliacs and regretted the terrible tragedy: that 89 hemophiliacs at the end of the 1970s and in the following years had been infected with HIV via their factor preparations before the danger of HIV infection was realized and preventive methods were developed. *Folketinget* and the government acknowledged and regretted that in the light of recent knowledge, measures taken in 1985 and 1986 had to be regarded as insufficient in certain respects. Nevertheless, they respected the High Court's judgment, which held that the relevant authorities had not acted negligently.

It was in this context that politicians endorsed a proposal of the Hemophilia Society's chairman that Denmark follow the German example by creating a fund for compensation and support of survivors of hemophiliacs and that they establish a medical insurance scheme to cover drugs. Action was swift. The DHS was immediately invited to negotiate with the Health Minister. Ultimately the government moved to create a hemophiliac fund of US$ 3.2 million on top of the *ex gratie* compensation already granted, initiate a medical injury insurance scheme to cover drugs in broad terms, and to ensure easier access to compensation than provided by the Product Liability Act. Finally, the DHS was offered representation in the NBH Blood Products Committee.[85]

Thus, with the exception of the demand that the authorities formally and explicitly accept responsibility for the infection of hemophiliacs with HIV, all of the Hemophilia Society's demands had been met. In a March 15 press release, the DHS noted its disappointment over the failure of the authorities to acknowledge the inadequacy of their response between 1984 and 1986.[86] Nevertheless, said the Hemophilia Society, the minister's February declaration was sufficient to bring the case to an end.

A year later, when the European Court of Human Rights issued its decision, it was able to draw some attention. The Danish Supreme Court's judgment of October 3, 1996, was barely mentioned in the press.

The Aftermath of Scandal

As a result of the "blood scandal," the Danish health system has become extremely sensitive to issues involving blood safety. The price to be paid by what initially appeared to be a salutary development is illustrated in the decisions surrounding hepatitis C and HTLV I/II viruses.[87]

Shortly after hepatitis C was identified in 1989, several Danish blood banks initiated trial screening programs. Subsequently, other blood banks expressed a strong interest in undertaking such screening. But county health authorities, responsible in Denmark for blood bank activities, were unwilling to allocate the necessary funds for such enhanced screening. If the NBH were to require such efforts, the cost would fall on the central state budget. The NBH was reluctant to take that step, at least in part, because of the quality of the early HCV tests.

The quality of the test for hepatitis C had improved markedly in early 1991, and a TV show about HCV infection produced a minor media frenzy. These two factors led the National Board of Health to recommend the introduction of anti-HCV screening, despite the fact that heat treatment had already reduced the risk to hemophiliacs significantly. Indeed, for the Board of Health, HCV was viewed as essentially a problem for transfusion recipients who receive whole blood, which was not heat treated.

From this perspective, it became necessary to resolve the question of *when* blood products should be derived exclusively from screened blood. The NBH was concerned that imposing a requirement that all blood products be based on HCV-screened blood would result in the destruction of valuable raw material and a consequent shortage of blood products. Politicians saw the situation differently. They favored a rapid introduction of screening for coagulation factor: Repetition of the HIV saga was to be avoided at all costs. The cost of withdrawal of unscreened product from the market in March 1992 was $4.2 million.[88]

Questions of cost also surfaced over the introduction of screening for HTLV I/II. The matter had been analyzed on several occasions by the Danish Society for Clinical Immunology. HTLV had not been detected in Scandinavia, transmission was difficult, and the clinical consequences of HTLV infection were limited (very rare cases of cancer), so there were no well-founded arguments for screening. In early 1994, the detection of a single case of HTLV in donor sera caused Sweden to introduce HTLV screening on a trial basis for a year. Immediately thereafter, the first case was detected in Denmark.[89] An extremely media-savvy member of the opposition, who was a doctor, exploited Danish media attention on HTLV and demanded the introduction of screening.[90] The Social Democratic Minister of Health chose to ignore the NBH recommendation and introduced anti-HTLV screening from April 1, 1994, even though it had been statistically estimated that all Danish blood donations would have to be tested over a period of 30 to 60 years before one case of cancer could be prevented. For the minister of health it would have been a no-win situation to oppose the politically cost-free standpoint of the opposition member that blood should be 100 percent safe. After the first two years, the cost of the HTLV screening was estimated at US$ 4.8 million, the equivalent of approximately 600 hip operations (waiting lists for hip operations have been considered a major problem in the Danish health care system for a long time). Given these costs and the medical risks, the NBH suggested canceling the screening or limiting screening to only new donors. Only in mid-1997 did the Minister of Health relent and accept a policy of screening new donors only. Interestingly, the DHS never expressed its opinion on HTLV screening, and its chairman has questioned its justification.[91]

Conclusion

The Danish "blood scandal" had a legal as well as a political dimension. In strictly legal terms the scandal evaporated before judicial scrutiny. Politically the story was very different. The political dimension permitted the DHS not only to obtain the largest *ex gratie* compensation ever granted to a patient group in the history of the Danish health system, but also to ensure (1) introduction of medical injury insurance in Denmark that makes it easier for patients to obtain compensation for injury sustained through treatment in the Danish health system and (2) great sensitivity to issues involving blood safety among health officials. "Cold" cost-benefit analyses have lost legitimacy—in particular, when politically elected officials must calculate the population's tolerance for risk as one parameter of the analysis. The result has been more exacting standards of safety in blood therapy. The question posed by this attainment is clear: Has safety been achieved at a reasonable cost? A clear question, but one that cannot be discussed as part of public discourse in Denmark because it would inevitably result in a discussion of the establishment of priorities. And prioritizing in health care is taboo in Danish political culture.

NOTES

The following persons were interviewed for and/or have commented on the manuscript in the period June 1996 through September 1997.

Andersen, Terkel. Member of the Board of the Danish Hemophilia Society 1981–1985; Chairman of the Society since 1985.

Bacher, Theis. Director of the Blood Bank at Slagelse Hospital; member of the Board of the Danish Hemophilia Society at various times during the last 20 years; Danish Hemophilia Society representative on the National Board of Health Blood Products Committee since 1995.

Brockenhuus-Schack, Anne. Freelance journalist.

Christensen, Jens Peter. Associate Professor, Aarhus University School of Law.

Dickmeiss, Ebbe. Head of the Department of Clinical Immunology, Copenhagen University Hospital.

Eriksen, Poul Birch. Radio Journalist, Danish Broadcasting Corporation.

Jørgensen, Jan. Head of the Blood Transfusion Centre at Aarhus University Hospital since 1971; head of the hospital's Department of Clinical Immunology since 1988; chairman of the Danish Hemophilia Society Medical Committee 1976–1986.

Loiborg, Steen. Head of Office, Ministry of the Interior.

Melbye, Mads. Professor, the National Serum Institute.

Nielsen, Kurt Anker. Novo Nordisk.

Sandberg, Eva. Head of Division, Medicines Control Office, Danish Medicines Agency.

Schall Holberg, Britta. Former Minister of the Interior.

von Magnus, Michael. Head of Division D, National Board of Health.

The DHS has given me access to their archives, and Information Officer Jo Gudmand-Høyer has helped me find my way through them. Annette Andersen has provided secretarial assistance and Karen Prehn library assistance. The editors, Eric Feldman and Ron Bayer, have commented thoroughly on the manuscript.

I am grateful to all of them.

E. A.

1. Although hemophiliacs are not the only actors in the blood field with an interest in HIV and AIDS, their efforts to influence Danish AIDS policy has been *the* central effort. Therefore, the struggle of hemophiliacs for acceptance of their demands and wishes in Danish AIDS policy will be the axis of this chapter's analysis of the Danish blood system's response to AIDS.

2. *Betænkning nr. 907/1980 om organisering af indsamling og fordeling af blod samt fremstilling af blodfraktioneringsprodukter. Betænkning fra det af Indenrigsministeriet den 11. februar 1977 nedsatte blodproduktudvalg.* København, 1980, p. 119.

3. *Ibid.*

4. Danmarks Bløderforening, *Danmarks bløderforening gennem 25 år—en forenings arbejde på godt og ondt: 1970–1995.* København: Danmarks Bløderforening, 1996; interview, Terkel Andersen.

5. A 6.25 exchange rate has been used to convert Danish kroner into US$.

6. *Ekstra Bladet* (November 22, 1983), "Jern-Britta sjakrer med liv og død."

7. *Ekstra Bladet* (November 22, 1983), "Skal penge afgøre om bløderne skal leve."

8. Interview, Theis Bacher; interview, Jan Jørgensen.

9. Interview Theis Bacher; interview; Jan Jørgensen.

10. M. Melbye, R. Madhok, P. S. Sarin, G. D. O. Lowe, J. J. Goedert, K. S. Froebel, R. J. Biggar, S. Stenbjerg, C. D. Forbes, R. C. Gallo, and P. Ebbesen, "HTLV-III Seropositivity in European Haemophiliacs Exposed to Factor VIII Concentrate Imported from the USA," *Lancet* II (1984), pp. 1443–1446.

11. Sundhedsstyrelsen, *Retningslinier ved optræden af erhvervet immundefekt syndrom (AIDS).* København: Sundhedsstyrelsen, maj 1983.

12. U 1996.1574 (*The Weekly Courts Report* with reprints of the High Court's and the Supreme Court's decisions in the hemophilia compensation case); H. Jørgensen. "AIDS—myter, skræmmemiddel og homopolitik," *Pan*, 30 (1983).

13. *Sundhedsstyrelsens redegørelse til indenrigsministeriet om sygdommen AIDS.* København: Sundhedsstyrelsen, Juni 1985.

14. Interview, Mads Melbye.

15. M. Melbye, R.J. Biggar, J.C. Chermann, L. Montagnier, S. Stenbjerg and P. Ebbesen, "High Prevalence of Lymphadenopathy Virus (LAV) in European Hemophiliacs," *Lancet*, II (1984), pp. 40–41.

16. M. Melbye, R. Madhok *et al.*, *op.cit.*

17. Interview, Terkel Andersen.

18. Interview, Mads Melbye.

19. A. Brockenhuus-Schack and P. Birch Eriksen, *AIDS—mellem linjerne.* (København: Sommer & Sørensen, 1988), p. 7.

20. March 13, 1985, letter from the Danish Hemophilia Society to Interior Minister Britta Schall Holberg re AIDS prevention in hemophilia treatment.

21. Interview, Terkel Andersen.

22. Interview, Jan Jørgensen.

23. U 1996.1588–89.

24. U 1996.1574.

25. Interview, Jan Jørgensen.

26. June 15, 1985, letter from the Danish Hemophilia Society to Interior Minister Britta Schall Holberg re prevention in hemophilia treatment; July 29, 1985, letter from the Danish Hemophilia Society to the Parliamentary Committee on Municipal Affairs.

27. U 1996.1580.

28. U 1996.1573.

29. May 7, 1985, letter from the Ministry of the Interior to the Danish Hemophilia Society.

30. U 1996.1589.

31. June 15, 1985, letter from the Danish Hemophilia Society to Interior Minister Britta Schall Holberg re prevention in hemophilia treatment.

32. *Sundhedsstyrelsens redegørelse til Indenrigsministeriet om sygdommen AIDS.* København: Sundhedsstyrelsen, June 1985.

33. *Beretning* 1988, pp. 86–87.

34. June 24, 1985, cover letter from the National Board of Health (signed by Director Søren Sørensen and Head of Division Michael von Magnus) to the Ministry of the Interior.

35. June 18, 1985, letter from the National Board of Health to Professor Flemming Kissmeyer, Aarhus Kommunehospital.

36. *Beretning* 1988, p. 93.

37. Interior Minister Schall Holberg's copy of *Sundhedsstyrelsens redegørelse til indenrigsministeriet om sygdommen AIDS*, p. 28.

38. June 25, 1985, letter marked "private" from Interior Minister Britta Schall Holberg to National Board of Health Director Søren Sørensen.

39. July 29, 1985, letter from the Danish Hemophilia Society to the Parliamentary Committee on Municipal Affairs.

40. U 1996.1574.

41. *Beretning* 1988, p. 99.

42. *PRESS* (No. 23, October 1987), "Britta Schall sendte dem ud i mareridt: Spillede russsisk roulette med 350 mennesker," p. 11, p. 59.

43. M. Eide & G. Hernes, *Død og Pine! Om massemedia og helsepolitikk.* Oslo: FAFO, 1987.

44. *Politiken* (July 24, 1985), "AIDS og bløderne."

45. Interview, Terkel Andersen.

46. *Beretning* 1988, p. 107.

47. *Ibid.*, p. 104.

48. *B.T.* (July 3, 1985), "AIDS i donorblod: Vi kan alle blive smittede."

49. *Ekstra Bladet* (September 3, 1985), "Læger spøjtede AIDS ind i døende."

50. J. W. Kingdon, *Agendas, Alternatives, and Public Policies* (Boston: Little, Brown & Co., 1984).

51. R. W. Cobb and C. D. Elder, *Participation in American Politics: The Dynamics of Agenda-Building* (Boston: Allyn & Bacon, 1972).

52. A. Brockenhuus-Schack and P. Birch Eriksen, *op.cit.*, p. 56.

53. E. Albæk, "Denmark: AIDS and the 'political pink triangle,'" in D. L. Kirp and R. Bayer, eds., *AIDS in the Industrialized Democracies: Passions, Politics and Policies* (New Brunswick: Rutgers University Press, 1992), pp. 281–316.

54. *Ekstra Bladet* (September 14, 1985), "Britta ønsker lig på bordet."

55. O. P. Kristensen, "The logic of political-bureaucratic decision making as a cause of government growth," *European Journal of Political Research* 12, (1980), pp. 349–264.

56. *Beretning* 1988, pp. 109–17.

57. *Ibid.*, pp. 135–36.

58. *Ibid.*, pp. 137–38.

59. *Ibid.*, p. 264.

60. *Ibid.*, pp. 9–10.

61. *Gentofte Kriminalrets dom af 29.11.1989 i sag 443/1988.*

62. *Beretning om tjenstlig undersøgelse mod overlæge Poul Hansen, overlæge Michael von Magnus, overlæge Henning Sørensen, overlæge Niels Axelsen, administrativ direktør Jacob Tørning og afdelingschef Jens Overø.* Afgivet den 28. April 1989. København.

63. U 1996.1595.

64. European Court of Human Rights. *Case of A. and Others v. Denmark (60/1995). Judgment of 8 February 1996.*

65. *Ekstra Bladet* (February 9, 1996), "Terkels store sejr."

66. *Ekstra Bladet* (February 9, 1996), "En blodtud til systemet."

67. *Ekstra Bladet* (February 9, 1996), "Terkels store sejr."

68. U 1996.1577.

69. Report from Danish Hemophilia Society re compensation to HIV-infected hemophiliacs, April 1987.

70. B. von Eyben, "Lægeansvar," in *Medicinsk Etik*, ed. D. Andersen, C. E. Mabeck and P. Riis (København: FADL's Forlag, 1985), p. 219.

71. *Indenrigsministeriets bekendtgørelse nr. 581 af 2. september 1987 om godtgørelse til HIV- smittede blødere.*

72. *PRESS* (No. 23, October 1987), "Britta Schall sendte dem ud i mareridt: Spillede russsisk roulette med 350 mennesker."

73. As for transfusion patients, there are today 26 registered cases of HIV transmission at Danish hospitals; only one patient has been infected since the introduction of anti-HIV screening on January 1, 1986 (see E. Dickmeiss, "Smittemarkørundersøgelser af donorblod," in A. Svejgaard, E. Dickmeiss, and J. Ingerslev, *Kliniske immunologi 1970–1995: Den hvide side.* Dansk Selskab for Klinisk Immunologi, 1995, p. 72). The total number of registered cases in Denmark is higher because it includes patients infected abroad.

74. *Sundhedsministeriets bekendtgørelse nr. 313 af 14. juni 1988 om godtgørelse til HIV-smittede blødere m.fl. og HIV-positive transfusionssmittede m.fl.*

75. Danmarks Bløderforening, *op.cit.*, p. 25.

76. *Jyllands-Posten* (October 24, 1992), "Navne på ansvaret."

77. *Ekstra Bladet* (October 30, 1992), "Britta gjorde grin med menneskeliv."

78. *Ibid.*

79. *Weekendavisen* (October 30–November 5, 1992). "Drop den sag."

80. *Aarhus Stiftstidende* (October 30, 1992), "Professor: Bløderanmeldelse absurd."

81. *Jyllands-Posten* (October 28, 1992), "Ekspert: Blødernes straffesag står svagt"; *Berlingske Tidende* (October 28, 1992), "Svært at anklage tidligere minister."

82. November 3, 1992, letter from attorney Jørgen Jacobsen to Minister of Justice Hans Engell.

83. October 15, 1993, letter from public prosecutor H. Bech Hansen to attorney Jørgen Jacobsen.

84. *B.T.* (February 15, 1995), "Samfundet har et moralsk ansvar."

85. February 22, 1995, press release from the Ministy of Health re the political consequences of the compensation case.

86. March 15, 1995, press release from the Danish Hemophilia Society.

87. E. Dickmeiss, *op.cit.*

88. E. Sandberg, "Introduction of Hepatitis C Testing: Regulatory Aspects," *Quality and Safety of Plasma Products*, pp. 87–89. Proceedings from the 3rd EPFA/EAPPI Regulatory Affairs Symposium. Zeist, the Netherlands: Medical Forum International, 1997.

89. E. Dickmeiss, *op.cit.*

90. *Politiken* (January 22, 1994), "HTLV 1: Ny dødelig virus på vej."

91. Interview, Terkel Andersen.

6

Blood "Scandal" and AIDS in Germany

Stephan Dressler

It was not until late 1993 that the safety of the German blood supply attracted the attention of the general public and the media. The discovery that the Koblenz-based company UB Plasma had used blood and plasma that had been improperly screened for HIV antibody shocked the German public and led the federal minister of health, Horst Seehofer, to open an official inquiry into what was widely perceived as a "scandal."[1] Such reactions were late in coming, given the fact that press accounts of the effect of HIV contamination of the blood supply had appeared years earlier. In 1991, the mass circulation *Der Spiegel* had in "Der Tod Aus der Spritze" (Death by Injection) noted that half of Germany's hemophiliacs, almost 2000 men, had been infected through HIV-contaminated clotting factor.[2] The *Sueddeutsche Zeitung*, in "Scandal or Just a Sad Story," had made clear that those dependent on the blood supply had been infected as a consequence of circumstances that were not inevitable. More than tragedy was involved.[3]

As early as 1981, when AIDS was first reported,[4] Federal Health Office officials (*Bundesministerium für Gesundheit*), physicians from hemophilia treatment centers, and representatives from pharmaceutical companies and blood banks had discussed the possible transmission of an infectious agent via blood and blood products. From the perspective of 1999, it is still not easy to determine which of the steps taken in the epidemic's early years were appropriate. In 1982, when the first transfusion-associated case of AIDS was reported in the United States, it was even more difficult. The etiologic agent responsible for the new disease had yet to be isolated and characterized. The risk of transmitting AIDS through blood and blood products was uncertain. No one could have known the extent to which blood transfusion services and the blood products industry would be affected by AIDS. Such ambiguity stood at the beginning of more than a decade of discussions, proposals, and attempts to reduce a possible risk to the blood supply.

Background

Red Cross, Pharmaceutical Companies, Hospitals: Blood Providers

A variety of institutions and producers provide blood and blood products in Germany. Erythrocytes, thrombocytes, and other blood products used for transfusion are supplied mainly by governmental institutions (e.g., city blood banks, *kommunale Blutspendedienste*) or not-for-profit organizations. Commercial companies, organizations such as the Red Cross, and blood transfusion centers at university hospitals and other large hospitals operate the whole-blood collection and distribution system. In general, there is no payment to whole-blood donors, but plasma donors may receive remuneration (approximately 30 to 60 DEM, or US$20 to 40 as of 1996) as compensation for their time. Many in Germany do not consider this "payment."

After World War II, the German Red Cross began providing services related to the protection of the general population in case of catastrophe or war. For this purpose, the Red Cross received DEM 2 million from the federal government in 1952.[5] Since then, the German Red Cross has operated blood banks. The Red Cross processed more than 2 million blood donations in 1984,[6] and today produces an estimated 4.5 million blood products annually. It considers its services humanitarian aid, which means the blood banks are operated as charitable, nonprofit institutions. Blood products are sold on a cost-recovery basis, with prices including all costs for personnel, materials, and buildings.[7]

Larger hospitals, university hospitals, or specialized clinics sometimes run their own blood banks and produce products to meet local needs and requirements. In Berlin, for example, blood banks at university hospitals provide specialized products like blood components for rare blood groups. Several Red Cross blood banks in Berlin produce the more commonly used products.

The pharmaceutical industry is active in the field of plasma-derived products, such as clotting factor concentrates or prothrombin. The 1996 edition of the directory on drugs and medicinal products lists more than ten industrial producers of factor concentrates, anticoagulants, and hemostatics.[8] Once a product is approved for marketing, health insurance generally covers the cost of treatment if no less expensive product is available.

According to a recent survey, German blood donors are not homogeneous.[9] Whether commercial companies rely on particular groups of individuals for plasma donation, such as homeless persons or drug users seeking compensation, is not known.

Legal Aspects of Blood and Blood Products

Under Germany's federal constitution (the *Grundgesetz*), health and health-related issues lie within the authority of the *Länder* (the states), and the regulatory power of federal authorities (including the Federal Ministry of Health and its agencies) is limited to certain issues that are delegated from the *Länder* to the federal authorities. The Federal Ministry of Health controls various federal institutes, such as the Federal Health Office and the *Paul-Ehrlich-Institut* (PEI), and is the supervisory authority for federal health offices. Whenever a health-related decision is required for the nation as a whole and the Federal Ministry of Health is involved, other federal agencies counsel the Ministry and prepare the scientific background for its policy decision.

Indicative of the division between the federal authorities and the *Länder*, the Paul-Ehrlich-Institute and the Institute for Pharmaceutical and Medicinal Products, for example, may license blood products or new drugs for marketing, but the direct control of production facilities is under the authority of the state where the producer is based.

Before responsibility for blood and blood products was clearly regulated in 1994 as a consequence of the HIV/AIDS scandal, the former Federal Health Office was responsible for identifying health risks for the general population (including risks by drugs, medicinal products, and blood products) and for taking adequate preventive measures. Not only did the Federal Health Office control the approval of new drugs, but it had regulatory authority in the post-marketing period. Such authority was thought to ensure that newly approved drugs did, in fact, demonstrate a positive risk-benefit ratio. A central feature of postmarketing control was the obligation of physicians to report possible adverse effects of pharmaceutical products to the commission on pharmaceutical substances (*Arzneimittelkommission*) of the Federal Medical Council. With that authority, the Federal Health Office could have halted the distribution of HIV-contaminated blood products in 1984.[10]

Several doctrines of German law complement this regulatory regime in securing the safety of blood products. Liability for blood-related injury or illness is governed by the Medical Preparations Act (*Arzneimittelgesetz*), the federal law governing the production and distribution of medicines, and through the German Civil Code (*Bürgerliches Gesetzbuch*). These laws require a clear demonstration of causation between a product, its use, and a possible injury or illness. The plaintiff bears the burden of proof of establishing beyond a reasonable doubt that a given product caused an injury. Plaintiffs cannot be awarded damages unless they meet that heavy burden. This standard would, in years to come, pose enormous difficulties when those affected by HIV-contaminated blood and blood products turned to the courts.

Hemophilia in Germany

There are an estimated 3500 to 6000 hemophiliacs in Germany.[11] Approximately 2500 to 3500 of them require substitution therapy with coagulation factors; 50% to 75% of these hemophiliacs were infected. Anticoagulant treatment enriched with factor VIII was widely available in Germany from the early 1970s through specialized hemophilia treatment centers, hospitals, ambulances, or physicians in private practice.

Seventy-five percent of hemophiliacs who need treatment receive their care at home.[12] Clotting factor is stored in home refrigerators, and patients typically keep a supply that lasts approximately six months. Health insurance covers the entire expense, and physicians are not constrained with regard to the product or dose prescribed[13] as long as the prescription is medically indicated. This broad clinical authority permitted the use of high doses of coagulation factor in the treatment of hemophilia, for physicians as well as patients felt that such treatment was necessary to enable hemophiliacs to lead normal lives and enjoy leisure-time activities such as sports and travel. Doses varied; however, the average German dose of 4 to 4.5 international units of factor VIII per capita per year far exceeded the amount of factor VIII used in other European countries or the United States.

The German Hemophilia Society is an organization for people with bleeding disorders and their relatives. The majority of its members suffer from hemophilia A or B or from von Willebrand's disease (lack of factor VIII R: Ag).[14] Self-described as a "self-help organization," the group has always involved physicians who treated hemophilia in its leadership — they even served on the society's board of directors. In later years, that intimate linkage would be subject to criticism by those who saw in the relationship of trust with physicians, health officials, and the pharmaceutical industry the source of a deception with fatal consequences.[15] But it was as an organization involving physicians that the German Hemophilia Society influenced blood policy before, during, and after the HIV/blood crisis. In the early 1980s, the society would confront the risk of AIDS in a way that, in retrospect, profoundly mistook the potential for disaster.

The umbrella organization of AIDS service organizations in Germany, *Deutsche AIDS-Hilfe*, did not play a major role in the context of HIV/AIDS and blood. Indeed, the HIV-infected hemophiliac Karl Caspari, describing a "cartel of silence," has claimed that AIDS-Hilfe organizations are dominated by homosexual men and drug addicts, who do not understand the problems of hemophiliacs.[16] However, local AIDS-Hilfe organizations vary considerably. For example, the AIDS-Hilfe in Bonn included on its staff Oliver Köppchen, an HIV-infected hemophiliac who later worked on the German parliament's commission established to investigate the blood scandal and who provided a variety of counseling services for hemophiliacs.

Import Dependency

In contrast to West Germany, East Germany (the former German Democratic Republic, GDR) was quick to aim for national self-sufficiency of blood and blood products. Formally and officially, blood donation was declared a humanitarian act reflecting the demands of socialist morality. But behind this ideology were economic motivations. Convertible foreign currency was limited in the socialist GDR, and imported blood products, as well as other Western pharmaceutical products, were not generally available. An ironic consequence of this scarcity-imposed limitation was the protection of East German hemophiliacs from the fate that would befall those in West Germany. In 1986 and 1987, only five of the estimated 1300 East German hemophiliacs were known to be HIV-infected. Those few infections were caused by imported, HIV-contaminated blood products and did not influence the general epidemiology of HIV and AIDS in the GDR.[17] The history of HIV infection among hemophiliacs in Germany is thus the history of the West German blood system.

In the 1970s and 1980s, the Federal Republic of Germany, West Germany, imported most blood products. Indeed, when the possibility of using the national blood supply for the production of coagulation factor concentrates was first discussed in the early 1980s, representatives from the pharmaceutical industry and self-help organizations for hemophiliacs argued that national resources were insufficient to meet the demand. Such warnings were fueled by fears that shortages would have a profound impact on the hard-won normalization of life that accompanied the treatments of the 1970s. Even though imported plasma products had been responsible for a high incidence of hepatitis B among hemophiliacs, clearly an adequate supply of such medication was considered more important than product safety. Thus there was profound resistance to change.

At a public hearing in November 1983, when the risk of AIDS transmission through coagulation factors was already evident, a hemophiliac patient and representative of a German hemophilia association strikingly declared that hemophiliacs would rather risk getting AIDS than abandon the advantages of modern high-dose substitution therapy.[18] Although a lack of information might explain the failure of patients to appreciate the danger of AIDS, it is remarkable that guidelines for the treatment of hemophilia A and hemophilia B, published by the Federal Health Office in June 1985, demonstrated a similar misperception. These guidelines, based on the results of a working group on "Standardization of Use of Factor VIII- and Factor IX Concentrate," mention post-transfusion hepatitis as an adverse effect of clotting factors and declare that the risk of transmitting AIDS through clotting factors is "very low, according to the current state of knowledge . . . and based on the available data."[19]

Hepatitis B and Plasma Products

Not only was the risk of AIDS underestimated, but the thrall of the factor concentrates that had so transformed the lives of hemophiliacs led to a too sanguine response regarding the risk of hepatitis. The risk of hepatitis A and B virus transmission via blood factors was recognized early in the course of hemophilia treatment. It was also known that the risk of hepatitis infection increased when high doses of coagulation factors were used in substitution therapy,[20] and that plasma products derived from large donor pools carried a relatively higher risk.[21] Pharmacological or chemical methods for inactivating the hepatitis virus (especially hepatitis B) were not available until February 1981, when the first heat-treated factor VIII product, manufactured by Behring, was licensed in Germany.

The use of plasma products from smaller donor pools, and a domestic plasma supply, would have helped to prevent hepatitis B infections among many German hemophiliacs. The prevalence of hepatitis B in Germany is much lower than the prevalence in countries from which factors were imported. This should have been reason enough for pharmaceutical companies and regulatory agencies to restructure the blood and plasma system. But those in positions of responsibility did not react, or reacted inappropriately; the majority of (West) German hemophiliacs were infected with hepatitis B. For these patients, the introduction of heat-inactivated factor VIII and the approval of an anti–hepatitis B vaccine in the 1980s came too late: 66% of the hemophilia population already suffered from chronic liver disease.[22] From 1978 to 1987, hepatitis B–linked cirrhosis caused 18% of deaths among West German hemophiliacs. Only severe hemorrhage exacted a greater burden, accounting for 47% of deaths.[23]

Both hemophiliacs and their physicians considered hepatitis B infection the price of normalization. They did not realize that protection against hepatitis B virus would have an impact on the general safety of blood products and would prevent transmission of other infectious agents. Indeed, there was no thought about the possibility of a new virus, and discussions about heat-inactivated coagulation factor focused solely on hepatitis B. When the heat-inactivated factor became available in 1981, it was twice as expensive as regular factor. German health insurance refused reimbursement for those hemophiliacs already seropositive for hepatitis B. Furthermore, heat-treated factor—which was rendered less active during processing—was in very short supply. Had the supply been greater, and had insurers taken a different course, much of the HIV infection among German hemophiliacs could have been prevented. Ten years later, this lost opportunity would assume central importance in both the parliamentary investigation of the AIDS scandal and in the litigation brought by HIV-infected hemophiliacs.

Blood and AIDS

Learning about AIDS and Blood

The West German Federal Health Office reacted promptly to the December 1982 report by the U.S. Centers for Disease Control suggesting the possibility of transmission of AIDS through blood transfusion. A newly established working group composed of virologists and specialists in internal medicine and infectious diseases immediately published an alert on AIDS that mentioned the possibility of blood-borne transmission.[24] In August 1983, the Federal Health Office published an AIDS summary for physicians that indicated that recipients of coagulator factor and other blood products were at risk.

Until late 1984, however, when the Federal Ministry for Health started a general information campaign on AIDS, the problem went almost unnoticed in the general public. Those most concerned were gay men and their physicians, who had learned through their private connections to the United States about the new health threat. Public concern about AIDS was slow to take shape; it was not until 1987 that debate about the new epidemic threat reached a peak. In these early years, hemophiliacs and transfusion recipients did not play a major role in public discussion about AIDS. It was not until 1993 that they would emerge as a critical force.

Epidemiology of HIV and AIDS in Germany

Epidemiologically, West Germany has long been considered a Pattern I country, according to the World Health Organization definition, with the spread of HIV infection predominantly among homosexual men and injecting drug users. As of March 31, 1997, 16,138 AIDS cases had been reported in Germany, with 9521 cases reported among homosexual and bisexual men, and 2041 cases in injecting drug users. Five hundred and twenty-nine hemophilia associated cases and 276 cases linked to blood transfusions have been reported. Fifteen years after AIDS was first diagnosed, heterosexual transmission remains infrequent, though it is continuously increasing. Official statistics indicate 752 cases from heterosexual transmission.[25]

In contrast to West Germany, East Germany (GDR) was considered a Pattern III country where few HIV infections occurred. Only 271 AIDS cases have been reported from the former communist state as of March 1997.[26]

Only since 1987 has the law required the reporting of anonymous, positive HIV antibody tests to the Robert Koch-Institute. That data reveals a total of 78,085 HIV infections,[27] of which 1857 are among hemophiliacs and 539 among those who had received blood transfusions.[28]

These data indicate that approximately 50% to 75% of hemophiliacs who received treatment with coagulation factor were infected with HIV.[29] The majority of transfusion-associated infections and infections among hemophiliacs occurred before October 1985 and before mandatory HIV antibody testing for blood and blood products was introduced.[30] Some data suggest that the majority of infections among hemophiliacs occurred in one year, 1984.[31]

The first AIDS cases in transfusion recipients and hemophiliacs were diagnosed in October 1983. By 1984, seven hemophiliacs with what was then called "full-blown AIDS" were diagnosed, and for the first time the AIDS problem was discussed at a national conference on hemophilia.[32] One year later, the national hemophilia conference was told in an opening address that viral infections were now playing a major role in the care of hemophilia patients. "As a consequence of widespread . . . antibody testing," the audience was told "we have been confronted with the disillusioning fact that a large proportion of our still symptom-free patients are infected and possibly even contagious."[33]

In the light of this emerging epidemiological picture, what steps were taken? Which opportunities were forgone?

Blood: Measures Taken

As early as January 1983, Germany's Red Cross, as the largest national supplier of blood, introduced measures to exclude donors at risk for AIDS from the donor pool. People with weight loss, lymph node swellings, or other clinical signs were excluded. The efficacy of these measures was, of course, limited, because only persons with overt symptoms could be detected. Six months later, in June 1983, most Red Cross leagues in Germany started to exclude people who belonged to "high-risk groups" (e.g., intravenous drug users, homosexual men) from blood donation. Other blood banks and transfusion centers followed. When the HIV antibody test was licensed in April 1985, most transfusion service centers introduced it before it became mandatory on October 1, 1985.

In Germany, as elsewhere, antibody testing was remarkably effective in securing the safety of the blood supply. The rate of HIV infections before introduction of HIV antibody testing was 7.35 per 1 million blood transfusions, and has been estimated to be between 0.51 and 1 per 1 million since October 1985.[34]

Although confidential self-exclusion procedures, which informed blood donors through a leaflet that AIDS/HIV could be transmitted through blood and blood products and asked those who considered themselves at risk to withdraw their donation, were not made mandatory until July 1987, some transfusion service centers and blood banks asked blood donors to fill out questionnaires and to declare that they did not belong to a "risk group" more than two years earlier.[35]

Autologous blood transfusions were encouraged as an approach to reducing the risk of transfusion-associated infections, despite the limited circumstances in which they might be used. Introduced in Germany in the late 1980s, and promoted by authorities and consumers' organizations, autologous transfusion is still not available nationwide. Nevertheless, when the Federal Center for Health Education published a brochure on autologous blood transfusion in August 1994, it sought to underscore the importance with which it viewed the practice through a foreword prepared by Horst Seehofer, the federal minister of health.[36] The possibility of reducing the risk of blood transfusion–associated infections by reducing the reliance on transfusions attracted far less attention.

Blood: Measures Not Taken

A number of steps that might have been taken to secure the blood supply were thwarted because of institutional resistance to measures that would have incurred cost or required changes in conventional approaches to managing the blood donor system. In June 1984, the Federal Health Office announced that a hepatitis B core antibody test would become mandatory as a surrogate HIV marker on January 1,

1985. The proposal to introduce such testing was based on the belief that the test could be used as an indirect marker for the risk of infection by other sexually transmitted diseases. The blood industry objected. The introduction of the surrogate test, it was asserted, would not only be of limited utility in securing the blood supply from the risk of AIDS but would entail the burden of an expensive laboratory procedure. Reflecting the influence of the industry, the Federal Health Office withdrew its proposal.

The HIV antibody test, which became available in April 1985, was not made mandatory for blood until October 1, 1985. Remarkably and with still unknown costs in terms of infections that might have been averted, blood that was already "on the shelf" was neither tested nor withdrawn.

Finally, despite the fact that it had become clear that a number of at-risk individuals had turned to blood donation as a way of obtaining an antibody test without the potential burden of counseling, it took years to mandate the system of confidential donor exclusion that would have permitted the withdrawal from the donor pool of infected blood units that did not have detectable levels of antibody.

Coagulation Factors: Measures Taken

Many of the measures taken to secure the general blood supply contributed to improving the safety of coagulation factors. But additional steps were clearly required. Concern about the extent to which hemophiliacs were at risk was of sufficient magnitude by the end of 1983 that the *Bundesgesundheitsamt* commenced a regulatory procedure aimed at confronting the dangers associated with factor VIII concentrate (factor IX remained unexamined). As part of that process, a hearing was convened on November 14. Demonstrating the seriousness with which the session was considered, representatives from Alpha, Armour, Beecham, Behringwerke, Eurim, Hoechst, Hormonchemie, Intersero, Immuno, Medac, Mérieux, Nordisk, Rhône-Poulenc, Schering, Schwab, Serlac and Travenol/Cutter pharmaceutical companies, as well as from the federal association of the pharmaceutical industry (*Bundesverband der Pharmazeutischen Industrie*, BPI), participated, as did representatives of several Red Cross leagues and hospitals.[37]

From the industry's perspective, it was essential to minimize the extent to which factor concentrate could be viewed as a vector for an as yet to be identified agent responsible for AIDS. It is thus not surprising that its representatives adopted the most conservative posture in interpreting the available data. Despite the fact the first case of AIDS in a hemophiliac had been diagnosed in October, the BPI spokesperson declared that there was no "*proven* AIDS case among hemophiliacs" in Germany.[38] Further, he denied the possibility that factor VIII concentrate could cause AIDS.[39] More strikingly, Dr. Johann Eibl of Immuno asserted that AIDS was not caused by an infectious agent.[40] In the face of such resistance, the director of the Federal Health

Office, Professor Karl Überla, sought to convey a balanced picture at the session's end. While careful analysis of the risk-benefit ratio of the continued use of factor VIII was essential, he was certain that its benefit to hemophiliacs ultimately would be demonstrated.[41] Nevertheless, he suggested that measures be taken to enhance the safety of concentrate. Seven months before the Federal Health Office was to make its ill-fated proposal for hepatitis B core testing, he suggested that screening of donors would enhance the safety of concentrate. Furthermore, he called for the improvement of plasmapheresis units.

On June 8, 1984, the Federal Health Office issued an Administrative Decision based on the results of the November hearing. The nearly six months between the hearing and the decision illustrates the typical pace of administrative procedures in Germany. The Federal Health Office demanded that blood products include a declaration of the country of origin, information about the size of the donor pool, the process of donor selection, and a warning regarding the possible transmission of AIDS.[42] Factor concentrates were to be used only in the treatment of severe hemophilia.

The government planned to introduce these measures on September 1, 1984, but almost all regional Red Cross blood banks and many producers of blood products objected to the guidelines. So outraged were two Red Cross leagues that they filed a complaint against Professor Überla, whom they accused of misconduct and endangering the general public.[43] Their objections were based on the argument that limiting the use of factor VIII concentrates to the treatment of severe hemophilia would interfere with the therapeutic freedom of physicians. It was also argued that knowing the country of origin, pool size, and number of donors would not improve product safety. Stunningly, objections were also raised to the proposed warning that the use of factor VIII could cause AIDS. In the second half of 1984, the opponents of the proposed regulations still asserted that there was no evidence for the possible transmission of AIDS via factor VIII![44]

Although the complaint against Überla was rejected by the Federal Health Office, it did result in significant modifications in the proposed regulations. An amended decision was issued by the Federal Health Office on December 12, 1984. The use of factor VIII concentrate was no longer limited to severe forms of hemophilia, and indication of the country of origin and production information was not to be required. Products consisting of pooled plasma could be imported, and only products derived from pools of more than 20 single donations would have to be tested for quality and safety before marketing.[45] Beginning March 1, 1985, producers of coagulation factors would have to declare whether their product had undergone a viral inactivation procedure and, if so, which method was used. These alterations were received with a feeling of relief not only by pharmaceutical companies, but by hemophiliacs and their physicians as well. Treatment could continue as usual.

Only with regard to the issue of viral inactivation of factor concentrate did the urgency of the situation have some impact. After extended discussion, a decision was made to require the use of heat-inactivated factor as of February 1985. Indeed, the absence of an appropriate sense of urgency is best reflected by policy regarding HIV-antibody testing of all blood donations—the single most important measure that could have been taken to protect hemophiliacs—which was not made mandatory until six months after its availability in April.

Coagulation Factors: Measures Not Taken

The Federal Health Office first published a warning about the possible risk of HIV infection through blood products (especially factor VIII) in December 1982. Appearing in *Bundesgesundheitsblatt*, a scientific journal edited by the office, the warning was directed toward physicians rather than patients, the general public, or groups at risk.[46] Most physicians and hemophilia specialists did not inform their patients about the possible risk of AIDS, believing that transmission of AIDS through blood was an insignificant risk for hemophiliacs.

In June 1983, the decline of T helper cells in German hemophiliacs was reported at a symposium in Frankfurt.[47] The risk of blood products could no longer be denied. But most hemophiliac patients continued to receive inadequate information. As late as 1985 some physicians told their patients that the risk of AIDS was only minor in comparison to the risk of life-threatening hemorrhage.

During these first years of the AIDS epidemic, when evidence of the fact that hemophiliacs were at risk became ever clearer, there was virtually no discussion about the possibility of dose reductions in factor concentrate. From the perspective of a decade later, it would appear that such a move would have had a salutary impact on German hemophiliacs who were treated with high doses of concentrate, but physicians believed that only such dosage levels would permit their patients to live the normal lives to which they had become accustomed.

The furor produced by the June 1984 recommendations of the Federal Health Office has been noted, as has the six-month delay in mandatory HIV screening. The consequence of the failure to impose a recall of potentially infected blood and blood products—an authority available to the Federal Health Office—was far more tragic for hemophiliacs than it was for those dependent on blood transfusions. Whole blood has a short shelf life, whereas factor concentrate can be stored for much longer periods. Based on the erroneous assumption that only a small, untested supply of blood products was being held by patients, the office did not appreciate the fact that many hemophiliacs involved in home care had typically stored a six-month supply of coagulation factor in their own refrigerators.[48] Had such products been recalled, there is little doubt that many infections could have been averted.

The Aftermath of Infection

Individual Claims

In the early 1960s, Germany experienced the biggest drug-related scandal in its history: 2000 children of mothers who had taken thalidomide during pregnancy were born with severe limb defects, including complete amelia, and associated heart and organ malformation. After prolonged civil litigation, the pharmaceutical company Gruenenthal, the producer of thalidomide, (sold under the name Contergan), was required to pay pensions to the children, to carry the cost of medical treatment, and to pay compensation.

When 20 years later the first HIV-infected hemophiliacs considered bringing legal claims against producers of coagulation factors, they learned that the legal situation with regard to blood and blood products differed in many respects from the thalidomide case. First, it was unclear whether blood and coagulation factor concentrates were considered pharmaceuticals or biological products, to which the law concerning pharmaceutical products would not apply. Second, it was extremely difficult to establish the clear causal relationship between the use of a specific blood product and HIV infection, required by German law. Most hemophiliacs had been treated with products from different producers, and each producer sought to demonstrate that the weight of evidence was insufficient to implicate its product. Finally, the HIV antibody test was not available until April 1985, so it was virtually impossible to determine the exact date of infection with HIV, if the infection occurred before that date. As a consequence, it was impossible to establish a clear relationship between the use of a given product on a given date and the transmission of infection.

Given these difficulties, it is not surprising that even well-informed individuals delayed bringing claims against producers of coagulation factor concentrates, or against physicians who had administered the products. But for the vast majority of hemophiliacs, who were poorly informed, the very idea that they had been placed at risk by their physicians and the clotting factor on which they were so dependent was late in coming.

Claims began to mount in 1985/86. In response, the pharmaceutical companies' insurers offered a settlement to infected hemophiliacs of 70,000 DEM (US$ 47,000) each; 30,000 DEM for the cost of medical and nursing care, 30,000 DEM (US$ 20,000) to compensate loss of income, and 10,000 DEM (US$ 7,000) for estimated funeral costs. Given the nature of such cases, the expenses associated with litigation (100,000 DEM US$ 67,000) at a minimum), the years involved before such cases are brought to a conclusion, and the fact that the majority of hemophiliacs believed that time was running out, many accepted the offer. In so doing, they relinquished all other claims for damages against pharmaceutical companies and gave up the opportunity to use the courts to compel the companies to acknowledge their legal responsibility.[49]

In 1986, a hemophilia patient who had rejected the offer of compensation sued two physicians working at Germany's largest hemophilia treatment center at Bonn University. The case makes clear the obstacles that confronted those who would seek to hold both institutions and individuals accountable for the infection of hemophiliacs. For more than two years it was impossible for the litigant to find a physician who would offer an expert opinion on his behalf in court. Potential experts were either personal friends of the most senior of the physicians against whom the suit was brought, or had cooperated closely with the Bonn center, or had filed applications for employment at the Bonn center. Even the Medical Council of Germany could not identify an appropriate witness.[50] As a result of these and other difficulties, no physicians have been prosecuted for treating patients with HIV-tainted blood products. In 1993, civil litigation was commenced against employees and civil servants from regional health authorities. It was unsuccessful because of the difficulty of amassing evidence demonstrating that they had reacted inappropriately to the risk of HIV infection through blood products.

In contrast to the legal difficulties regarding blood products, some cases involving transfusion-associated HIV infection have resulted in clear judgments. Nevertheless, such cases also encounter difficulties. One such case involved a regular blood donor who tested positive for HIV in 1985. A Hamburg hospital traced transfusion recipients who had been treated with blood from this donor in 1984, when a test had not yet been available. For a period of six months, a commission discussed whether these recipients should be contacted and offered HIV antibody testing. Ultimately it decided to do so. A female patient who received blood from this donor was found to be HIV-infected. She had transmitted HIV to her husband, who then sued the hospital for compensation. The case went to the Federal High Court of Justice where it was decided in 1986. The husband received 1,000 DEM (US$ 670) monthly as compensation for damage on the grounds that transmission of HIV might have been prevented if the hospital had excluded members of high-risk groups for AIDS from blood donation and had warned transfusion recipients after the infection in donors was discovered. In addition, the hospital was required to pay all costs related to the HIV infection.[51] On the other hand, the wife did not receive any compensation, because the possible risk of HIV infection through blood could not have been completely eliminated at the time when she had received the transfusion.[52]

Ten Years After: The German Parliament Investigates the HIV/Blood Scandal

Despite the years of litigation and a number of newspaper accounts of the infection of hemophiliacs and transfusion recipients, no formal investigation of what had occurred in Germany was undertaken until the scandal of October 1993, when UB

Plasma's failure to screen for HIV was made public. The scandal underscored the inadequacy of the prevailing regulatory regime. Although UB was under the regulatory authority of Rhineland-Pfalz region, the company's misconduct had been discovered by the Federal Health Office only because of a routine examination of positive HIV test results. Thus, it was simply by chance that the illegal activities of UB Plasma were uncovered. While the efforts of the Federal Health Office were repaid by its dissolution at the end of 1994,[53] its discovery led to the establishment by the German parliament of an investigation commission on HIV/AIDS, whole blood, and blood products. Such a commission had been demanded since February 1992 by the German Social Democratic Party, but it was only in the wake of the UB Plasma scandal that the political system was forced to respond. On October 24, 1993, the commission, composed of members of parliament, was asked to find answers to a broad spectrum of questions; these involved the extent to which the blood-borne infections had been the result of policy and regulatory failures and entailed the violation of German law. The commission was also to address the liability of federal agencies, pharmaceutical firms, and treating physicians. Finally, it was to examine the question of whether there was adequate financial and social support for individuals infected through blood and blood products as well as for their families.[54]

The almost 700-page final report of this commission was released in November 1994. It included a detailed official chronology of HIV and blood-related events and concluded that pharmaceutical companies, physicians, blood banks, hospitals, and the Federal Health Office—thus, the Federal Republic of Germany—shared responsibility for the HIV infection of many hemophiliacs, PPSB (prothrombin) recipients, and recipients of other blood and plasma products. Recommendations were broadly framed, bringing within their scope not only blood product safety and the issue of compensation of HIV-infected recipients, but matters bearing on pharmaceutical substances and medicinal products more generally.

Despite the apparent condemnation of the state and the blood establishment, the report was remarkable for how little it threatened the status quo. Indeed, the report could have had as its preamble an observation made seven years earlier by Professor Hans Rüdiger Vogel, executive director of the BPI, the federal association of the pharmaceutical industry. In 1987 he had, not surprisingly, underscored the importance of resolving the scandal of blood and AIDS in Germany in a way that did not threaten the interests of the blood industry.[55] This perspective informed the long-awaited commission report.

The commission generally voted for changes that could simplify the process of establishing proof or gathering evidence, but did not make recommendations that would have had a major impact on pharmaceutical companies. While endorsing the notion of compensation, the report provided nothing by way of a discussion of the central issue of the sums that would be considered adequate in the light of the claims of those infected with HIV. Nor did it propose new regulations regarding compensation and regulation for future blood-borne pathogens.

The weakness of the commission's findings was a function of its composition. The majority of commission members were drawn from the Christian-Democratic Party and its Bavarian sister-party, the Christian-Social Union, which, together with the Liberal Democrats, formed the ruling coalition. The commission clearly avoided voting on issues that would have exerted pressure on the governing parties. More critical proposals made by the Social-Democratic and Green representatives could not garner the necessary support.

Despite the weakness of the report, the Federal Ministry of Health moved to establish a foundation to compensate those infected through blood and blood products. Established in 1995, it was based on voluntary financial contributions from pharmaceutical companies, the Red Cross, the states, and the Federal Republic, which fought a prolonged battle over which parties would contribute, and at what level.[56] Bayer AG, Immuno GmbH, Baxter Deutschland GmbH, Behringwerke AG, Armour Pharma GmbH, and Alpha Therapeutic GmbH were to pay a total of 90.8 million DEM (US$ 54 million) over a four-year period, beginning in 1995. The Red Cross was to pay 9.2 million DEM (US$ 5.4 million), the federal government was to contribute 100 million (US$ 59 million), and the states were to provide 50 million DEM (US$ 29.5 million).[57] Persons infected with HIV through contaminated blood or blood products before January 1, 1988, were to receive a monthly payment of 1,500 DEM (US$ 2,500); those with AIDS a payment of 3,000 DEM (US$ 1,770).[58] Wives and children of HIV-infected hemophiliacs were also to receive 1,000 DEM (US$ 590) monthly for between five and 25 years.[59] Prior payment on the basis of the compensation scheme of the mid-1980s did not bar access to the foundation's funds. Those who accepted the foundation's funds were, however, required to waive all further claims against the donors.[60]

Those who sought to pinpoint responsibility for the infection of hemophiliacs and blood transfusion recipients were dissatisfied with the foundation. Established on the principles of humanitarian aid and solidarity, it sidestepped the issue of fault. The German Hemophilia Society objected to the fact that payments by the foundation were not considered compensation or reparation, but humanitarian support.[61] The society was also critical of the fact that those infected with HIV through blood or blood products after January 1, 1988, received no payment, and expressed concern that the funding of the foundation was inadequate.[62] The foundation was also the target of criticism by some members of the investigation commission who advocated a model similar to the Contergan foundation, which receives continuous support from industry, government, states, and physicians. But the lure of the proposed payments is clear. As of 1997, 1000 individuals had applied to the foundation for the promised aid.

Ultimately, the establishment of a flawed, possibly underfunded, foundation can be explained by the politics of an electoral moment. With a campaign under way for the Bundestag it was clearly advantageous to the Christian Democratic Party to capitalize on the appeal of a foundation based on humanitarian principles, one that could provide immediate assistance to the victims of the HIV/blood scandal.

Securing the Blood Supply in the Future

Improvement of Safety

The HIV infection of German hemophiliacs is a tragedy for which nobody has been found legally responsible. Physicians, pharmaceutical companies, and the health authorities all played a role in this tragedy, and all share responsibility for what occurred. But if in the past federal agencies failed to control the infectious risks of blood, blood products, and plasma-derived products, they now bear the burden of taking responsibility for the future safety of blood and blood products.

The history of HIV infection through blood and blood products, and especially the history of HIV infection among the hemophiliac population in Germany, suggests that it is critical to have *one* national agency with adequate authority and power to handle all issues related to the safety of blood and blood products. It is evident that non-cooperation and competition among agencies working on state and federal levels does not provide an optimum level of safety for recipients of blood and blood products. Since July 1, 1994, the Federal Paul-Ehrlich-Institute near Frankfurt has been responsible for the safety of blood and blood products. The Institute is responsible for the licensing of laboratory tests and vaccines, thus it seemed reasonable that it also handles blood and blood products, which pose similar problems.

In addition to federal institutions and state offices, a working group on blood and blood products has been established at the Robert Koch-Institute of the former *Bundesgesundheitsamt*. This working group first convened in September 1993 and has the mandate to provide expert advice to the federal and state governments, and their health offices. Members of the working group include federal and state experts, representatives from the pharmaceutical industry, blood banks, and external experts.[63]

As a result of the HIV/AIDS scandal, German self-sufficiency in blood and blood products has emerged as a central goal. Where the prevalence of pathogenic threats such as HIV is low, such self-sufficiency can preclude the importation of threats to the blood supply.

The history of HIV has shown that the emergence of new viral diseases is possible, and has demonstrated that safety demands great caution even before all relevant scientific data and evidence are at hand. It also underscores the importance of mandating newly developed screening tests — even at some cost — to detect old viral threats. Even before the HIV/AIDS affair was over, a new scandal appeared, demonstrating the consequence of the failure to move swiftly. Many hemophiliacs, transfusion recipients, and women in the former GDR who received anti–D antigen immunoprophylaxis with a serum product (who now seek government compensation[64]) were infected with hepatitis C because the available antibody test was not mandated in a timely fashion.

Additional Measures under Discussion

As laboratory medicine continues to develop, new tests and diagnostic techniques such as the polymerase chain reaction (PCR) or branched DNA (bDNA) become available. These tests raise new controversies, such as whether PCR testing of blood and blood products should be mandatory. There are several concerns: first, very few HIV infections—if any—would be detected with PCR that would not have been diagnosed with a conventional ELISA HIV antibody test. Therefore, the PCR method would not increase significantly the safety of blood and blood products. Second, the costs of PCR are high, and the price for blood products would rise considerably if PCR were introduced. Third, PCR can produce false-positive results, inaccurately suggesting the presence of HIV infection. Thus positive PCR results would require confirmatory tests. With a high number of false-positives and the necessity of discarding positive units, a severe shortage in blood could develop. Despite the potential costs, PCR remains under discussion, reflecting the legacy of concerns that emerged during the blood scandal.

Because a universal surrogate marker for clinically "silent" viral infections does not exist, what tests should be used to reach the highest level of safety, and at what cost? Those will be the central questions that federal health officials will have to confront in the wake of the AIDS disaster.

Finally, German physicians have come to recognize that because absolute safety of the blood supply is unattainable, concern for patient welfare dictates a reconsideration of the extent to which blood transfusions are relied on in clinical practice. The era of medical practice within which the indications for blood transfusion were overly broad has come to an end. A more conservative posture in this regard may be facilitated by the use of drugs such as erythropoietin, but at costs that are not insignificant.

Conclusions

The history of HIV/AIDS, blood, and blood products in Germany is complex. It has kept lawyers, courts, politicians, and those affected busy more than 10 years after most infections occurred. Now, however, the general public is inclined to forget the HIV/AIDS blood issue. On the surface, the scandal is over. But premature peace comes at a price.

As long as pharmaceutical companies place the safety of their products second to sales figures and market shares, and as long as government agencies and politicians are lax about product safety, another scandal can be foreseen. It could be caused by Hanta, Calices, or hepatitis C virus, or by an as-yet-unknown infectious agent. And in Germany, a new scandal does not necessarily require a new infectious agent. In 1996, for example, a German news magazine described how the pharmaceutical producer Alpha bribed physicians and sold factor IX concentrate that was not approved by the Paul-Ehrlich-Institute.[65] The article implied that corruption among hemophilia-treating physicians could result in the use of unsafe products. An "old" infectious agent—HIV—and a new scandal.

The HIV/AIDS blood scandal in Germany resulted in a compromise between regulatory agencies and pharmaceutical companies, and between pharmaceutical companies and those who were infected through their products. The scandal has been officially settled and "pacified,"[66] which was the declared aim of the Federal Minister for Health, Horst Seehofer. Sadly, although there have been some changes, they have not been fundamental. Within this context, it would not be unreasonable to anticipate that, as a consequence of compromise and inaction, economic interests will again overcome ethical concerns for patients—opening the way to another disaster for patients treated with blood- or plasma-derived products.

NOTES

1. The use of the word scandal follows the usage in German newspapers and journals, which labeled the affair a scandal. S. Dressler, Superseehofer. Moderne Zeiten im Gesundheitswesen. *Blätter für deutsche und internationale Politik.* 39. Jahrgang 1994, Nr. 1, 23–27. p. 24.

2. *Der Tod aus der Spritze,* quoted in Archiv fuer Sozialpolitik (ed.): Pressedokumentation HIV/AIDS und Blutspende/Blutprodukte in der BRD 1991–1992. Frankfurt 1993, p. 16, 17. Cf. also the introduction in E. Koch, Meichsner, 1, 1993, p. 9.

3. *"Skandal oder nur eine 'traurige Geschichte'?" Sueddeutsche Zeitung,* November 18, 1991, quoted in Archiv fuer Sozialpolitik (ed.): Pressedokumentation HIV/AIDS und Blutspende/Blutprodukte in der BRD 1991–1992. Frankfurt, 1993, p. 16, 17.

4. "Pneumocystis Pneumonia—Los Angeles." *Morbidity and Mortality Weekly Report,* 30 (1981), pp. 250–252.

5. G. Müller-Werthmann, *Konzern der Menschlichkeit: Die Geschäfte des Deutschen Roten Kreuzes,* (Hamburg: Hohenheim-Verlag, 1984).

6. G. Müller-Werthmann, p. 168. This figure illustrates the size of the Red Cross—operated blood banks in (West) Germany in the early years of HIV/AIDS. Precise figures on the number of blood products produced and/or distributed by Germany's Red Cross or, more important, on donations and donors in earlier years are not available, but it may be estimated that the number of donations was similar in 1980.

7. Müller-Werthmann, p. 172.

8. Cf. Rote Liste 1996, 48. Hämostyptika/Antihämorrhagika.

9. M. A. Koch, B. Schwartländer, W. Kirschner, "Blutspender als Sentinelpopulation

für sexuell übertragbare Krankheiten-Ergebnisse einer soziodemographischen Untersuchung und Befragung zum Sexualverhalten," *Gesundh-Wes*, 55 (1993), pp. 504–513.

10. Abschlussbericht, p. 146.

11. W. Schramm, and J. Schulte-Hillen, "Todesursachen und Aids-Erkrankungen Hämophiler in der Bundesrepublik Duetschland (Umfrageergebnisse Oktober 1994)," *25 Hämophilie-Symposium Hamburg 1994*, ed. I. Scharrer and W. Schramm (Berlin, Heidelberg, New York: Springer, 1996), pp. 7–17.

12. H. Egli and H. H. Brackmann, "Die Heimselbstbehandlung der Hämophilie. Erfahrungen bei 130 Patienten," *Deutsches Ärzteblatt*, 59P (1972), pp. 3143–3146.

13. K. Schimpf, "Should Clinical Freedom Be Constrained in the Name of Self-sufficiency? *Blood Coagulation and Fibrinolysis*, (1994) 5 Suppl. 4, pp. S47–49.

14. U. Braun, "Die HIV-Infektion durch Blutprodukte aus der Sicht der Deutschen Hämophiliegesellschaft," *HIV-Medizin: Möglichkeiten der individualisierten Therapie* ed. H. Jäger (Landsberg: Ecomed, 1994), pp. 417–419.

15. E. R. Koch and I. Meichsner, *Böses Blut. Die Geschichte eines Medizin-Skandals. Aktualisierte und erweiterte Neuausgabe*. Mit einem Vorwort von Horst Seehofer (Hamburg: Hoffmann und Campe, 1993).

16. *Ein Kartell des Schweigens*. Interview with Karl Caspari, an AIDS-infected hemophiliac, on responsibility of physicians and pharmaceutical companies. Source: Archiv fuer Sozialpolitik (ed.): Pressedokumentation HIV/AIDS und Blutspende/Blutprodukte in der BRD 1991–1992, Frankfurt, 1993, p. 30.

17. W. Kiehl and D. Altmann, "AIDS und HIV-Infektionen im Gebiet der ehemaligen DDR," *AIDS und HIV-Infektionen* ed. Hans Jäger (Landsberg: Ecomed. [Loose-leaf collection, supplement 6, 4] 1991), pp. 1–18.

18. Marcus 1993, p. 6. Cf. also Abschlussbericht, p. 35. Later, hemophilia organizations argued that they were not aware of the risk at this time, because physicians did not provide adequate information about the risk of HIV/AIDS transmission at that time. In 1983, the majority of hemophilia physicians had not yet informed their patients about the possible risk of AIDS through blood products or clotting factors.

19. Bundesgesundheitsamt, ed., *Klinik und Therapie der Haemophilie A und B. Indikation und Therapie mit Faktor VIII-und IX-Kozentraten* [Clinical course and treatment of hemophilia A and B. Indication and therapy with factor VIII and factor IX concentrates], Bundesgesundheitsblatt 28 (June 6, 1985).

20. W. Weise, Hepatitisübertragung durch therapeutische Substanzen menschlichen Ursprungs. Bundesgesundheitsblatt 22;6/7:1979. Weise W. Lessons from other Infectious Agents. *AIDS: The Safety of Blood and Blood Products* ed. J. C. Petricciani, I. D. Gust, P. A. Hoppe, H. W. Krifnen. Published on behalf of the World Health Organization by John Wiley & Sons: Chichester, New York, Brisbane, 1987, pp. 117–121.

21. With regard to other infectious agents, W. Weise, former director of the Robert Koch Institute, postulated as late as 1985, "Blood services and commercial companies should be obliged to declare the quality of the original material, the size of the pool, the source of the plasma, the geographical origin of the donors, and the number and quality of the screening tests used for prevention and the transmission of infectious diseases." W. Weise, 1987, p. 121.

22. Abschlussbericht, p. 44.

23. G. Landbeck, "Therapiebedingte Infektionen bei Hämophilen. Entwicklung und derzeitiger Stand der Erkenntnisse; Todesurachenstatistik 1978–1984." *2. Rundtischgespräch Therapiebedingte Infektionen und Immundefekte bei Hämophilen. 15. Hämophilie-Symposion*

Hamburg 1984, ed. G. Landbeck and R. Marx (Berlin, Heidelberg, New York: Springer 1986), pp. 7–14.

24. H. J. Weise and J. L'age-Stehr, "Schnellinformation: Unbekannter Krankheitserreger als Ursache von toedlich verlaufenden erworbenen Immudefekten? [Alert: Unknown agent as cause for fatal acquired immune defects?] *Bundesgesundheitsblatt*, 25 (December 12, 1982), p. 408.

25. O. Hamouda, L. Voss, A. Siedler, et al. AIDS/HIV 1995. Bericht zur epidemiologischen Situation in der Bundesrepublik Deutschland zum 31. 12. 1996. Berlin: Robert Koch-Institut; RKI-Hefte 13/1996.

26. Robert Koch-Institut Quartalsbericht I/97, table 5.

27. Robert Koch-Institut Quartalsbericht I/97, table 12.

28. Robert Koch-Institut Quartalsbericht I/97, table 13.

29. According to a survey at the 1995 Hamburg hemophilia meeting, 1366 hemophiliacs were infected with HIV. W. Schramm and J. Schulte-Hillen, "Todesursachen und AIDS-Erkrankungen Hamophiler in der Bundesrepublik Deutschland (Umfrageergebnisse Oktober 1995)," *Hämophilie-Symposium Hamburg 1995*. ed. I. Scharrer and W. Schramm. (Berlin, Heidelberg, New York: Springer) (in print). Quoted from Robert Koch-Institut Quartalsbericht III/96, p. 16, Cf. Hamouda et al. 1996, p. 17. These figures are lower than the estimate of 1857 infected hemophiliacs that is often used. The discrepancy may be accounted for by the fact that the lower figure is based on a survey of hemophiliac treatment centers. Not all hemophiliacs are treated in such settings.

30. Robert Koch-Institut Quartalsbericht I/96, table 13. (The report on the third quarter 1996 does not give the detailed figures on the time of infection.)

31. V. Erfle, R. Hehlmann, W. Mellert, et al., "Prevalence of Antibodies to HTLV-III in AIDS Risk Groups in West Germany," *Cancer Research*, 45 (9 Suppl.) (1985), pp. 4627s–4629s.

32. Landbeck, 1986, p. 9.

33. Landbeck, 1987, p. 1.

34. W. A. Flegel, K. Koerner, F. F. Wagner, et al., "Zehn Jahre HIV-Testung in den Blutspendediensten," *Deutsches Ärzteblatt*, 93 (1996), pp. A-816–821.

35. Examples of leaflets which were distributed to the blood donors are reprinted as document 77 and document 78. Abschlussbericht, p. 344–345.

36. Seehofer, Horst; Vorwort. In: Bundeszentrale für gesundheitliche Aufklärung (BZgA): Die Eigenblutspende. Köln: August 1994, p. 1.

37. Abschlussbericht, p. 132.

38. Abschlussbericht, p. 133.

39. Abschlussbericht, p. 133. The complete statement is published in the report as document 72 (Statement by the Federal Association of the Pharmaceutical Industry, November 14, 1983), pp. 330–332.

40. Abschlussbericht, p. 133.

41. Abschlussbericht, p. 135.

42. Cf. Abschlussbericht, p. 137, and Dokument 73 (Bescheid des BGA zur Abwehr von Arzneimittelrisiken-Blutgerinnungsfaktor VIII-haltige Humanarzneimittel vom 8, Juni 1984) p. 33, Marcus, 1993, p. 5.

43. "Dienstaufsichtsbeschwerde gegen den Praesidenten des BGA wegen des Verdachts auf ungesetzliche Amtsfuehrung durch gemeingefaehrliche und fachlich unqualifizierte Eingriffe in die gesundheitliche Versorgung der Bevoelkerung." (Disciplinary complaint

against the president of the Federal Health Office, based on the suspicion of illegal tenure of office due to dangerous and professionally unqualified intervention in the health care of the population) filed by the Red Cross leagues Nordrhein and Westfalen/Lippe on 26 June 1984. Cf. Abschlussbericht, p. 138; Koch, Meichsner, p. 85.

44. Cf. Abschlussbericht 2.4.2.4.5 Widerspruchsbescheide vom 12, Dezember 1984, p. 141.

45. Abschlussbericht p. 143. Cf. also Document 74 (Widerspruchsbescheid des BA zur Abwehr von Arzneimitteln — Blutgerinnungsfaktor VIII-haltige Humanarzneimitttel vom 12, Dezember 1984), pp. 338–342.

46. Weise, L'age-Stehr, 1982.

47. U. Marcus, "Die HIV-Epidemie bei deutschen Blutern — eine Chronologie," *AIDS Nachrichten aus Forschung und Wissenschaft*, 4 (1993), pp. 1–10.

48. A similar lag between the availability of a test and its mandatory introduction occurred with the hepatitis C antibody test, which was available in 1990 but not made mandatory until April 25, 1992.

49. M. Teichner, "AIDS, Ethik und Recht aus anwaltlicher Perspektive," *AIDS und Ethik*, ed. S. Dressler and K. M. Beier (Berlin: Edition Sigma 1994 [Ergebnisse sozialwissenschaftlicher AIDS-Forschung Band 13]), pp. 155–161.

50. Abschlussbericht, pp. 268, 206, 208.

51. Cf. *Der SPIEGEL*: Ahnungslose Ärzte. 4 March 1991; *Frankfurter Allgemeine Zeitung*: Krankenhausträger haften bei AIDS. 12 May 1991. In: Archiv für Sozialpolitik (ed.) *Pressedokumentation HIV/AIDS und Blutspende/Blutprodukte in der BRD 1992–1993*. Frankfurt, pp. 8–9.

52. Teichner, 1994, pp. 156–157.

53. Dressler, *op. cit.*

54. For the complete list of questions, cf. "1.2.1 Untersuchungsauftrag" in: Abschlussbericht, pp. 13–14.

55. Koch, Meichsner, 1993, p. 140.

56. Gesetz über die Humanitäre Hilfe. (HIVHG), 5.

57. HIVHG §2.

58. HIVHG § 16(1).

59. HIVHG § 16(2).

60. HIVHG § 20.

61. U. Braun, "Das Gesetz über die humanitäre Hilfe für durch Blutprodukte HIV-infizierte Personen (HIV-Hilfegesetz) aus Sicht der Deutschen Hämophiliegesellschaft," *AIDS. Management der Erkrankung*, ed. H. Jäger (Landsberg: Ecomed, 1996), pp. 370–372.

62. HIVHG § 14.

63. Mitteilungen des Arbeitskreises Blut des Bundesgesundheitsamtes. [Announcements by the working group blood from the Federal Health Office] Bundesgesundheitsblatt 36(12) (1993), p. 542.

64. "Hepatitis-C-Infizierte fordern Entschädigung von Bundesregierung," *Deutsches Ärzteblatt*, 93 (45) (November 8, 1996), C-2048.

65. M. Krischer, "Das alpha Komplott," *FOCUS*, 26/1996, (June 24, 1996), p. 20–30.

66. Horst Seehofer, Foreword in: Koch, Meichsner, 1993, p. 8.

7

Blood, Bureaucracy, and Law

Responding to HIV-Tainted Blood in Italy

Umberto Izzo

July 16, 1982, is a date that will long be remembered by the world's bleeding disorder community. The Centers for Disease Control (CDC) announced that three hemophiliacs treated with factor VIII had died as a result of *Pneumocystis carinii* pneumonia, which was linked to a new deadly disease called AIDS.[1]

One day earlier, the most prominent authorities of the Italian blood system met in Rome at the "first focus panel on the national blood plan." The director of the Italian Superior Health Institute (ISS) presented his proposal to solve the chronic shortage that had always affected the Italian blood system.[2] Only in passing did he note the failure of health authorities to effectively regulate blood plasma.[3] Tragically, his warning went unheeded.

In 1982, blood experts were concerned for good reason about the adequacy of the blood and plasma supply. In the early 1980s, the Italian supply of whole blood could meet only about two thirds of estimated demand. The shortage of plasma was, if anything, more striking: 95% was imported. In addition to the financial burden of reliance on imports, there was concern that factor VIII production might be subject to unanticipated shortages of raw material. No one predicted the danger of import dependency if a new viral threat appeared in the world's bloodstream. Aware of their inability to impose adequate controls on each batch of imported blood, experts put their faith in American regulations.[4]

In the crucial summer of 1982, Italy's blood system was structurally inadequate. It was governed by regulations codified 15 years earlier, before the advent of factor concentrate for hemophiliacs. Inspired by a tradition of bureaucratic centralism, these regulations ignored certain cultural and clinical features of the early history of the Italian blood system.

The Italian Blood System in Historical Perspective

In the first decades of the twentieth century, the few Italian hospitals that provided blood transfusions relied on lists of paid suppliers. The price of such blood was high; a single transfusion often cost the equivalent of several months' wages.

The first initiative to promote voluntary blood donation was prompted by the enthusiasm of a Milanese physician, Davide Formentano, who in 1927 organized a group of unpaid donors around his hematological practice. This undertaking led, two years later, to the official foundation of AVIS (Italian Voluntary Blood Association), the first association of its kind in Italy. The original goals of AVIS were to satisfy the growing need for blood by organizing a network of regular donors under ongoing medical supervision, to fight the commercial blood trade, to spread the idea of blood as a natural and anonymous gift, and to enhance scientific knowledge of transfusion practices. These principles have continued to inform the development of Italian voluntary blood donor organizations.

Supported by the pioneers of Italian transfusion medicine, AVIS quickly developed in the northern regions as a unique example of a civic and secular association in a society still deeply imbued by Catholic clericalism. Soon the spontaneous growth of voluntary blood donation was endangered by the regulatory plan with which the fascist regime sought to structure the public health administration. Mussolini himself unsuccessfully called upon Formentano to add the letter F (for fascist) to the acronym of the association.

The drama of the Second World War heightened the altruistic spirit of blood donation, despite the fact that fascist law recognized the role of professional donors who earned a living by selling blood. After the war, the new Italian government attempted to restructure the blood system. A monopoly over blood collection was granted to the Italian Red Cross, which was then the only nonprofit health organization officially recognized by the government. This was viewed as a threat by AVIS, and after a few years of political pressure the Red Cross's legal monopoly over the sector was abrogated. AVIS was recognized by the government as a nonprofit public institution devoted to the spread of the culture of voluntary blood donation.

For nearly twenty years, regulatory silence on blood-related matters prevailed. Nevertheless, this was also an era of important change. It witnessed the emergence of cooperation between donor associations and the first transfusion centers, which, by the end of the 1940s, were being organized by major hospitals.[5] AVIS, which today is still the leading Italian nonprofit organization for the voluntary collection of blood, structured itself territorially. A strong presence in the local community became the pattern that promoted a slow but steady diffusion of voluntary blood donation. Following the AVIS example, smaller organizations of blood donors started to operate, some with religious affiliation, others with the aim of serving the needs of large hospitals.

The absence of national policy explains the uneven development of the blood system. The entire health care system lacked central coordination; even the establishment of the Health Ministry in 1958 left the blood sector substantially unregulated.[6] In the north, towns like Turin could boast the existence of blood collection centers organized as replicas of American blood banks, but in the south the situation was far from satisfactory. Indeed, the "gift philosophy" toward blood has always been more accepted in the north than in the south, where notions of group loyalty did not foster the giving of blood by anonymous donors to anonymous recipients.[7] The persistence of a north/south divide on attitudes toward blood donation, reflecting more general regional differences, poses a major problem for Italian blood policy. In that context, a particularly vicious black market in *oro rosso* (red gold) flourished in the 1960s.[8] Even today, in the north blood is considered a community resource, whereas in the south it belongs to the family.

After years of unregulated development and change, the stage was set for a new regulatory regime. A strong call for the introduction of uniform standards and regulations was made by both physicians and representatives of the voluntary blood donor associations, a call that was consonant with the increasing institutional control that the Italian government was imposing on the National Health Service.

Blood and Bureaucracy

Following an intense and lengthy debate in the legislative arena, the "Collection, Preservation, and Distribution of Human Blood Act" came into force in 1967.[9] This law, and the set of ministerial decrees that supplemented its general provisions, regulated virtually every aspect of the Italian blood system for 23 years. At that moment, the "juice of life"[10] became a matter of state, justifying the Health Ministry's supervision of its collection, processing and distribution. Above all, this long-awaited state intervention marked the beginning of a never-ending stream of complex regulations.

Following a tradition of public administration that dates back to the fascist era, the blood system was hierarchically organized. Provincial blood boards were appointed by the Health Ministry as local agencies with the task of administering blood collection and distribution. The broad composition of these boards reflected the view that blood administration was a matter of public interest and, therefore, had to be democratically supervised by a wide range of representatives from "civil society." No wonder, then, that these provincial bodies were conceived as small parliaments, where, in addition to blood experts and delegates from the blood donor associations, there were representatives of the army and even of the local health workers' labor unions. The obvious result was administrative elephantitis, which greatly impaired the efficiency and decision making of these bodies.

The system, conceived according to the "rule of legal bureaucracy,"[11] could not discern local differences in attitudes toward blood donation. As a result, the act, which established identical local structures throughout the country, created a system incapable of balancing inter-regional differences in blood collection. To encourage blood donation, the act stipulated that employees giving their blood would receive one day of paid leave, for which the employers were reimbursed by the state.[12]

The Kafkaesque bureaucracy of the newly established system was characterized by a detailed set of second-level regulations. Legal provisions itemized the standard pieces of furniture for transfusion centers and stipulated that to obtain plasma for fractionation no more than 12 flacons of blood could be pooled. These technical regulations quickly became obsolete, revealing the rigidity of a system out of mesh with the dynamic process of scientific development.

In 1972, the system was further complicated when the state transferred a significant portion of its legislative and administrative functions to the regions, applying, at last, a constitutional provision that had existed since the adoption of the post-war Constitution of 1948. As a consequence, the health sector was gradually decentralized, and the newly established regional councils acquired an important role in the administration of the health care system. This transfer entailed a delicate period of transition during which the complex system of checks and counter-checks, typical of the Italian centralized ministerial bureaucracy, had to be coordinated with the new regional order.[13] By 1978, guidelines regulating blood transfusion, supply and manufacturing once again emphasized national standardization.[14] Not until 1990 was the system structured according to regional autonomy.[15]

The Unheeded Lesson: The Trilergan Case

It was against this backdrop that startling advances occurred in the treatment of hemophilia in the 1970s. The response of the Italian state to these developments and to the first signs of danger that they suggested revealed how unprepared Italy would be when the threat of HIV emerged a decade later. In 1974, a large number of users of Trilergan, an anti-allergenic drug, developed hepatitis B (estimates advanced by the press at the time indicated between 150 and 500 cases[16]). The complex relationship between Trilergan's local manufacturer and the international trade in blood products would, in retrospect, provide a microcosm of the problems associated with clotting factor for hemophiliacs. The drug was produced by Crinos, an Italian pharmaceutical company, and contained gamma-globulin provided by an Italian blood derivatives producer, the Istituto Sieroterapico Milanese Serafina Belfanti, which had, in turn, imported the immunoglobulins from the American company Armour Pharmaceutical.[17]

The Health Ministry, in charge of ordering the immediate seizure of the drug when the first cases were reported, responded slowly. Seizure was ordered eight months after the marketing of the drug. No accurate administrative inquiry was ever conducted to determine what had gone wrong in the institutional control system intended to preserve the safety of blood products. The Trilergan case rapidly disappeared from the press headlines. In the mid-1970s, the risk of viral contamination from blood products was considered an inevitable inconvenience. Hepatitis was deemed a serious but acceptable risk when compared to the great therapeutic potential of blood products derived from large donor pools.[18]

Several lawsuits brought against Crinos held legally accountable both the Italian pharmaceutical companies and the American supplier of the hepatitis-tainted gamma globulins. From a broader policy perspective, however, a timely analysis of the 1974 events would have taught Italian health authorities that existing controls prescribed for the safety of blood products — and especially imported raw blood — were mere formalities. The records of the legal proceedings revealed that the Italian importer had followed ministerial prescriptions then in force, but American gamma globulin proved to be infected, despite FDA certification. These findings should have produced a call for a careful review of the entire control system to ensure the safety of blood products. Future regulations should have been conceived in order to guarantee that each batch of blood derivatives was effectively tested. But nobody at the time realized the importance of modifying the central elements of blood product safety regulations.

Three years after the Trilergan mass contamination case, the Health Ministry finally drew its conclusions. Transfusion centers and the pharmaceutical industry were required to test each blood donation (regardless of its therapeutic use) for HBsAg by means of a third-generation method. These measures were issued by means of a mere *circolare*,[19] underlining the fact that public officials considered the safety of blood products a secondary concern.

These provisions, although late in coming, were appropriate for the challenge posed by hepatitis B, and their protective rationale might well have been relied on in the face of a new viral threat. But instead they were construed narrowly. The tragic events of the following decade would make clear the consequence of such shortsighted, inflexible policy making.

The Advent of HIV: Inaction in the Face of Awareness

The first cases of *Pneumocystis carinii* pneumonia and Kaposi's sarcoma in Italy were reported in 1982; in 1984 the first AIDS case was reported.[20] As Italian health officials became aware of the potential threat of AIDS to the blood supply, they failed to act. In May 1983, for example, a newsletter published by the Superior Health Institute included an article on AIDS that described the American reports of AIDS in hemophiliacs and focused on the link between the use of commercial factor concentrate made from large pools of donors and the new disease. The article clearly stressed that recipients of cryoprecipitate faced a lower risk of viral contamination because these blood products were obtained from small donor pools.[21] No recommendations or strategy for protecting hemophiliacs followed.

One month later, the Committee of Ministers of the Council of Europe, which included a representative of the Italian Ministry of Health, met in Strasbourg to adopt a common platform to prevent AIDS transmission from infected blood products. The warnings to the national health authorities of the member-states could not have been more explicit:

> wherever possible avoid the use of coagulation factor products prepared from large plasma pools: this is especially important for those countries where self-sufficiency in the production of such products has not yet been achieved.
>
> inform attending physicians and selected recipients, such as hemophiliacs, of the potential health hazards of hemotherapy and the possibilities of minimizing these risks.
>
> provide all blood donors with information on the Acquired Immune Deficiency Syndrome so that those in risk groups will refrain from donating.[22]

Although the text of the resolution was promptly translated and appeared in an Italian journal published for blood transfusion physicians, the Ministry of Health still failed to issue an official warning or set of policies to safeguard the blood supply.

Months later, when an expert panel submitted its proposal for a national blood plan to the Minister of Health, its findings, together with a warning about the risks of AIDS transmission through blood,[23] languished in the ministerial in-tray. Influential medical journals continued to recommend giving hemophiliacs "all the factor they need, on demand, for treatment of hemorrhages and elective surgery."[24] Even when, in 1984, the ministry issued a set of measures and recommendations to control the spread of AIDS among intravenous drug users and to protect health care workers from exposure to the blood of patients,[25] it remained silent on the blood supply itself.

It was in this context, but without much notice, that the first decree authorizing the marketing of a dry-heat-treated factor VIII concentrate produced by Immuno appeared in December 1984. Other companies received authorization in the next months.

Much effort would have been required to facilitate the distribution and consumption of safer, heat-treated concentrate to Italian hemophiliacs, given the institutional and economic factors that impeded the rapid uptake of the new factor preparations. Heat-treated factor concentrate, on average, is five times more expensive than untreated factor. Switching to the new product would entail a financial burden for hospitals and pharmacy administrators. Furthermore, they had every temptation to liquidate already purchased, untreated stock before using the more expensive preparations. Finally, it would have been necessary to recall stores of untreated factor kept in the refrigerators of hemophiliacs living far from health facilities.

When in March 1985 members of the Italian Hemophilia Foundation (IHF) received a therapeutic handbook edited by the Scientific Committee of the *Fondazione*, the message was mixed. The handbook expressed concern over the first dramatic findings in the United States. It stated, however, that the HIV retrovirus rarely developed into full-blown AIDS. The data sought to minimize fear:

> [O]nly one hemophiliac in 1,000/2,000 has full-blown AIDS in the USA and other European countries; on the other hand, cases among non-hemophiliacs in Italy amount to no more than 20/30, as compared with 200/300 in other European countries similar in size to Italy, like England, France and Germany. It would seem, then, that the Italian hemophiliac has greater defensive powers, and it is to be hoped that this tendency will be confirmed!

To the question, "[W]hat can the hemophiliac do to protect himself from AIDS?" the handbook answered:

> [The hemophiliac] may, or will soon be able to, screen his/her serum for [HIV] by means of commercial kits that will be available in a few months time and are already

available in some centers. It must be recognized, however, that it is still not clear whether the presence of antibodies, detected in about half of the hemophiliacs treated with more than 20,000 I.U. in our center, signals the actual presence of the virus in the blood, or whether it is, rather, a sign of a remote contact or, maybe protection. . . .

Finally, to the question, "[W]hat are 'treated concentrates'?" the pamphlet reported that the first results obtained using dry-heat or high-pressure methods to inactivate the AIDS retrovirus were encouraging.[26] It ended:

[O]n the basis of this data we can give a set of important messages to the Italian hemophiliac: AIDS has still not appeared in Italy; the risk of new concentrates is lower than old ones, or maybe even nil. Therefore, there is no reason to abandon, reduce or, at any rate, change the treatment programs and the concentrate dosages that have proved able to transform the hemophiliac condition from a state of dependence and permanent frustration to a condition of autonomy and free expression of individual capacity.

That spring the same message appeared in the IHF newsletter, this time with a firm reprimand against the "unjustified alarm" provoked in the hemophilia community by the inaccurate news about a hemophiliac AIDS case.

The Abbot test for HIV was approved by the FDA in March 1985, and the use of the kit was authorized by the Italian Health Ministry the following month. At the end of May, the IHF organized a press conference in Milan.[27] It announced the imminent wholesale availability of the ELISA test and urged hemophiliacs to use only dry-heat-treated factor. At the same time, Pier Mannucci, director of the Scientific Committee of IHF, reasserted that contamination among the Italian bleeding disorder community was small. Both warning and reassuring, the message invited hemophiliacs to undergo a closer follow-up of their antibody status and stated that to test positive did not mean that AIDS would develop. After 15 years of relentless improvements in the treatment of hemophilia, it was hard to yield an entrenched ameliorative posture.[28]

Finally, in mid-1985, after years of inaction, the Italian government took steps to secure the blood supply. On July 17, 1985, the Health Ministry issued a *circolare* introducing basic precautions against HIV contamination of blood and blood products. This ministerial communication provided for antibody testing of blood donors and recommended that the test be introduced quickly. It also recommended that groups at risk should not be permitted to donate blood, although it did not suggest the exclusion of individuals only suspected of belonging to high-risk groups. The *circolare* was sent to pharmaceutical companies, stressing the need to use pasteurization in the factor concentrate production. Significant as it was, the *circolare* never appeared in the legal bulletin and was not legally binding. Not until the promulgation of a law on April 29, 1987, did the safety measures become a clear legal obligation.[29]

Even when the Italian government acted, its patchwork of regulations revealed fragmented institutional decision making, stifled by bureaucracy. The use of treated factor concentrate, for instance, was recommended by the Ministry of Health in July 1985. Not until the next *circolare* of July 1986 did the ministry mandate that all plasma products be made from negative-testing single units of plasma, and that pool production be subjected to wet-heat treatment.[30] Not until May 1988 did the ministry order the withdrawal of stocks of factor concentrate that had not been subject to wet treatment.

Body Counts: The Epidemiological Impact of Contamination

Estimating the impact of HIV infection among those exposed to blood and blood products in Italy is difficult. First, the effort to estimate the rate of infection among hemophiliacs is complicated by uncertainty regarding the number of those afflicted with clotting disorders. In the 1970s, for example, when there was a need to draw political attention to hemophilia, advocates estimated that as many as 10,000 individuals suffered from the disease. A few years later, a more sober analysis reduced the estimated prevalence to 4000.

Not until 1988 did the ISS publish the first national report on HIV infection among those with hemophilia. These data were published in a report that sought to provide a message of reassurance by comparing the Italian rates of infection with those that prevailed in France and Germany (Table 7-1).[31]

The data were indeed striking. Although it became clear that Italy was not an exception to the international HIV/blood tragedy (637 HIV-positive hemophiliacs), its rate of contamination (22.8%) appeared far lower than the rates in France and Germany. In Germany, where patients were treated with the same American-plasma-derived concentrate as in Italy, this difference was explained by the higher doses of factor VIII used in the early 1980s, when most infections occurred (84,000 I.U./patient/yr. vs. 25,000 in Italy). For France, where the average use of concentrate had been slightly lower than in Italy (22,000 I.U./patient/yr.) the study suggested that reliance on French domestic plasma had contributed to the higher rates of infection.

More careful scrutiny casts doubt upon the assumptions that underlay this sanguine characterization of the Italian situation. German and French reports are restricted to individuals with hemophilia A and B, whereas the Italian data include 650 patients with von Willebrand's disease and 171 "other" bleeding disorders. By so inflating the denominator, the comparative rate of infection was misleading. A 1990 survey by the Istituto Superiore di Sanita of 2839 hemophiliacs provides a more accurate picture; 26.75% of those with hemophilia A, and 47% of those with hemophilia B, were found to be infected. Although reducing the discrepancy between Italy,

Table 7-1. Comparison of rates of infection among hemophiliacs in Italy, France, Germany[*]

	Total Number of Hemophiliacs Surveyed	Hemophilia A and B Combined		Hemophilia A		Hemophilia B	
		AIDS Cases	HIV Cases	AIDS Cases	HIV Cases	AIDS cases	HIV Cases
Germany	2,476	148 (6.0%)	1,172 (47.4%)	131 (6.1%)	1,024 (47.6%)	17 (5.2%)	148 (45.6%)
France	2,445	58 (2.4%)	1,038 (42.3%)	40 (1.9%)	903 (36.9%)	18 (4.6%)	136 (35.0%)
Italy	2,792	57 (2.0%)	637 (22.8%)	36 (2.2%)	476 (28.7%)	20 (6.4%)	138 (44.1%)

[*]Minor errors in tabulation appear in the table as originally published.

Germany, and France, these levels still suggested that Italy avoided the high level of infection that occurred in other industrialized nations.

A host of unresolved questions emerge from the data, none of which have been subject to official study. However the differences between national rates of infection are explained, the level of infection in Italy was clearly not the consequence of far-sighted measures taken by Italian health authorities in the years when the world's hemophiliacs were being exposed to HIV infection.

Data on the level of infection of blood transfusion recipients is even less satisfactory than that available for hemophiliacs. No systematic look-back program has been attempted to identify blood transfusion recipients with HIV infection. An unpublished 1993 analysis from the ISS suggested a figure of around 700.[32] Some have suggested a more accurate estimate would be twice that high. What is known is that as of 1996, 381 individuals with AIDS had acquired their infection through transfusion.[33]

Victims' Awareness: Perceiving an Iatrogenic Defeat

Until late 1985, Italian hemophiliacs were repeatedly assured that not only was their level of HIV infection relatively low, but that the presence of antibody to HIV might have little clinical significance. Italy was no different from other nations where scientific uncertainty rendered predictions about the fate of those who were antibody-positive difficult. Some suggested that as few as 10% would go on to develop AIDS.[34] What happened within the hemophiliac community when those who were infected began to appreciate the significance of their diagnosis?

In 1987, the hemophilia newsletter, EX, began to publish obituary notices. Anonymous letters would announce the deaths of hemophiliacs in local communities. In June 1987, a notice about the death of Frank Schnabel, the president of the World Federation of Hemophilia, ignited concern. Aware that they had been exposed to a fatal virus, hemophiliacs lost confidence in the scientific experts who had until then been viewed as bringing about radical improvements in their lives. Profound strain gripped the community that had emerged over the prior 15 years. Those infected experienced feelings of rage and desperation. Those spared infection sought to distance themselves from the community that was now synonymous with fear and death. Ultimately, even infected hemophiliacs rejected their membership in a "hemophiliac community."

As late as 1987, the IHF and its network of provincial and regional associations were united in representing what was taken to be the common interest of hemophiliacs. For instance, beginning in 1985, the IHF pressed regional health authorities to obtain separate hospital care for hemophiliacs with full-blown AIDS. Some regions, like Lombardy,[35] provided the necessary financial support on the assumption that those with hemophilia-related AIDS had unique needs.

News of the first claims for compensation brought by hemophiliacs in other countries began to circulate among Italian hemophiliacs in 1987.[36] The community was bewildered. Most of its members had never engaged in activism. They were kept informed by IHF bulletins, paid annual dues, and sometimes played a part in local associations. But the task of engaging politicians and public institutions[37] was the prerogative of the executive committee of the IHF. Protected by the legal rules of the *Fondazione*, the leadership had not changed since the IHF was established in 1969.

In this context, it became crucial to devise a strategy to support a claim for compensation. That strategy, according to the IHF leadership, had to be informed by the central importance of safeguarding the privacy of infected hemophiliacs, because the stigma associated with AIDS was their preeminent concern. In the absence of protections that were to come ultimately from the AIDS Act of 1990,[38] hemophiliacs feared the discrimination that would follow from being known as plaintiffs in a lawsuit. Accordingly, the IHF favored an accommodationist approach that would establish a dialogue with institutions and establish political contacts with those who might support the hemophiliac claim in parliament.

Angelo Magrini, president of the Piedmont Hemophiliacs Association based in Turin, was not convinced by the IHF's political line. For him it was time to act and, if necessary, to protest loudly. It was time to capture the individual rage of those who had been betrayed by blood. Not only hemophiliacs but blood transfusion recipients had to join hands in the struggle for compensation. Any means that would shed light on the tragedy and rally public opinion had to be employed.

This clash of strategies led, in the summer of 1988, to the founding of the *Associazione dei Politrasfusi Italiani* (Italian Multi-Transfused Association, the API). There was a strategic reason for setting up a common representational identity based on the drama of contamination, despite important differences that existed between hemophiliacs and transfusion recipients. Presenting a larger "social bill" would amplify bargaining power with politicians and institutions. By broadening the class of afflicted, it would be possible to attract the media, which were to be extensively utilized by the API. Above all, a united front could capture a key element in the lay person's perception of HIV-tainted blood contamination. Blood transfusion recipients, unlike hemophiliacs, were not (and could never have been) a class. Every individual, in the course of his/her life, might be confronted with the prospect of becoming a transfusion recipient: a woman after a cesarean birth, a teenager after a motorbike accident, any person undergoing a surgical operation. In the tragedy of HIV-contaminated blood, blood transfusion recipients were the "everyman." The universality of risk provided the basis for the rhetorical challenge, "It could happen to any of us." It was a rhetorical challenge that the API would use in its quest for compensation and the demand for improved blood safety.

The Compensation Claim in the Italian Political Arena

Approaching parliament has never been difficult in Italy. With more than 900 Italian deputies and senators, even small local pressure groups do not encounter much trouble in finding an available ear.[39] As comparative analyses report, the volume of statutes introduced each year by Italian legislators finds no equal in other Western democratic legislative bodies, with the notable exceptions of the U.S. Congress and the Swedish Riksdag.[40] This fertility, though, comes at a price: the quality of the proposed bills. The diminutive term *leggine* is commonly used in Italy to indicate the plethora of "proposals" resulting from its fragmented and narrow-gauged law-making. The great majority of *leggine* become mired in the parliamentary agenda and never become law.

The role of Italian political parties is critical in the legislative process.[41] Faced with thousands of private member bills, but wary of major programmatic legislation, the parliament is impenetrable without the mediation of political parties. Legislative success is further improved when a proposal is promoted by the executive.[42]

In this context, the IHF and API began to seek political contacts in the Roman corridors of *Montecitorio* and *Palazzo Madama*. The two groups followed different strategies. The IHF relied on its well-rooted tradition of advocacy for Italian hemophiliacs. To a certain extent, the "official" identity of the organization smoothed the way of the IHF toward law-makers. This was not the case for the API, which needed to build its representational role before members of parliament. The media helped facilitate the introduction of legislative proposals.

"*AIDS: Infected Because of the State's Negligence*," the first story of institutional failure supporting the hemophiliac's claim for compensation, appeared in early 1989 in *La Stampa*, a Turin newspaper with national circulation.[43] A few months later, a leading Italian news magazine, *Panorama*, published "*AIDS from the State*,"[44] which told the sad story of 11-year-old Rocco Mico, the Italian "Ricky Ray" who died of AIDS in 1987. That summer, *Panorama* fanned the flames of scandal by incorrectly reporting that 70% of Italian hemophiliacs were already contaminated.[45] Such press preceded by months the first initiatives introduced into the Italian Parliament on behalf of hemophiliacs.

A first legislative proposal was presented in the senate at the end of 1989 by proponents acting on behalf of the IHF.[46] The draft envisaged a no-fault compensation scheme to recover damages suffered only by hemophiliacs or other consumers of pharmaceutical products derived from blood. The Italian State was culpable for having delayed the enactment of the National Blood and Plasma Plan, asserted the proposal's preamble. If implemented in a timely fashion, as the IHF had demanded since the 1970s, the plan would have made national self-sufficiency possible, avoiding import dependency and HIV contamination of factor concentrate recipients. Instead, hemophiliacs received concentrate " . . . almost totally obtained from plasma of American mercenary donors." The preamble further noted that other European countries already compensated hemophiliacs, and that France was preparing to compensate.

The need for a no-fault compensation plan was based on a specific legal consideration. The injured parties had, as a class, been compelled to consume state-guaranteed, lifesaving medicines included in the National Drug List. Furthermore, hemophiliacs could not recover from pharmaceutical companies under the newly enacted Product Liability Act of 1988, for the statute barred action for products marketed before that date. As a result, a state-financed fund administered by an *ad hoc* agency was seen as the only equitable solution. The agency was to act as an insurer of first resort that could then seek recourse against those who had manufactured and distributed contaminated products. In this way, HIV-infected hemophiliacs would avoid the hardship of piecemeal litigation against pharmaceutical companies, which would necessitate the identification of the precise timing of infection and the concentrate brand responsible for transmitting the virus.

Damages were to be awarded according to standards applied by courts in personal injury claims. In case of death, awards could be made to the spouse, the parents, or the children of the injured. A time limitation of 90 days from filing of the administrative claim to the fund was prescribed for the examination of the record, with an additional 60 days for the payment of the awards. The legal architecture of the IHF bill was similar to that which was to be endorsed by the French compensation plan in 1991.

Totally different in its philosophy was the bill introduced in the House of Deputies on the API's behalf in February 1990. The preamble referred to the state as "unmindful," and "insensitive," and contained a vibrant indictment of Italian blood system regulations, which had been left unmodified for 20 years. The Italian Health Authority was also denounced for delaying heat treatment of factor concentrate and mandatory screening of plasma donations.

Armed with these facts, the bill advanced claims on behalf of an array of individuals exposed to HIV via body fluids: hemophiliacs, blood transfusion recipients, dialysis patients, and organ transplant recipients. The legislative aim was twofold: prevention for the future and compensation for the past. A national commission for the assistance and protection of multi-transfused subjects was proposed to establish measures to prevent the possible recurrence of viral contamination, as well as to grant compensation to those infected by HIV. Damages were to be awarded on a lump-sum basis: approximately $200,000 initially, a further $200,000 at the time of the claimant's death to the spouse, parents, or children. In July, 1990, proponents amended the API bill.[47] Reference to organ transplant recipients and dialysis patients disappeared, but the range of victims was extended to include those with hepatitis C infection.

The proposals put forth both by the Hemophilia Foundation and the API encountered an array of obstacles. First, each would have entailed heavy—although unspecified—financial burdens for the treasury. Second, despite a flourishing welfare tradition,[48] the issue of compensating victims of iatrogenic disease was completely new to the Italian political agenda. Third, while in other nations the proposals might have been viewed as the appropriate expression of pressure group politics, in Italy they generally were considered an unacceptable effort to use the legislative process for narrow "personal advantage."[49] Finally, the ideological neutrality of the bills—both the IHF and API proposals gained support from legislators on the left and the extreme right as well as from the parties of the governing coalition—also presented difficulties. Bills with such broad support lack the partisan support necessary to move legislation through the Italian system.

Stumbling into Legal Arguments: On How the Legal Process Can Ease a Political Struggle

On June 22, 1990, the Italian Constitutional Court issued a landmark decision with important implications for compensation of victims of HIV contamination. The court declared unconstitutional a 1966 Act mandating anti-polio vaccination, because it did not provide just compensation for those injured as a consequence of the inoculation.[50] The court ruled that individuals who suffered the consequences of risks inherent to vaccination had a claim on the state because of the burdens they had been forced to bear. The court asserted that such compensation was required by the Italian Constitution, which protects the health of each individual as a fundamental right. This was not a matter of tort, the court held, because the state, in this case, could not be deemed legally accountable for the breach of a duty of care. Furthermore, the deterrent function inherent in tort law was not relevant in a case where injury was the unavoidable consequence of mandatory therapeutic treatment. Rather, it was a matter of indemnification.[51] Damages were to be quantified as if they had been awarded in an ordinary personal injury claim, taking into account medical expenses, lost income, and pain and suffering. Then the award was to be equitably reduced to reflect the lack of negligence on the part of the state.

For the first time, the legal system imposed on the state the obligation to serve as the social insurer for a particular class of disabled people.[52] Although not formally binding on parliament, the court's ruling opened the way to lawsuits against the state filed by the many individuals with polio-related claims. Large damage awards resulting from the Constitutional Court ruling would have overwhelmed the state budget. Parliament was thus confronted with the need to develop a legislative solution.

With a remarkable sense of timing, three weeks after the Constitutional Court decision, a group of deputies presented a bill aimed at establishing a general compensation plan for all victims of diagnostic or therapeutic interventions, including hemophiliacs and blood transfusion recipients.[53] This proposal, drafted by expert jurists, was far more ambitious than those proposed by the Italian Hemophilia Foundation or the *Associazione dei Politrasfusi Italiani*. Strikingly, it had been drafted by jurists who sought to systematize the Constitutional Court ruling.

The core of the proposal was a concept of individual "biological wealth." The legal foundations of this concept, the bill's preamble explained, were to be found in the case law that followed a 1986 landmark decision of the Constitutional Court on the legal notion of "biological damage." It led to Italian law increasing damage awards in personal injury cases, assigning a *per se* value to individual health, apart from the loss of earning capacity. The jurists' proposal envisaged the establishment of a national scientific commission with the task of drawing up uniform criteria for the safety of therapeutic and diagnostic interventions and equipment, and the quality of drugs, blood and other human materials; an effective administrative decentralization of the blood system; the classification of blood as a product in order to apply the 1988 Product Liability Act to HIV-tainted blood related claims; and the establishment of a national fund under the Health Ministry's supervision, which was to act as an insurer of first resort for individuals who had been treated at a public health facility or had been administered a drug included on the National Drug List.

By 1990, the number of legislative proposals supporting the hemophiliacs' claims for compensation was probably greater than in any other industrialized nation. Nonetheless, there was only limited press coverage and the issue was not the focus of public attention. No national commission examined the causes and circumstances of contamination. Even the number of potential claimants was unknown. Still, the issue of compensation was added to the agenda of the Italian legislature. The scope of the claim to compensation expanded exponentially once it was before parliament. What started as a claim by hemophiliacs extended to those infected with HIV through blood transfusions. It was but a short step to include those infected with hepatitis C. Ultimately, there was a leap to compensation for all victims of therapeutic and diagnostic intervention. This expansion occurred without a conceptual resolution of why victims of iatrogenic disease or disability should be compensated.[54] Nor had the more "trivial" issue of how such a scheme would be financed been confronted.[55]

The Claim for Compensation in the "Maelstrom" of the Italian Law-Making Process

The story of the enactment of the Italian compensation plan provides insight into the dynamics, the "maelstrom," of the Italian legislative process. The government, in fact, ignored all the above noted legislative proposals. In so doing, it ignored the protests of both the IHF and the API until June 1991, the month when the International AIDS Conference was held in Italy, and thousands of AIDS specialists, activists, and the world's media converged on Florence.

It was not surprising that on June 16, 1991, four days before the opening of the conference, Health Minister Francesco De Lorenzo wrote a letter to the API president announcing that the drafting of a bill providing compensation was almost concluded.[56] Assuring his personal commitment, he pledged that the act would be promulgated. A public-private solidarity fund with a financial contribution from pharmaceutical companies of 0.025% of their total revenue from the sale of drugs included in the National Drug List was envisaged.[57]

Easy propaganda in view of international media coverage at the Florence meeting? Fear of noisy protests by hemophiliacs during the meeting? Maybe both. The draft promised in June 1991 by the Health Minister mysteriously changed when the act finally came into force in February 1992. We shall never know if pharmaceutical companies would have wished to contribute to the compensation plan promised by De Lorenzo, who in 1993 was jailed for corruption.

What the minister had solemnly promised to the hemophiliac community became, in its final version, nothing more than a badly amended variant of an old and preliminary 1986 draft to compensate victims of vaccination-related injuries.[58] It was buried in the ministerial archives until the Constitutional Court ruling of 1990 forced the issue of vaccine injury onto the legislative agenda. The result was a jumbled statutory text. Despite the fact that the legal, biostatistical, and economic foundations of no-fault plans differ according to the kind of personal injury being addressed and the context within which the injury occurs,[59] the new legal scheme merely grafted the issue of HIV-contaminated blood onto that of vaccine-related injuries.

Passed the day before the end of the 10th legislature of the Italian Republic,[60] the compensation bill was amended by each parliamentary chamber.[61] In February 1992, a crisis in the government coalition compelled the president to call for new elections. With hemophiliacs angered by endless delays, the approval of hybrid legislation was a compromise that avoided further delay until the next elections.[62]

The classes of injured parties entitled to compensation under the act share nothing other than a common listing in the statute. They include those injured by mandatory vaccinations who suffered permanent disabilities, as well as those who suffered from permanent disabilities resulting from contact with such injured individuals; recipients of HIV-tainted blood or blood products; post-transfusion hepatitis victims; health care workers infected by HIV as a result of workplace exposure; health care workers suffering from permanent injuries as a consequence of nonmandatory vaccinations designed to prevent workplace hazards; and those with permanent disabilities resulting from nonmandatory vaccinations for reasons of work or travel abroad.

The financial burden of this scheme is borne by the national treasury, but involves much less money than was demanded by hemophiliacs. A monthly life pension amounting to about $700 (equal to that paid to disabled ex-servicemen) is to be paid to claimants starting the month following filing of the claim. In the event claimants should die, a lump sum of approximately $35,000 is to be awarded to relatives, but only if they were financially dependent on the deceased.

A time limit of 10 years from the actual diagnosis of the HIV infection is established for filing a claim (reduced to three years in the case of infection from hepatitis), which does not preclude filing separate tort claims. For those already infected by the date of enactment of the act, there is a shorter, three-year time limit. The onus is on the claimant to furnish medical documentation to establish when, how, and from which transfusion event or concentrate administration the HIV contamination stemmed. Ironically for hemophiliacs, who have always been army-exempted, military medical commissions were appointed for evaluating the causal link between the use of factor concentrate and infection.

Politically, the act did not meet the blood victims' expectations: the financial relief offered was insufficient to cover the everyday needs of those with HIV. Not surprisingly, both the API and the IHF soon expressed their dissatisfaction. The lump-sum award set to compensate the death of victims of blood contamination was renamed by those representing hemophiliacs a "mite from the State."

After three years of protest by the API and the IHF, the Italian government amended the act, issuing in August 1995 a decree-law that raised the lump-sum payment to approximately $100,000.[63] The decree also introduced other positive amendments for the beneficiaries of the act. The lump sum was to be paid to the relatives of the deceased even if they were not financially dependent on the original claimant. The life pension and the lump sum in case of death were independently awarded to spouses infected through sexual intercourse with a contaminated partner, and to children contaminated during pregnancy or birth. Claimants who suffered from more than one disease (as in the case of dual contamination by HIV and HCV) were to receive supplementary awards. The administrative task of evaluating claims was given to civil health facilities instead of military medical commissions. These changes were made permanent in 1996 when new provisions became law.[64]

One last twist occurred in the tale regarding compensation, and once again it was driven by events surrounding vaccine injury. In April 1996, in a petition by a plaintiff injured by anti-polio vaccine in the 1960s, a claim was made for compensation from the moment of injury. The Italian Constitutional Court upheld the petition and declared unconstitutional the provision of the 1992 Act, which established the starting point of pensions as the moment when the injured party filed his/her claim. The court maintained that such a limitation conflicted with its 1990 ruling regarding polio and with the constitutionally protected right-to-health. Such retroactive payment, taking into account interest rates and adjusted for inflation, would increase the treasury's burden enormously. To date, a petition has not been filed by the HIV-infected beneficiaries of the 1992 Act. Should such an application be made, it appears that, on the basis of the equality clause of the Constitution, claimants could receive their pensions from the time when HIV infection supposedly occurred.

While national budgetary constraints due to integration of the European monetary system have caused the Italian Government to consider cutting welfare programs, legal process surrounding compensation has pressed in the opposite direction. Five years after its enactment, the 1992 compensation scheme has become a time bomb for the Italian treasury. In March 1997, the press reported the government's inability to find budgetary resources for paying claims brought under the 1992 Act.[65] Such fiscal constraints have, at least in part, informed the sorry tale of the act's implementation.

A pivotal justification for no-fault compensation plans is the assurance of quick relief to victims of misfortune, enabling them to by-pass uncertain litigation,[66] making available what would have been litigation-related transaction costs to beneficiaries.[67] It had been anticipated that the initial "meager" compensation of the 1992 Act would be counterbalanced by the efficient administrative handling of the claims filed, guaranteeing a prompt and effective response to those who could benefit from financial support.

At the end 1992, the Health Ministry had received 2045 claims, of which only 886 received *prima facie* examination.[68] No claimants had been called for medical examination by the commissions in charge of evaluating the causal validity of the claim. Although the act set a time limit for claimants, it did not impose a time limit on the Health Ministry for settling claims quickly, and claimants were legally defenseless given the unavailability of an administrative law-based cause of action for speeding the ministerial review. The no-fault plan management followed the fuzzy logic of the Italian bureaucracy: only in November 1993 did the Health Ministry create an *ad hoc* bureau, which in the maze of ministerial departments and subdepartments had exclusive responsibility for the administration of claims based on the act. By then, the number of claims had risen to 3412, and no claimants had yet received a *lire* from the state. The *ad hoc* bureau demonstrated a singular incapacity to act expeditiously. In May 1995, 2511 claims had been dealt with, and a number of heirs had received financial relief (604 claimants had died by that time). At the same time, the number of claims received by the *ad hoc* bureau had risen to 20,140. By April 1, 1996, 26,978 claims had been made, with 3408 pensions and 514 lump-sum payments awarded, for an expenditure of 171,966,164,290 lire (approximately $110 million) by the treasury. Such delayed payments were, of course, one way of confronting the dire implications of meeting the obligations of the compensation scheme.

Meanwhile, for the many waiting claimants, the only option available for securing their rights is to file a claim before the European Court of Human Rights. Perhaps it will be the Strasbourg judges who will hold the Italian government accountable for denying justice on the basis of Article 6 of the European Convention, which prohibits unreasonable delay of legal proceedings. It is in France that the final chapter of the never-ending saga of the Italian compensation plan may be written.[69]

Turning to the Courts: Tainted-Blood Litigation

The quest for a public compensation scheme represented but one aspect of the struggle of those infected with HIV through the blood supply. A second dimension of that struggle involved litigation. In 1989, the IHF, before potential claims were extinguished by the statute of limitations, with the support of the Italian Lawyers Association for Human Rights Protection, urged HIV-contaminated hemophiliacs to address a letter to the health minister and to pharmaceutical companies claiming damages and reserving the right to sue. By then it was clear that hemophiliac contamination was a case of mass tort in which the legal and factual elements of each claim could be deemed common to the entire class of potential plaintiffs.

Painfully aware that the Italian legal system does not provide for a procedural instrument comparable to the American class action system, lawyers close to the hemophiliacs' organizations sought to devise a common litigation strategy for the class. But such an effort confronted a number of obstacles. First, it would have been extremely difficult, if not impossible, to gather information from hundreds of potential plaintiffs spread throughout the country, and to counsel them to sue those responsible for their contamination before a single tribunal. Second, in the face of the many personal dramas that had taken shape in the aftermath of infection with HIV, there was a singular common fear: being forced to identify oneself publicly in court as an HIV-infected hemophiliac. Despite these obstacles, it might still have been possible to open discussions with potential plaintiffs about ways to limit the personal costs that could be incurred during protracted litigation against powerful defendants. But this course was not so readily available. The "loser pays all" rule usually applies in Italy, and rules of professional conduct prohibit the use of contingency fees. Lawyers are also prohibited from recruiting clients. A letter or a telephone call through which a lawyer attempts to reach potential clients, informing them of the possibility of suing, would be considered advertising and contrary to bar regulations.

These considerations help to explain why there are so few lawsuits pending before the Italian courts as a consequence of HIV contamination. Nevertheless, two antagonistic organizations—API and IHF—have fashioned litigation on behalf of their hemophiliac clients.

The API supported two lawsuits filed in 1990 before the Genoa Tribunal. In January, API announced it had filed against Italy's Sclavo and Austria's Immuno Corporation. The complaints were also brought against the Health and the Internal Affairs ministries. Plaintiffs in both cases were parents of hemophiliac children who had died of AIDS. In *Rocco*,[70] one of the two cases, it is alleged that Sclavo was liable for marketing AFC without warning consumers about the viral risk entailed. The government authorities are accused of not having appropriately regulated the product before issuing authorization for sale and for not having carried out effective control and verification measures on the risk of contamination in the postmarketing period. At the heart of this case are two questions: Should the production, importation, and distribution of drugs be considered a dangerous activity, thus shifting the burden of proof, in Italian law, to the defendants? Second, had Sclavo taken all due precautions to prevent the transmission of HIV infection?[71]

The legal principles that should guide the court in this matter were established in the litigation surrounding hepatitis B contamination in the 1970s—the landmark *Trilergan* case. In 1987 the *Corte di Cassazione* issued the final word on the central legal issues of that case: all activities subject to regulation for the purpose of protecting public safety and having an intrinsic potential dangerousness are subject to the standard of strict liability prescribed by the Civil Code. In addition, the court held that defendant companies in *Trilergan* were obligated to undertake all measures that might have reduced the risk of contamination, even when such measures were not mandated by the state and when such measures were viewed within the scientific community as providing only a *possible* means of reducing hazard.[72]

The Italian Hemophilia Foundation's lawsuit before the Rome tribunal has focused solely on the liability of the state, claiming that it failed for 20 years to establish an efficient blood and plasma collection system. It was that failure that set the stage for the mass infection of hemophiliacs when the state compounded its error by failing to impose regulations to prevent the spread of HIV through blood products. The IHF suit, despite the *Trilergan* precedent, did not seek recovery from the producers of factor concentrate.

This legal action, involving 340 plaintiffs and years of preparation, may represent the largest single lawsuit brought before an Italian court. Plaintiffs have asked the court to do what has never been done in Italy—to hold the state accountable for its failure to act or legislate.[73] To make their case, plaintiffs have asserted that by enacting the compensation plan of 1992 the state implicitly acknowledged its responsibility for infecting hemophiliacs. Whatever its outcome, this case represents a powerful political statement regarding the failure of the state at a moment when those with bleeding disorders might have been protected against a life-threatening infection. Given the political force of the case, it is noteworthy that the IHF-sponsored case did not seek to hold accountable those responsible for the production of AFC—the pharmaceutical companies.

Despite the particular and urgent nature of these claims, both the Genoa and Rome actions were, as of late 1998, still pending. Considering the controversial issues at stake, this is not surprising. In Italy, an ordinary tort lawsuit requiring expert witness testimony may take 4 to 8 years to come to a decision.[74]

The Blood System Reform of 1990

In addition to the issue of compensation, the tragedy of HIV-tainted blood contamination forced the Italian parliament to end more than a decade of fruitless legislative debates and bring about a radical reform of the national blood system. The system's inability to ensure the nation an adequate supply of blood and plasma exposed Italy to an international iatrogenic catastrophe. In May 1990 the Italian blood system received its long-awaited general reform.[75] As a consequence, all transfusion facilities and blood product production centers are under the control of the National Health System. Blood collection was henceforth to be based solely on periodic voluntary blood donations, and the general principle that blood donation and distribution should be completely non-remunerative was affirmed. Selling the *oro rosso* became a crime in Italy, and specific criminal punishments were established to deter violations of the new act's provisions. Blood and its components were not to be considered a source of profit and were declared tax-exempt. The cost of blood collection, fractionation, preservation, and distribution were to be charged to the National Health Fund budget. In rejecting the market, planning and institutional coordination became central to the new system. This is especially true with regard to the reform's complex scheme of management for the collection and manufacture of blood and blood products.

The new system has had an impact on the adequacy of the blood supply. In 1995, AVIS alone provided 1,415,288 units of whole blood, out of a total national need estimated at 2,400,000 units. At long last Italy has almost achieved self-sufficiency in blood, although occasionally deficits still occur in the south. The gap between north and south may yet be overcome if the system manages to achieve a higher level of coordination.

With regard to plasma self-sufficiency, the regulations of 1990 have not produced the desired results. The national supply of plasma has more than doubled since the 1990 Act, but is still far from achieving the total autarchy sought by reformers. In 1992, Italy produced 180,000 liters of plasma to meet a national need of 1,200,000 liters. By 1996, the figure had risen to 400,000 liters. The machinery for producing Italian AFC has encountered significant obstacles, largely due to the bureaucratic logic imposed by the reform.[76] There is no financial incentive for the north-south transfer of surplus plasma.

Finally, reforms in the blood system have sought to create new policy-making procedures to enhance the capacity of the Ministry of Health to promulgate safety regulations and standards in response to emerging threats to blood safety. The centralization of power in the Ministry of Health represents an attempt to overcome the paralysis that gripped the previous system.[77]

New rules for blood safety still rely on ministerial authorization, but at least for UE-member countries, their own national authorization is considered equivalent to Italian certification.

In addition, a new transfusion practice standard has been specified by ministerial decree. Close attention is paid to donor selection. Informed consent has been introduced to heighten the donors' sense of responsibility and to ensure a more successful medical interview prior to donation.[78] The preventive testing of donors for syphilis, HBaAG, HIV, HCV and HIV2 is now mandatory.[79]

Have these administrative and technical changes had an impact on the safety of the blood supply? A 1997 study calculated the likelihood of infection by a whole-blood unit testing negative for HIV, HCV, and HBV as 1 in 245,000, 1 in 8,000, and 1 in 63,000.[80] These changes, largely the product of technical innovations, have brought the risk of transfusion-associated AIDS to an end. Only the future will tell whether the new system has sufficient flexibility to respond to the first signs that a new pathogen threatens the blood supply.

Conclusion

The Italian conflict over HIV-tainted blood demonstrates how the response to a global tragedy can be shaped by a society's political values and legal traditions. From this perspective we can begin to understand the contradictions revealed by the Italian response to the tragedy of an HIV-infected blood supply. Although the rate of HIV infection among Italian hemophiliacs is lower than in any of the other nations discussed in this volume, only Italy has elected to provide government compensation to victims of hepatitis C–tainted blood in addition to those infected by HIV. The roots of that decision, the extent to which bureacratic delays affected the interests of claimants, and the source of funds for those who were to be payed all reflect the specificity of Italian political culture.

What ultimately drove the Italian response to the claims of those infected with HIV was the legal process surrounding the indemnification of the victims of polio vaccination–related injury. Parliament acted in the absence of any careful, official study of the dimensions of the iatrogenic disaster surrounding HIV, and thus it passed legislation without due consideration of the legal and financial implications of its decision.

What followed marked the Italian experience as unique. The experience of other nations will be remembered for the heat of the social conflicts, the breadth of the political scandal, the severity of the criminal charges brought against political officials, and the drama of apologies by ministers in the wake of the HIV disaster. Italy will stand out because the state bureaucracy took years to disburse the promised compensation, adding insult to injury for dying beneficiaries.

With more than 30,000 administrative claims brought under the compensation scheme and the cost of each filing escalating because of amendments to the law, the Italian treasury alone now confronts the burden of skyrocketing compensation expenses. Unlike other industrial nations with long-established welfare traditions, where the state sought to spread the cost of compensation to other actors, such as insurance funds or pharmaceutical firms, Italy turned to the budget. In so doing, it repeated a pattern of resolving social conflicts by recourse to the deep pockets of the state.

NOTES

Many people helped me write this chapter. I cannot mention all of them here. I would like to thank Ronald Bayer, Eric Feldman, and all the friends in blood. Thank you for the encouragement and all the precious teachings. A special thanks is for Ugo Mattei, Roberto Pardolesi, and Roberto Caso, without whom I would not be writing this acknowledgment.

1. Centers for Disease Control and Prevention (CDC), "Pneumocystis Carinii Pneumonia among Persons with Hemophilia A," *Morbidity and Mortality Weekly Report*, 31 (1982), p. 365.

2. F. Pocchiari, "Il Problema Sangue: Proposta di Soluzione," paper delivered at the "Giornata di Studio sul Piano Nazionale Sangue, Rome," July 15, 1982, *La Trasfusione di Sangue*, 4 (1983), p. 274.

3. Pocchiari, *ibid.*, 283.

4. P. Mannucci, "Availability of Plasma Fractions for Therapeutic Use in Italy" — Proceedings of the International Conference on Plasmapheresis 82, Milan, 27–28 May 1982, *La Ricerca in Clinica e Laboratorio*, 13 (1983), p. 1.

5. G. Reali, "La Storia della Medicina Trasfusionale," *La Trasfusione di Sangue*, 2 (1995), p. 72.

6. Law, March 13, 1958, n. 296.

7. G. Clerico, "Raccolta e Allocazione di Sangue: Donazione, Mercato ed Intervento Pubblico," *Rassegna Giuridica della Sanità*, IV, (1994), p. 140.

8. "(S)ometimes blood black-marketeers loiter at the entrance to the transfusion center, waiting to contact the patient's relatives. After negotiating a price they present themselves as friends of the patient. For us it is not easy to determine whether they are engaged in illegal transactions . . . ," see N. Scarano, "Il Dramma della Raccolta di Sangue" [The Blood Collection Drama], *Nel Mese*, 2 (1966), p. 11.

9. Law, July 14, 1967, n. 592.

10. P. Camporesi, *Il Sugo della Vita: Simbolismo e Magia del Sangue* (Milan: Edizioni di Comunità, 1984), reissued as *The Juice of Life* (New York: Continuum Publications, 1995).

11. This formula summarizes what Joseph LaPalombara has perfectly explained to non-Italians: ". . . Italy is a lawyer's paradise, and not just because Italians admire forensic skills. A prevailing lawyer's mentality dictates that all possible contingencies regarding public policies must be anticipated and codified. This means that people are forever in search of what nuance "The Law" will or will not permit . . . one has the impression that without the *Gazzetta Ufficiale*, which publishes weekly updates of the country's many legal codes, the country, or at least most of its institutions and transactions, would simply fall apart." J. LaPalombara, *Democracy Italian Style* (New Haven and London: Yale University Press, 1987), p. 209.

12. Law, July 13, 1967, n. 584.

13. S. Cassese, "The Higher Civil Service in Italy," in *Bureaucrats & Policy Making: A Comparative Overview*, E. Suleiman (ed.) (New York and London: Holmes & Meier, 1984), p. 66.

14. Law, December 23, 1978, n. 833.

15. On the uneven capacities of administration displayed by regions under the regionalism plan implemented in Italy in the early 1970s, see F. Spotts, T. Wieser, *Italy: A Difficult Democracy* (Cambridge: Cambridge University Press, 1986, 26) and the analytical study of R. Putnam, R. Leonardi, R. Nanetti, *La Pianta e le Radici: Il Radicamento dell Instituto Regionale nel Sistema Politico Italiana* (Bologna: El Mulino, 1985).

16. P. Guzzetti, "E il controllo? Dopo" [Controls when? Afterwards] *Panorama* (October 16, 1975).

17. For a medical discussion of the Trilergan case, see F. Petrilli et al., "Hepatitis B in Subjects Treated with a Drug Containing Immunoglobulins," *Journal of Infectious Diseases*, 2 (1977), p. 95.

18. See, for instance, P. Mannucci et al., "Asymptomatic Liver Disease in Hemophiliacs," *Journal of Clinical Pathology*, 28 (1975), p. 620.

19. Health Ministry *Circolare*, 24 July 1978, n. 68. It is important to note that a *circolare* is conceived to be an internal communication between superior and inferior administrative bodies. If it contains an order, this applies only to the administrative office to which it is directed, and not—as in the case of a law—to whoever is in a position to abide by the rule. As an administrative act, a *circolare* is not required to be published in the Italian Official Bulletin. With respect to rule-making, this suggests that a *circolare* cannot ensure uniform and prompt implementation of mandatory measures, especially when they are directed at health facilities spread out across the country and embedded in a highly hierarchical administrative system.

20. G. Rezza, "Epidemiologia dell'AIDS in Italia," F. Dianzani, G. Ippolito, M. Moroni eds., *Il Libro Italiano dell'AIDS* (Milan McGraw-Hill Libri Italia, 1994), p. 3.

21. ISIS, *Medicina nel Mondo 19/83*, n. 19, May 14, 1983, pp. 11–12.

22. June 23, 1983: Ministries Committee of the European Council Recommendation n. R (83) 8. This document made reference to two previous recommendations issued by the same international body: the R (80) 5 (recommending the implementation of plasmapheresis obtained from voluntary blood donations; stressing the risk of viral infections from pools composed of plasma from different regions; recommending that member states should create national registers of coagulopathic subjects) and the R (81) 14 (dealing with the general prevention of infectious diseases transmitted by the trade in blood and blood products among countries; urging member-states to consider the epidemiological situation of the country of origin when importing blood and blood products).

23. See *Proposta di Piano Sangue Quinquennale*, Ministero della Sanità—Centro Studi, December 1983.

24. P. Mannucci et al., "Abnormalities of Lymphocyte Subset Are Correlated with Concentrate Consumption in Asymptomatic Italian Hemophiliacs Treated with Concentrates Made from American Plasma," *American Journal of Hematology*, 17 (1984), p. 167.

25. Health Ministry Circolare of June 25, 1984, n. 48, and of August 25, 1984, n. 65.

26. P. Mannucci, L. Montagner et al., "Absence of Antibodies to AIDS Virus in Hemophiliacs Treated with Heat-treated Factor VIII Concentrate," *Lancet* (February 2, 1985).

27. The conference echoed in the headlines of the time: "Contro l'AIDS Arriva 'Elisa' un Nuovo Test per le Trasfusioni" [To Fight AIDS Elisa Arrives, a New Transfusion Test], *La Repubblica*, May 31, 1985; "Milano Decide: Test per I Donatori" [Milan Decides: Test for Donors], *Il Secolo XIX*, May 31, 1985; "AIDS, Ricercatori Milanesi: 'Immotivato il Panico'" [AIDS, Milanese Researchers: "Unmotivated Panic"], *Il Manifesto*, May 31, 1985;

"Nuovi Controlli nelle Trasfusioni per Limitare I Rischi" [New Controls on Transfusions to Limit the Risks], *Il Corriere della Sera* June 11, 1985.

28. This stance may be understood in terms of Rene P. Fox's "scientific magic," that is: "[that attitude which] helps physicians to face problems of uncertainty, therapeutic limitation and meaning by ritualizing optimism . . .," "The Human Condition of Health Professionals," R. Fox (ed.) *Essays in Medical Sociology: Journeys into the Field* (New Brunswick, NJ: Transaction Publishers, 1988), p. 581.

29. See Law Decree, April 29, 1987, n. 166, November 7, 1997.

30. Health Ministry *circolare*, July 16, 1986, n. 47, November 7, 1997.

31. A. Gringeri, P. Mannucci et al., "National Survey of Human Immunodeficiency Virus Infection in Italian Hemophiliacs: 1983–1987," *La Ricerca in Clinica e Laboratorio,* 18 (1988), pp. 275–280.

32. Letter of July 29, 1993, by N. Schianaia from ISS (source: Italian Multi-transfused Association).

33. ISS, *Aggiornamento dei casi di AIDS notificati in Italia al 30 settembre 1996,* Rome, 9:12 (1996).

34. This prediction was made in a hemophiliac newsletter, see *Ex,* 12:8, August 1985.

35. "Second Regional Plan for the Fight Against Aids," *Bulletin of the Lombardy Region* (June 1, 1988).

36. See, *Ex,* 14:7, July 1987, 6, reporting the news that British hemophiliacs were being invited to sue pharmaceutical companies responsible for distribution of tainted-AHF.

37. D. Kirp, "The Politics of Blood: Hemophilia Activism in the AIDS Crisis," in E. Feldman and R. Bayer (eds.) *Blood Feuds: AIDS, Blood, and the Politics of Medical Disaster* (New York: Oxford University Press, 1999).

38. Law 5 June 1990, n. 135. Among a set of measures for the prevention and the fight against AIDS, the Act provided anti-discriminatory rules for individuals testing HIV-positive and introduced a specific prohibition against the public disclosure of data concerning the seropositive condition.

39. For this prerogative of Italian democracy, see G. Pridham, "Parliamentarians and Their Constituents in Italy's Party Democracy," in V. Bogdanor (ed.), *Representatives of the People?: Parliamentarians and Constituents in Western Democracies,* (Aldershot, UK; Gower, 1985), p. 158; Barnes, *Representation in Italy: Institutional Traditions and Electoral Choice,* (Chicago: University of Chicago Press, 1977), p. 12.

40. The International Centre for Parliamentary Documentation of the Inter-Parliamentary Union, *Parliaments of the World: A Comparative Reference Compendium* (Aldershot, UK: Gower, 1986), p. 909.

41. In these terms, S. Tarrow, "Italy: Crisis or Transition?" *Italy in Transition: Conflict and Consensus* ed. Lange, Tarrow (London: Cass Pub. 1980), p. 178.

42. On the supremacy of executive-promoted legislation in European democracies, see E. Page, *Burocrazia, Amministrazione, Politica: un'Analisi Comparata* (Bologna: Il Mulino, 1990), p. 89 [*Political Authority and Bureaucratic Power: A Comparative Analysis* (Knoxville, TN: University of Tennessee Press, 1985)]

43. "AIDS, Malati per Colpa dello Stato", LA STAMPA (February 15, 1989).

44. G. Milano, "AIDS di Stato" in PANORAMA, (April 2, 1989).

45. G. Milano, "Solo Sangue DOC" [Only controlled denomination origin blood], *Panorama* (June 18, 1989).

46. Bill proposal n. 2019, December 19, 1989, Senators Corleone and others.

47. Bill proposal n. 4928, July 3, 1990, Deputies Caria and others.

48. LaPalombara, *op cit.*, p. 54.

49. R. Putnam, *The Belief of Politicians: Ideology, Conflict and Democracy in Britain and Italy* (New Haven-London: Yale University Press, 1973), p. 228.

50. Corte Costituzionale, June 22, 1990, n. 307, *Foro. Italiano* 1, (1990), p. 2694.

51. Conceptually the court ruled as if the injured was subject to a taking for public utility. As Stephen Munzer would put it: ". . . [S]ome may find bizarre that anyone would even imagine that such laws take private property. But if persons have property rights in their bodies, then government action adversely affecting these rights might be a taking. If there were a taking, then the government might have to pay compensation or even abandon its action . . . ," "Compensation and Government Taking of Private Property," *Compensatory Justice: NOMOS XXXIII*, ed. L. Chapman (New York, New York University Press, 1991), pp. 195–198.

52. See G. Ponzanelli, "Lesione da Vaccino Antipolio: che lo Stato Paghi l'Indennizzo!" Il *Foro Italiano*, I, (1990) 2697.

53. Bill proposal, n. 4964, July 12, 1990, Deputies Bernasconi, Rodotà, Violante, and others.

54. As J. Stapleton notes (in *Disease and the Compensation Debate* (New York: Oxford University Press, 1986) "(U)ntil there is a re-evaluation of such fundamental issues as why, if at all, the disabled should be treated preferentially over victims of other misfortunes, there will not be much gained from formulating detailed designs for schemes and benefits. The daunting lesson to be learned from a disease focus is that the 'compensation' debate is fundamentally and disturbingly more complex than we have generally assumed." p. 183.

55. See A. Klein, "A Legislative Alternative to 'No Cause' Liability in Blood Product Litigation," *Yale Journal on Regulation* 12 (1995) 107, 115.

56. Published in the API bulletin, *Emonews* (September 1991), p. 3.

57. Financing, at least in part, of a loss-based compensation system with premiums paid by potential injurers is considered an efficient solution in EAL terms: see K. S. Abraham and L. Liebman, "Private Insurance, Social Insurance, and Tort Reform: Toward a New Vision of Compensation for Illness and Injury," *Columbia Law Review*, 93 (1993), pp. 75–91.

58. Draft bill n. 3730 presented to the House of Deputies and to the Senate on May 7, 1986.

59. See S. McLean (ed.), *Compensation for Damage. An International Perspective* (Dartmouth: Aldershot—Brookfield, 1993).

60. Law, February 28, 1992, n. 210.

61. See P. Farber and D. Frickey, *Law and the Public Choice. A Critical Introduction* (Chicago-London: University of Chicago Press, 1991), p. 153.

62. See *Parliamentary Reports*, Senato della Repubblica, discussion of January 30, 1992.

63. Law Decree, August 28, 1995, n. 362. Law decrees—"the pragmatic answer to serious bottlenecks in the Italian representative system," according to LaPalombara (*quoted above*, 115)—are promulgated by the executive and may lose effect if not ratified by parliament within two months. Until such definitive approval they can be reenacted by the government, often with significant amendments, thus having a puzzling effect on the certainty of the law.

64. See Law, July 25, 1997, n. 238.

65. In the remand judgment, the plaintiff of the constitutional case was awarded more than $1.2 million. See Pretura Firenze, October 10, 1996, *Manichi v. Ministero della Sanità*.

66. P. Atiyah and P. Caine, *Accidents, Compensation and the Law* (London: Weidenfeld and Nicholson, 1987).

67. Abraham and Liebman, *op cit.*

68. All the data regarding the implementation of the compensation plan have been provided to this writer by the API, after a fruitless official request submitted to the Italian Health Ministry in May 1996.

69. As early as the X v. *French Government* decision of March 31, 1992, the European Court of the Human Rights condemned the French government for unreasonably delaying the administrative action brought by a HIV-contaminated hemophiliac under the French compensation plan.

70. The plaintiff is the father of the "Italian Ricky Ray," whose sad story was told in the only book that—to date—has outlined a story of the hemophiliac contamination in Italy. See G. Milano and P. Mico, *Puoi Correre Rocco. Sangue e AIDS: Cronaca di uno Scandalo Italiano* [You Can Run Rocco. Blood and AIDS: Chronicle of an Italian Scandal] (Rome: Pensiero Scientifico Editore, 1995).

71. The strict liability standard introduced by the 1988 Product Liability Act does not apply to events occurring before its promulgation, thus the claim is brought under the special liability clause in article 2050 of the Italian Civil Code: "(W)hoever causes injury to another in the performance of an activity dangerous by its nature or by reason of the instrumentalities employed, is liable for damages, unless he proves that he had taken all suitable measures to avoid the injury." See M. Beltramo, G. Longo, J. Merryman, *The Italian Civil Code* (New York-London: Oceana, 1969), p. 503.

72. Cass. 15 July 1987, *Il Foro Italiano* I, (1988), 144. As one legal scholar noted, the Trilergan case rule clearly places the development-risks liability on pharmaceutical companies. See D. Caruso, *Quando il Rimedio e. Peggiore del Male: Emoderivati Infetti e Responsabilità Civile, Il Foro Italiano* I, (1988), pp. 144, 152.

73. The Italian legal system historically encompasses the civil law private/public law dichotomy. Accordingly, the government's liability for failing to legislate must confront the fact that public bodies are subject solely to a duty to act fairly towards citizens. This duty does not give rise to a subjective right; but rather to (what is technically defined as) a "legitimate interest." The operational consequence is that in Italian law a tort claim for unlawful acts or omissions by the government has been barred much as a similar action would be in the common law tradition: according to the "king can do no wrong" privilege, and the resulting government (or "sovereign") immunity from private tort claims J. R. Robertson, "The Effects of Consent Decrees on Local Legislative Immunity", *University of Chicago Law Review* 56 (1989), 1121. In the hemophiliac case, an attempt has been made to present a tort claim based on a subjective right inferred from the constitutional right to health. It stresses that the administrative supervision of the Health Ministry in the health sector is eventually addressed to protect a subjective right of the citizens. Arguments to support this theory may be inferred by the common law doctrine of "specific detrimental reliance" (i.e. the duty to continue past warnings which have induced reliance by the plaintiff), M. Woodall, "Private Law Liability of Public Authorities for Negligent Inspection and Regulation," *McGill Law Journal* 37 (1992), p. 83.

74. The "biblical" duration of the Italian civil proceedings has been already condemned in 785 claims presented by Italian plaintiffs before the European Court of Human Rights, see "Processi Lenti, il Record Italiano" [Slow Trials, the Italian Record], *Il Sole 24 ore*, April 9, 1997.

75. Law May 4, 1990, n. 107.

76. See G. Aprili, M. Marchiori, "Autosufficienza Regionale nel Settore degli Emoderivati: l'Esperienza Veneta," *La Trasfusione di Sangue*, 38 (1993), p. 238.

77. See A. Flores, "Alcune Considerazioni e Riflessioni sulla Legge n. 107," *La Trasfusione di Sangue* (1991), p. 674.

78. See L. P. Comoglio, "Consenso Informato e Profili di Responsabilità nelle Donazioni di Sangue," *Il Foro Italiano*, V, (1992), p. 363.

79. HCV screening was made compulsory in July 1990. Mandatory testing for HIV2 virus followed in December 1992.

80. See G. de Stasio, *Rischio Residuo da Trasfusione nel 1997*, paper delivered at the course *Sicurezza del sangue e dei suoi prodotti: emovigilanza; indicazioni cliniche alla trasfusione*, organized in Rome on June 26–29, 1997, by the European School of Transfusion Medicine.

8 HIV-Contaminated Blood and Australian Policy
The Limits of Success

John Ballard

Australia's approach to AIDS was different from that of other countries, and much of the difference developed around the issue of blood control. During the formative stage of policy making on AIDS, from 1982 to 1985, awareness of risk to the supply of blood and blood products varied critically in industrial societies among those responsible for making policy choices. In the United States, the issue of risk and appropriate response was publicly debated from the end of 1982, but elsewhere that debate was largely ignored. In Australia, however, with an exceptional measure of government responsibility for the blood supply, any risk had a political dimension. By 1984, once a virus was identified and tests indicated that Australian blood was in fact contaminated, there was a political imperative to respond quickly. Matched with scientific capacity, political concern ensured that Australia had its blood supply fully tested and the virus eliminated from blood products before other countries. Political mobilization on the issue of blood then flowed into proactive policies on AIDS education and prevention.[1]

Any account of the Australian response to HIV-contaminated blood must examine the shaping of the unique institutional arrangements that underlay a policy of self-sufficiency in blood and blood products and an exceptional measure of government responsibility. Following an elaboration of the historical development of these arrangements, this chapter provides an account of the events and decisions of 1982–85, with emphasis on the evolving perceptions of risk that broke through assumptions of a hermetic national system. Announcement of the death of three infants after infection by transfusion thrust not only blood safety but AIDS onto the political agenda in Australia at a time when other governments were inactive. Responsibility for infection then became a significant contested issue and the progress of claims for compensation is traced through the development of policy and legal strategies. Finally outcomes of the HIV contamination experience are mapped through the restructuring of the blood supply system and policies on screening for other sources of infection.

Historical Background

Australia has particular characteristics that have shaped its policies and institutions. Its geographical isolation placed a premium on self-sufficiency but was also seen to require close linkage with professional and technical developments in the heartlands of the English-speaking world. A relatively small population, 18.2 million, concentrated in state capital cities, made possible close internal networks of communication among limited professional communities. In addition, Australia's isolation and the absence of domestic capital made for a tradition of "colonial socialism," which gave legitimacy to a central role for government in a wide range of programs. These characteristics shaped the institutions and forces involved in making policy in the 1980s.

Under the constitution of Australia adopted at federation in 1901, responsibility for health was not specified and so remained with the states. Quarantine, seen as essential for the protection of Australian health and agriculture from external contamination, was identified as a federal function. However, it was not until 1909 that a Quarantine Act took effect and a Director-General of Quarantine was appointed, to become the nucleus for the federal government's Commonwealth Department of Health in 1921.

World War I provided the occasion for establishing the main institutions later involved in blood control. An Australian branch of the British Red Cross was launched at Government House nine days after the declaration of war to provide civilian support for the military.[2] The war cut Australia off from its traditional sources of vaccines and other bacteriological products, and this led in 1916 to the establishment in Melbourne of the Commonwealth Serum Laboratories (CSL),[3] which developed between the wars a capacity for producing blood grouping serum and blood products.[4] During the war, blood transfusion was used extensively in battlefield hospitals, made feasible by the recent discovery of blood groups.

Australian medical officers returning from the war extended blood transfusion to civilian practice, giving rise to the need for blood donor panels based at hospitals. Following the model of the British Red Cross Society, which took over the running of donor services in London in 1925, the Red Cross of Victoria established a Blood Transfusion Service in Melbourne in 1929. Donation was entirely voluntary, despite a brief experiment with a professional donor panel among medical students for private patients in 1938, and state laws were enacted against the sale of blood. Early in World War II the Red Cross took responsibility for collecting blood donations in all states; at the same time the development of blood storage technology made blood banking possible.[5]

World War II required greatly increased blood supplies and new institutional arrangements. The Australian Red Cross Society, separated from its British parent under a royal charter in 1941, provided blood and serum for the Australian military as well as civilians, working in close association with the Defence Forces and the CSL. Donation became a patriotic activity though, as early as 1936, public servants had been given leave for donation purposes. Under Red Cross auspices a National Emergency Blood Transfusion Service was established in 1941, together with a scientific advisory National Blood Transfusion Committee. At the end of the war the Commonwealth government rejected proposals that it finance a national Red Cross transfusion service arguing that, because blood transfusion was ancillary to hospital treatment, it was a state responsibility. The state Blood Transfusion Services (BTS) continued to operate under the umbrella of the Red Cross and coordination was maintained through the National Blood Transfusion Committee (NBTC), comprising the BTS directors and scientific advisers.[6]

In the postwar period, blood transfusion was regarded not only as an emergency measure but as a standard adjunct to surgery. Demand for blood and blood products rose rapidly, and the BTS became the most significant program within the Red Cross, accounting for roughly 80% of its financial turnover. The BTS also became increasingly dependent on government subsidies, with the Commonwealth adding to state contributions from 1954. From 1976 on, the federal and state governments covered capital costs of the BTS on a 50/50 basis, while operating costs were met 60% by state governments, with the Red Cross contributing the lesser of 5% of costs or 10% of its independent fund-raising, and the balance covered by the federal government. In practice the Red Cross contribution was typically 1% to 2% of total operating costs.

In response to a federal proposal in 1977 that this complex formula be replaced by funding under Commonwealth–state hospital funding agreements, the Red Cross argued that it was different from other health services as a national organization and one dependent on volunteer activity, "which must be seen to be independent of government authority."[7] The status of the Red Cross, fortified by the prestige accorded to its national and state officials, led to instructions from the prime minister that the Department of Health not pursue the proposal.

Despite the growing presence of the Commonwealth in health matters, particularly through its monopoly of income taxation and the establishment of universal health insurance, the six state and two territorial governments have retained primary responsibility for providing health services. Some measure of concerted policy and uniform standards is achieved through twice-yearly meetings of the ministers of health and their chief officials, and through the National Health and Medical Research Council (NHMRC) and its many committees, serviced by the Commonwealth department. The committees have brought together health officials with leaders in medical research and practice, provided advice on health and medical issues, and allocated research funds.

The Commonwealth continued to maintain as a statutory body the Commonwealth Serum Laboratories, which developed an international reputation for research, much of it in conjunction with the Walter and Eliza Hall Institute in Melbourne. With a record of rapid production of influenza vaccine and insulin before the war, it produced penicillin in 1944 to make Australia the first country with free civilian access. It produced pooled human serum in 1940 and dried plasma during the war in collaboration with the Red Cross. It followed closely overseas research on fractionation and in 1949, the Commonwealth government agreed to finance fully the production of fractionated plasma, supplied free to hemophilic patients through the Blood Transfusion Services and hospitals since large-scale production began in 1953. CSL began production of factor VIII as early as 1960 and contributed to the rapid series of product developments of the 1970s. Cryoprecipitate, extracted from plasma from a small number of donors, was produced by CSL until 1969–70, when the BTS themselves took over its production while CSL moved on to higher purity anti-hemophilic factor (AHF), requiring blood from up to 2000 donors.[8]

Until 1974 factor VIII concentrates were available in only limited amounts. A working party of the National Blood Transfusion Committee then determined factor VIII and IX supply needs, and in 1977 the NBTC agreed that the first priority of the BTS was the provision of an adequate supply of factor VIII. Yet by 1982, despite substantial increases in the production of AHF by CSL and cryoprecipitate by the BTS, supply was always below the recognized world standard of 2.5 units of plasma per head of population. Each state BTS sent fresh frozen plasma to the CSL for fractionation and received a share of blood products in proportion to its contribution, with detailed exchange and accounting among states to meet current requirements; New South Wales, in part because of its centralized blood collection and its specialist hospitals serving other states, was perennially in deficit.

Quality control of the Blood Transfusion Services and CSL was a statutory responsibility of the federal National Biological Standards Laboratories from the late 1950s, succeeded by the Therapeutic Goods Administration from 1967. In practice, however, BTS policy was set by the BTS directors at meetings of the NBTC, whereas CSL largely escaped external regulation and inspection.[9] This provided scope for suspicion to flourish between the BTS and CSL concerning the quality of collection and fractionation practices.[10] From 1982, CSL, considering the smaller states and territories to be producing a higher quality of plasma, did not pool their contributions with those of New South Wales and Victoria, while the Sydney BTS judged its own method of fractionation superior to that of CSL.

An epidemic of hepatitis B, which accompanied the spread of injection drug use during and after the Vietnam War, provoked new forms of medical mobilization and linkage that were in place before the arrival of HIV/AIDS. After discovery of the specific antigen for hepatitis B, testing of blood started late in 1969, and by September 1970 Australia's blood supply was the first to be fully screened. Hepatitis B sparked a revival of interest in infectious diseases, and staff at Fairfield Infectious Diseases Hospital in Melbourne tracked its early spread among drug users from Sydney, which was a major rest and rehabilitation center during the Vietnam War. Dr. Ian Gust, returning to Fairfield in 1969 from postgraduate virology research overseas, built an international reputation with his research on hepatitis A and B. The public impact of hepatitis was, however, never sufficient to mobilize political interest in a campaign for its eradication.[11]

Other forms of mobilization also shaped the capacity for response to AIDS. During the 1970s, gay community organizations developed within Australian cities, especially Sydney, with a lively gay commercial structure, community media, and close links with the West Coast of the United States. Political mobilization centered on the issue of decriminalization of homosexuality, which took place in some states during the 1970s but remained an issue in New South Wales and others. Sexually transmitted diseases rapidly increased within the communities, and by the late 1970s gay men were collaborating with medical research as hepatitis B cohorts. Especially in Sydney they also became a valued contingent of donors to the Blood Transfusion Services, which provided free and confidential testing for hepatitis B and syphilis.

People with hemophilia had no comparable capacity for mobilization and their links lay primarily through medical specialists on whom they were largely dependent for treatment and care. Bryce Courtenay provides an excoriating account of medical dominance, conservatism, and ineptitude in the treatment of hemophilia and of his efforts to obtain the right to home treatment years after its availability in the United States.[12] As early as the 1950s, a few people with hemophilia and their caregivers began to form state associations, assisted by medical specialists but not, as in the United States, under their control. A national Australian Haemophilia Federation was organized in 1979–80 linking groups in the three eastern states, primarily through the efforts of its first president, Jenny Ross of Melbourne, the mother of two sons with hemophilia.

AIDS and Blood

The announcement in the U.S. *Morbidity and Mortality Weekly Report* of June 5, 1981, of the first cases of what became known as AIDS was noted a few days later in the Sydney gay community's *Star*, though national and medical media coverage of AIDS appeared much later. Early research and news on AIDS in the United States were followed in Australia by several medical specialists and a few gay activists, and the federal Department of Health's *Communicable Diseases Intelligence Bulletin* published several notes on U.S. developments in AIDS. Australian communicable disease specialists, closely networked throughout the country, were accustomed to seeing new diseases—Legionnaire's disease, toxic shock—a short time after their appearance in the United States, but AIDS was seen as only a remote risk for Australia. Even the first overseas evidence of blood transmission in the latter half of 1982 raised limited concern, given Australia's self-sufficient blood system.

This situation changed rapidly early in 1983, at a time when debate on blood transmission was becoming heated in the United States. As early as February 1983, when AIDS was first mentioned at a Victorian meeting, Jenny Ross of the Haemophilia Federation asked for the introduction of donor voluntary deferral forms, but was told by a BTS representative that questions about sex would embarrass women donors and that Australia's blood supply was safe. The first diagnosis of AIDS in Australia was made in Sydney in December 1982 and was publicly reported in April 1983, despite continuing uncertainty about the case's meeting AIDS-defining criteria. It related to a gay visitor from the United States who told doctors at St. Vincent's that he had had sex with over 100 men in Sydney.

However, AIDS did not become a media and political issue in Australia until May 1983, when Dr. Gordon Archer, Director of the Sydney BTS, called publicly for homosexual men to avoid donation, declaring in a television interview that it was "a virtual certainty that AIDS was in the blood supply." The National Blood Transfusion Committee had decided to wait for firm U.S. Red Cross guidelines, but Archer had heard from the visiting director of an Oklahoma blood bank that it was implementing a US Public Health Service request for a voluntary deferral program, despite the absence of detected cases in Oklahoma. Archer decided to act unilaterally.

His statement was the first public labeling of high-risk groups — "Disease Fear Leads Red Cross to Ban Gays as Donors"[13] — and it brought a prompt response from a few gay activists in Sydney, who were frustrated in their attempts to persuade New South Wales politicians to follow other states in decriminalizing homosexuality. When Archer refused to meet with a deputation to discuss alternative strategies of blood safety, a small group picketed the BTS for a day, distributing leaflets — "Ban the Bigots not the Blood" — calling for surrogate blood testing for hepatitis B instead of group deferral. Two days later a meeting of gay groups discussed the threat from AIDS and from further stigmatization and organized an AIDS Action Committee, the first among committees organized by gay communities in each of the states. A consultation was then organized between Archer, the state Department of Health, and the AIDS Action Committee and agreed on voluntary deferral and on the need for confidentiality and collaboration.[14] Much later the picket was often invoked as evidence that "the gay lobby" had shaped blood policy,[15] but there were in fact other stronger influences.

The BTS directors in other states were reluctant to follow Archer's initiative. Not only were they concerned with potential loss of confidence in the blood supply and among donors, but there were also considerations of privacy, confidentiality, and possible concealment. Professor David Penington, chair of the NBTC, responded publicly by stating that there was no risk of contracting AIDS from blood, because Australia relied on voluntary donation. Nonetheless, after the South Australia BTS director returned from the United States later in May with the American Red Cross "Important Message to All Blood Donors" of March, the NBTC recommended on June 1 that information sheets with similar wording be issued at donation centers asking for abstention by sexually active homosexual or bisexual men with multiple partners,[16] intravenous drug users, and sexual partners of these people. The next day the Australian Red Cross issued its first public statement on the subject: although AIDS had been diagnosed in U.S. blood recipients, no case had yet been seen in Australia, where risk was greatly reduced by exclusive use of voluntary donors. Implementation of the NBTC guidelines was left to each BTS, and none of them proceeded to introduce screening measures beyond the distribution of pamphlets to donors, relying on voluntary self-exclusion.

At the national level, arrangements for planning and advice to governments and health facilities were set in place. At its meeting on June 8–9, 1983, the National Health and Medical Research Council (NHMRC) supported the Australian Red Cross statement and established an expert working party on AIDS chaired by Penington. On June 11 the *Medical Journal of Australia* published several papers on AIDS, with a leading article observing that

> It is now recommended that individuals at risk should not donate blood, while the risk to persons with haemophilia can probably be lowered by replacing pooled lyophilised factor VIII concentrate with single-donor cryoprecipitate—a formidable exercise.[17]

An Australian immunologist reporting on a U.S. symposium offered contrary advice in the same issue: "Avoidance of blood donation by high-risk groups is predicted to be ineffective and inappropriate."[18] When the NHMRC met again in October to accept recommendations from its working party on AIDS, it issued public advice that

> There is no evidence that blood products in Australia are at risk of transmitting AIDS, following precautions already taken by the Australian Red Cross Society. This matter is kept under close and constant review.[19]

Despite the initial flurry of action and a rapid rise in the number of reported cases, AIDS remained, as in other countries, a low-priority problem perceived as confined to self-contained peripheral groups. Although planning took place within the NHMRC working party and the AIDS Action Committees, there was little media or government attention. Once the virus was identified and methods were developed for culturing it (announced in the United States April 1984), it was relatively easy to develop diagnostic tests. A year of "phoney war" for Australia ended in July 1984 with announcement of a diagnosis of post-transfusion AIDS, confirmed by Jay Levy's new immunofluorescence assay at the Cancer Research Institute of the University of California at San Francisco. Ten days later Levy confirmed a positive test for one of the donors of the transfused blood, a gay man who was aware of the BTS warning but who did not consider himself promiscuous.[20] The announcement launched a spate of media coverage of AIDS and substantial mobilization of activity to prevent blood transmission of the newly confirmed virus.

In Sydney, already established as the Australian epicenter for AIDS, Archer spoke to a public meeting of gay men to explain the need for those with multiple partners to refrain from donation, and his BTS, with support from the AIDS Action Committee, began to require donors to sign a form stating that they were not a member of a risk group. Despite objections from the New South Wales Privacy Committee, the

BTS maintained use of the form. Having heard that some U.S. blood banks were introducing surrogate testing, Archer also arranged to import Belgian hepatitis B core antibody test kits and began surrogate testing in October as a further means of identifying donors in high-risk groups. In these actions he had more scope and resources for action than other BTS directors; unlike the other Services, Archer's was ranked as a hospital, could pay higher salaries and had a close relationship with the state Department of Health. In other states, deferred donor categories were broadened in public notices, but signed forms and surrogate testing were not adopted.[21] In Melbourne, however, the BTS began to send only plasma from women donors to CSL for fractionation.

Attention to AIDS developments in the United States was intense during this period. Links between Ron Penny of St. Vincent's Hospital in Sydney and Jay Levy in San Francisco had established early access to the immunofluorescence assay, which provided evidence of widespread infection among a Sydney gay cohort. At Fairfield Hospital in Melbourne, Ian Gust, who had heard Luc Montagnier's report on isolation of a virus at a WHO meeting in November 1983, had twice received from him viral material for research, but it had perished each time; CSL, seen as a commercial organization, had been unable to obtain material from Montagnier or CDC. Gust's colleague at Fairfield, Ron Lucas, had also become interested in AIDS after hearing French findings at an International Infectious Diseases Society meeting in 1983. He spent his sabbatical leave from July to November 1984 at CDC, where he was the only overseas visitor following AIDS issues. Opting to work on blood donor policy, he attended meetings of the CDC AIDS team and relayed developments in US thinking by telephone to Melbourne. In August Gust sent a laboratory specialist to CDC and the US National Institutes of Health to learn how to perform their tests and he returned with a jar of antigen; by September 16, Fairfield was able to test blood samples with the ELISA screen and an early confirmatory assay.

Meanwhile the Sydney BTS, where research had led to an alternative (Margolis) method of preparing factor VIII, pressed CSL as early as February 1983 to begin heat treatment of freeze-dried AHF, the standard CSL product. CSL experimented with heat treatment during 1983, but this reduced yield to unacceptable levels. On September 16, 1984, heat treatment to inactivate the AIDS virus was first discussed at the CDC in Atlanta and Lucas relayed CDC views as they developed. On October 18, a meeting of the National Blood Transfusion Committee's AIDS working group recommended that CSL introduce heat sterilization urgently and test all AHF supplies through Fairfield, which had enough antigen to conduct 10 to 15 thousand tests. The next day Fairfield's initial testing of stored sera from about 30 people using AHF found that one third were HIV-antibody-positive. Three days later, CSL received from CDC the news that heat treatment had proved effective in inactivating the virus, and the *MMWR* published CDC's recommendation of heat treatment another four days later.

A working party on heat treatment of factor VIII was convened by the Commonwealth Director of Public Health on November 2 at CSL. CSL had switched over to the Margolis method of factor VIII production from Sydney BTS; experiments showed that this product retained acceptable yield after 12 hours of 60°C heat, and it was agreed that this be applied forthwith. The meeting was the first to which the Haemophilia Federation was invited, and it was left to Jenny Ross of the Federation to notify individuals with hemophilia of the implications of the decisions taken. From November 5, 1984, all relevant blood products produced by CSL were heat-treated, although states and hospitals varied in their use or recall of previous stocks until March or April 1985. From November 12, all plasma received by CSL for pooling and fractionation was tested.

Despite increasing media coverage of AIDS, many of these developments drew no public attention, but in mid-November 1984, AIDS suddenly achieved prominence on Australia's political agenda. During September 1984 the Labor federal government had called an early election to extend the term it had won in March 1983. On November 15, two weeks before polling, the conservative Queensland government announced that tests confirmed three infants had died after receiving contaminated blood from a homosexual donor. Within 24 hours the Queensland Parliament passed legislation imposing criminal sanctions for false declarations by donors, and the prime minister appealed for calm in the midst of media hysteria. Headlines read "Gays Accused of Giving Blood out of Spite"[22] and a leader of the federal opposition declared that, "If it wasn't for the promotion of homosexuality as a norm by Labor, I am quite confident that the deaths of these three poor babies would not have occurred."[23]

The next day Neal Blewett, the Commonwealth Minister for Health, announced a program of urgent initiatives, pledging substantial funds for the production and supply of test kits as soon as they became available. Blewett's senior staff adviser, Bill Bowtell, had followed AIDS developments closely for several months despite preoccupation with a threatened strike by doctors over hospital fees. Overriding Department advice in favor of a meeting among public servants and medical specialists, Bowtell arranged an emergency meeting in Melbourne between Blewett and state health ministers and put forward proposals for exceptional arrangements to deal with the crisis. Despite resistance from Queensland, the ministers agreed on coordinated national action on AIDS and a uniform blood donor policy. The NHMRC Working Party of medical experts was reconstituted under Penington as the National AIDS Task Force, and a National Advisory Committee on AIDS (NACAIDS) was appointed, with membership from government, the health professions, the AIDS Action Committees (rebaptized AIDS Councils) and the Haemophilia Federation. The basis for a new kind of "partnership" in health policy making was thus laid, shifting from the traditional public health model favored by Queensland and Penington to a politically inspired health advancement model.

When the ministers met a month later, after Labor's reelection, to consider recommendations from the two advisory bodies, they adopted Task Force proposals to require signed donor declaration forms concerning risk activities and to recommend legal penalties for false declarations. The state ministers of health were initially reluctant to adopt legal penalties, but agreed that they could not offer less blood protection than Queensland. Federal support for BTS capital funding that had been sought for years by the states was forthcoming, and the Haemophilia Federation was quickly provided with funds for an office, newsletter, and care and counseling programs, and all persons with hemophilia and coagulation disorders were offered testing through Fairfield. Meanwhile blood donations had fallen off drastically, and one of the first priorities of NACAIDS was the recruitment of women donors.

A certain measure of the traditional rivalry between Sydney's and Melbourne's medical establishments existed between the teams at St. Vincent's and Fairfield hospitals. At the initial Melbourne meeting of ministers, Gust's access to CDC antigen meant that a National Reference Laboratory to conduct confirmatory testing was established at Fairfield, rather than at St. Vincent's, but both collaborated with three BTS laboratories under Gust's leadership as the only non-U.S. participants in the Food and Drug Administration's evaluation of five diagnostic test kits from October 1984 to January 1985. When Archer in Sydney sought to import Belgian ELISA kits, which arrived on Christmas Eve, they were blocked on quarantine grounds by the Commonwealth Department of Health, a decision having been taken to introduce only tests whose characteristics had been subjected to the collaborative evaluation.[24]

In January 1985, Bowtell persuaded Blewett and senior federal health officials to visit San Francisco, Atlanta, Washington, and London to observe AIDS programs at first hand. They returned determined to avoid repetition of the U.S. experience, having succeeded in obtaining from pharmaceutical companies a commitment to provide supplies of test kits. The results of the FDA evaluation were revealed early in March, and the Australian experience from participation in the exercise, together with a major logistical effort in the importing and distribution of kits, made possible the testing of all blood donations throughout the country by May 1, 1985, and the establishment of alternative testing sites. Blewett's first major parliamentary statement on AIDS, on April 23, explained the action taken. The harnessing of scientific expertise and political commitment had made possible a national proactive stance on AIDS.

Following Queensland's initiative in November 1984, all states enacted legislation making false or misleading declarations by blood donors an offense punishable by fine or imprisonment[25]; Australia has the only legislation in the world of this kind. From April 1985 to December 1996, out of 11 million donations tested for HIV-1-antibody, 87 were found to be positive.[26] Although several HIV-positive donors were found to be aware of their risk status, there were no prosecutions until a case arose in

Table 8-1. Australian cases of transfusion-
acquired HIV, by year of infection

Year of infection	Number (%)
Before 1981	12 (6)
1981	20 (11)
1982	32 (17)
1983	54 (29)
Jan–Nov 1984	51 (27)
Nov 1984 to May 1985	4 (2)
Not known	16 (8)
Total	189 (100)

Source: National Centre in HIV Epidemiology and Clini-
cal Research, *An Epidemiological Assessment of the HIV
Epidemic in Australia* (Canberra: Australian Government
Publishing Service, 1996), 118.

1993 in Victoria, leading to conviction, in which there was public evidence that the donor was aware of being HIV-positive.

No instance of HIV transmission from blood or blood products since April 1985 has been identified. Out of an estimated 1500 people with hemophilia/coagulation disorder in 1984,[27] probably 900 were treated with blood products during that year and altogether 264 people with hemophilia received HIV-contaminated blood products.[28] Although it is not possible in most cases to determine the date of infection of people with hemophilia, some of whom were treated with blood products as many as 20 times per year, studies of stored sera showed the developing prevalence of HIV antibody: 1981—0.0%; 1982—9.8%; 1983—11.9%; 1984—31.0%.[29]

A total of 172 blood-transfusion cases had been identified by the end of 1995, with dates of infection as shown in Table 8-1; in addition, four women received HIV through artificial insemination.[30] The numbers of Australian transfusion cases prior to 1985 are among the highest recorded in the developed world, but these numbers reflect in part the thoroughness of the look-back program initiated by Archer in August 1985[31] and of epidemiological reporting administered by the National Centre for HIV Epidemiology and Clinical Research.

The Aftermath of Infection

The major issues arising from contamination of the blood supply were those of compensation for those infected and the potential liability of the Red Cross and others. Part of the rationale in December 1984 for adopting signed donor declarations and legal penalties for false declarations was to provide protection for the Red Cross against liability. Insurance companies were quick to announce that they would no longer provide cover for claims against the BTS for transmission of HIV, and the Red Cross—previously opposed to blood shield legislation for fear of losing donors—would have been unwilling to maintain its blood services without immunity from claims or government indemnity. In May 1985 the health ministers agreed to indemnify the BTS for uninsured costs and damages arising from compensation claims for infection from donations prior to July 1985. The Commonwealth government, which controlled legislation for the Australian Capital Territory, then drew up the ACT Blood Donation (AIDS) Ordinance 1985 as model legislation to shield the Red Cross Society and hospitals as long as a signed donor declaration had been obtained and a sample of blood had been tested for viral antibodies with an approved test.

The Senate Standing Committee on Regulations and Ordinances, in the Commonwealth Parliament's sole attempt to deal with substantive matters of AIDS policy, argued that the Ordinance should be amended to protect the right to sue for negligence in the actual performance of approved procedures and for failure to apply recognized standards of practice in testing. After Blewett made the first ministerial appearance before the committee in its 53-year history, he agreed to these amendments and to a one-year sunset clause on the legislation, though the latter did not take effect.[32] The states, except for Queensland where other arrangements were made, each enacted similar but varying legislation during 1985 and early 1986,[33] and in March 1986 Blewett informed state health ministers that the Commonwealth would contribute 40% of all uninsured costs relating to claims of transmission before July 1985. The states were in a vulnerable position, for only Victoria and Tasmania had substantial external insurance, the others having little or relying on their own funds to cover liabilities.

Meanwhile the issue of compensation for infection through factor VIII was brewing. Jenny Ross of the Haemophilia Federation raised it at the first meeting of the National Advisory Committee on AIDS (NACAIDS) in December 1984, a month after contamination of factor VIII became known. A government working party was appointed in February 1985 to look into the legal and financial implications of blood transmission and advised that a compensation scheme was not feasible on the grounds that there were no precedents, that there were no estimates of the extent of blood transmission or of the amount of compensation needed, and that compensation would not limit future legal liability. Ross then took steps, with Commonwealth government advice and support, to reconstitute the Haemophilia Federation as the Haemophilia Foundation Australia, with capacity for education and care as well as for administration of a compensation and support scheme.

Early in 1986 a NACAIDS working group on compensation was established with Ross as chair, and in November NACAIDS unanimously supported its proposed scheme of no-fault compensation for those with medically acquired AIDS or AIDS-related conditions. Whereas other NACAIDS proposals were quickly taken up, this one met extended delays. Confronted with a campaign in Sydney by a group of women with "innocently acquired" AIDS through blood transfusion, the AIDS Councils began to oppose compensation for special groups and the Commonwealth government balked at a precedent applicable to other diseases. At a meeting with Blewett in November 1987, Ross was told that compensation for one group was not politically feasible, but that the government would consider a trust fund to cover the exceptional expenses of people with hemophilia and AIDS; a similar trust fund had just been established in Great Britain after a successful media campaign. Ross submitted detailed costing of expenses in January 1988 and the Haemophilia Foundation Australia surveyed its members' views on whether to support a similar public campaign, receiving contradictory results, with many worried about a negative image for hemophilia and reluctant to pursue litigation against their own lifeline.

The Commonwealth government's HIV/AIDS discussion paper of late 1988 canvassed the issue of no-fault compensation for all medically acquired illness and raised for consideration the Haemophilia Foundation's proposal for a trust fund,[34] but a further meeting with Blewett indicated that there remained substantial opposition within the government. After negotiation with Blewett's department, the foundation put forward in March 1989 its detailed proposal for a government seeding grant of $11.7 million for a Haemophilia Foundation Endowment Fund, but the grant was caught up in the drafting and budgeting of the first national strategy on HIV/AIDS, and in May the foundation appealed past Blewett to all cabinet ministers and began to receive media coverage for their campaign. By August 3, Ross wrote to Blewett conveying the foundation's "anger and frustration" and five days later she released the Foundation's first media statement:

> This event is the greatest single tragedy in the history of the Australian health service. People receiving a life saving treatment have been infected with a life taking virus. Governments normally step in on occasions of disaster such as fire or flood. Not so this time. Negotiations on this matter have dragged on for four years while between fifteen and twenty have died, others have become ill, and an increasing number of families struggle financially.

The campaign received widespread support, including a media statement from the Australian Federation of AIDS Organisations, composed of the AIDS Councils. When Blewett responded to Opposition questions in Parliament with the suggestion that those who had been infected through blood could have recourse to the courts, a further foundation press release attacked his shifting position.

The government was concerned to have bipartisan support for its national strategy, and Blewett's office arranged for Ross to see the prime minister, who was persuaded by her arguments concerning the special needs of those with both hemophilia and HIV infection. A week later, on the day the national strategy was presented to parliament, cabinet changed its position. On November 1, 1989, the government, emphasising that it was covering only financial assistance for the consequences of infection, not compensation for the fact of infection, announced the establishment of a trust fund of $13.2 million for the benefit not only of those with hemophilia, but of all persons with medically acquired HIV. In discussions with the states about the terms of the trust, the Commonwealth assured them that, unlike compensation schemes, payments under the trust would not affect Medicare payments; had future health insurance benefits not been guaranteed, any compensation awards were likely to be very much higher.

Under the Mark Fitzpatrick Trust, named for a Tasmanian boy infected by AHF who had been active in HIV education, payments were to be limited to assistance on the basis of need. However the trustees from the start determined that payment was recognition of the trauma and costs of HIV infection and so should be available to all eligible persons regardless of need. As of May 1996, the trust had 415 registrations and had paid out $11.4 million. Living registrants receive an initial payment of $2000 and, depending on the stage of progression of HIV and number of dependents, between $1380 and $11,040 annually, with a payment at death of $8600 for single registrants and $24,700 for those with dependents. Retrospective payments of $10 to $30 thousand were made to the heirs of those deceased at registration. Assistance was not dependent on the recipient's waiver of the right to pursue compensation through the courts, and this encouraged the great majority of those eligible to participate.[35]

The trust met the concerns of the Haemophilia Foundation, which remained neutral in subsequent litigation. However, it did not satisfy all people with hemophilia, nor those who had contracted HIV through blood transfusion. The majority (68%) of the latter were in New South Wales and many had been identified through the Sydney BTS look-back program. Unlike most of those with hemophilia, who had a lifelong history of illness and medical dependence, as well as earlier infection with hepatitis B, those infected with HIV from blood transfusion were angry at the perceived failure of the health system. They were often isolated, without the community support provided by the government-funded AIDS Councils and Haemophilia Foundation. One articulate Sydney woman, diagnosed with AIDS and concerned about the lack of information and services available for transfusion cases, went to the media and was joined by two other women in forming a vocal group of those with "innocently acquired" AIDS. They secured media and political support in their campaign and the state Department of Health established in 1987 a Transfusion-Related AIDS (TRAIDS) unit at Westmead Hospital. Initially a temporary expedient, the TRAIDS unit became a world model and its director a leading advocate for support services for transfused HIV/AIDS cases, and latterly for those with transfused hepatitis C. The TRAIDS group were dissatisfied with the limited assistance available through the Mark Fitzpatrick Trust and launched litigation for more substantial funds.

Two court cases had already reached judgment without an award of damages. The first suit against the Red Cross had been heard in Queensland in 1987 and was unsuccessful, on the ground that no test had been available at the time of transfusion in May 1983.[36] In a hemophilia case in New South Wales, although the court found the hospital, the Red Cross, and CSL all negligent in failing to warn of the risk of HIV transmission, it relied on testimony from a U.S. expert that, prior to a September 1983 publication in the *New England Journal of Medicine*, the risk of withholding AHF would have outweighed the uncertain risk of AIDS.[37]

The TRAIDS group then sponsored a suit in the Federal Court in NSW. In the case of *E v Australian Red Cross*,[38] the court, after hearing expert testimony from the United States and Australia, found that the Red Cross in October 1984 did not require surrogate testing and that its screening methods were adequate by the standards of the day. The court set a precedent in finding that, although the Red Cross was a trading corporation for purposes of the Trade Practices Act of 1974, its gratuitous supply of blood was not an act "in trade or commerce" even though it was reimbursed most of the cost. It was not, therefore, liable for defective products.[39]

At this point the Melbourne law firm Slater and Gordon entered the scene. Having specialized in worker compensation cases, it had become prominent in managing group claims, with successes on asbestos mining, the Dalkon Shield intrauterine device, and silicone breast implants, and a major setback on repetition strain injury. It had developed

> a reputation as a tough-talking firm, willing to take on controversial cases. It has also one of the highest public profiles, with regular commercial radio ads, and solicitors who are willing to give the media 30-second "grabs" on the hot legal topic of the week. With its "no win, no fee" policy, Slater and Gordon has been accused of courting publicity and helping push Australia towards an American-style litigation frenzy.[40]

Slater and Gordon arranged for a substantial number of writs to be issued for medically acquired HIV and brought suits from plaintiffs in other states to the Victorian courts, where jury trial was available in civil cases, on the grounds that Red Cross and CSL headquarters gave jurisdiction.[41]

Slater and Gordon chose for trial the case of PQ (all plaintiffs' identities were protected by court order). Commencing in the Victorian Supreme Court in August 1990, it proceeded for 87 sitting days, the longest civil jury trial in Australian history, with testimony from a large battery of overseas and Australian experts. Although the Red Cross and CSL were found to have acted in accordance with international standards, the hospital was found not to have fulfilled its duty to warn of the risks of AHF use in October 1984.[42] The plaintiff was awarded $870,000, including general damages of $500,000, as well as legal costs estimated at $3 to 4 million; defendants' costs were over $5 million; some lawyers involved in the case estimate total costs at $15 million, a sum greater than the endowment of the Mark Fitzpatrick Trust.

In *BC v Australian Red Cross Society*,[43] a court order mandated that the Red Cross disclose the donor's identity under conditions of confidentiality, expressing doubt that this would jeopardize the blood supply. The Red Cross wanted to appeal this issue in a better case, so *BC* was settled for $300,000, leaving open the question whether a donor could be sued for providing false or misleading information.[44] Then the BY case was filed after the PQ decision, presenting the defendants with a worst-case situation in which a junior doctor had prescribed AHF rather than cryoprecipitate for an infant in late 1984 when no specialist would have done so. Prior to trial, the hospital insurers agreed to a settlement against the advice of the government lawyers, and the Red Cross felt compelled to settle as well. The settlements, totaling $600,000, left potential CSL and Commonwealth liability unsettled.

The problem for Slater and Gordon had been to find defendants with sufficient funding. Doctors were covered by the Medical Defence Union, but it refused all negotiation, and hospitals were seen as vicariously implicated in any negligence by doctors. The Red Cross was the only party involved in all cases. It was concerned about the damage to its reputation from media publicity on the compensation trials, and its viability as a defendant depended on both Commonwealth and state indemnity. After the *E* case proceeded to full trial, in July 1990 Commonwealth and state finance and legal officers met with the Red Cross to set up mechanisms for cooperation in defending AIDS litigation and to apportion potential damages against the Red Cross. The Commonwealth, which was fully responsible for the CSL, agreed to cover 40% of the Red Cross indemnity while the states, responsible together with insurance companies for the hospitals, covered 60% of the Red Cross. The Commonwealth, particularly concerned to avoid class actions involving the non-meritorious, insisted that any settlement of claims be made on their legal merit and an estimate of their forensic risk (that high legal costs would outweigh settlement costs); its contribution was made dependent on its own evaluation of these considerations. The Commonwealth and New South Wales, which had most to lose, wanted judicial determination of negligence. Western Australia, with only 22 cases, felt that litigation would cost more than settlement; the state was its own insurer and so negotiated a separate arrangement, paying out $5.4 million in May 1991 and forgoing its Commonwealth contribution.

In March 1991, after the *BC* appeal was dismissed, a further meeting was held to assess the outcomes of litigation, alternatives to out-of-court settlement, and future insurance arrangements. Then in September 1991, in the aftermath of the *PQ* award and the BY settlements, a roundtable was held among the Commonwealth, the states, the Red Cross, and the insurers of the hospitals, anxious to avoid further divisions among the defendants. The insurers, led by a representative of Lloyd's of London, were eager to settle and considered that *PQ* could have been settled for $125,000. It was clear at this point that HIV cases were being treated differently from other cases of medical misadventure largely because the patients could be mobilized as a group, and in this respect Slater and Gordon played a crucial role.

To avoid further legal costs, a compensation scheme based on a chronology of risk was mapped out by Commonwealth, Red Cross, and insurer lawyers. Infection before December 1982 was considered to involve only token liability; from then to the end of 1983, there was possible failure to warn, and a small percentage of likely damages in a successful case was conceded, largely on grounds of forensic risk. From the end of 1983 to mid-1984, although risk was seen as unchanged, a higher measure of liability was admitted. For cases of transmission from mid-1984 to the implementation of HIV screening in April 1985, the highest measure of liability was admitted, on the basis of a combination of failure to warn and screen and, in fractionate cases, to heat. These percentages were applied to traditional damages for loss of earnings, pain and suffering, and costs; future medical expenses were assumed to be covered by Medicare.

Politicians were pressing for quick settlement to remove from the public agenda an issue on which they could be portrayed as uncaring. Following Western Australia, South Australia, also with a small number of cases, reached a settlement while negotiating with the Commonwealth, which reassessed the cases and provided 35%. The Victorian government was under pressure to resolve the issue before a state election. A team of Commonwealth, Red Cross, and insurance company lawyers assessed each of the state's 140 cases in negotiation with Slater and Gordon, setting a model that was later applied in each of the other states and territories. There was rapid and consistent settlement of cases as well as collaboration by Slater and Gordon in encouraging all potential plaintiffs to participate in the scheme. The look-back program was crucial in determining the date of infection; where this was uncertain, because of inadequate hospital records, the negotiating team worked on the balance of probabilities. During the Victorian negotiations, Slater and Gordon discovered a precedent for covering claims by relatives of dead patients for shock, distress, and nursing costs, and these were included thereafter.

Much the largest number of cases concerned New South Wales, where the Government Insurance Office was insurer for both the Red Cross and hospitals and was reluctant to follow the Victorian precedent. New South Wales was already set on a different trajectory due to political support mustered by the TRAIDS group for further compensation. During 1990–91 a committee of the New South Wales Legislative Council held extensive hearings on medically acquired HIV with substantial media coverage, providing the first political forum for a confrontation of views on the issues of compensation. The AIDS Council of NSW, which had developed collaborative arrangements with the TRAIDS office at Westmead hospital, argued

> that none of the issues identified are unique to people with medically acquired HIV. All people with HIV suffer from some or all of these issues. The issues are not resolvable by the payment of compensation to a particular group of the infected and affected;

only significant improvements in the level of services for all people with HIV and changes to the social and legal climate in which services are provided will resolve them.[45]

Both the Commonwealth and NSW governments opposed further special assistance, on the grounds that all Australians were entitled to income security and free health care and that extra benefits for any one group were inequitable. On the other hand, there was medical and legal testimony in favor of compensation. The committee divided 5 to 4, though not on party lines, in recommending a compensation scheme for the state estimated to cost $10.42 million. In doing so it avoided the problem of allocating responsibility, instead focusing on British and Canadian precedents for substantial compensation. The New South Wales government thereupon committed itself to establish a supplementary trust, but in the end agreed to a settlement scheme similar to that of Victoria, with its trust fund counted as part of its contribution to settlement costs.

Under the compensation schemes, a total of about $90 million had been paid out by May 1996 in exchange for waivers of rights to litigation; individual payments ranged up to $650,000. Only one plaintiff persisted with a claim in court; although the case was eventually abandoned in favor of settlement, it yielded a judgment that donors could be identified under a supervised procedure to provide information.[46] New Zealand has a national compensation scheme preventing litigation, but New Zealanders infected by CSL products held the possibility of suing in Victoria courts, so an extension of the Australian arrangements to cover this group was settled early in 1996. Papua New Guinea, which also used CSL products, had no identified cases of transmission by AHF.

Further Developments

In August 1985 a private blood bank for storage of autologous donations was launched in Sydney, based on refusal by the Sydney BTS to provide long-term storage and opposition by all BTS to directed donations. Amid much publicity, some of it critical of Red Cross blood safety, and with the support of leading medical and business figures, the blood bank was listed on the Sydney Stock Exchange in November 1986 and its stock increased in value from $1.10 to $15.70 in two months. A further month on, it was suspended from trading at $3.70 and the following day its founder and managing director was arrested for fraud and bankruptcy.[47] He was sentenced in 1993 to two years in prison.

The technology of blood testing improved substantially in the aftermath of early HIV experience.[48] The BTS introduced screening for HIV-2 in 1992, using a combination HIV-1/HIV-2 antibody detection kit that reduced the length of the "window period" (when donor blood is infectious but seronegative) from about 50 to about 25 days. The "window period" remains a focus of concern but, given the low donor prevalence of HIV, the BTS have not followed the U.S. and Canadian practice of adopting p24 antigen testing to cover a brief period before the formation of a detectable antibody; calculations show that a cost of $5 to $10 million per annum would be needed to prevent less than one case of donation per decade. At present, fewer than one donation in every 100,000 collected is antibody-positive, which is some 5 to 10 times lower than the rate in similar developed countries.

> Certainly in Australia the risk of HIV transmission through blood transfusion is already extraordinarily low. Ultimately, the community will need to decide how safe is 'safe enough', as it is likely that a zero-risk blood supply will be unobtainable, regardless of the procedures in place.[49]

Screening for hepatitis C was introduced in February 1990 as soon as test kits became available, shortly after their introduction in Japan and prior to licensing of the test by the U.S. Food and Drug Administration; the high cost of screening was undertaken in the light of experience with HIV compensation claims. Screening for HTLV-1 was also begun from 1992, but only after long negotiations; two states decided to screen for HTLV-1 and together with the Commonwealth provided funds, but other states proved reluctant. In each of these cases screening recommendations were made by the National Blood Transfusion Committee to the National Executive of the Australian Red Cross, which then issued instructions to the directors of the divisional BTS.

The large number of donors reactive to hepatitis C overwhelmed the counseling services of the BTS, which arranged to transfer a considerable share of their counseling to general practitioners. A national strategy for detection and management of hepatitis C was recommended by a NHMRC working party, which estimated that 150,00 to 250,000 Australians were infected[50] and the third national strategy on HIV/AIDS, issued in September 1996, extended its purview and three-year funding commitment to hepatitis C and to other sexually transmitted diseases. By 1997 a number of lawsuits had been filed for failure to warn of hepatitis C infection before the introduction of blood testing. Slater and Gordon claimed that 1000 had received hepatitis C in blood transfusions in Sydney between 1985 and 1991, and perhaps a total of 2500 nationally.[51] The prospect of a rerun of the HIV compensation history became likely.

There has been a 25% decline in blood collections in Australia since 1984, particularly since 1989.[52] Despite the fact that Australia is a low user of red blood cells and factor VIII in comparison with northwest Europe, there are increasing shortages of red cells. Part of the decline in donations is considered in the BTS to be due to their own defensive practices in response to litigation and regulation, including lengthy donor interviews and increased donor rejection. The resultant delays have reduced attendance by repeat donors, on whom the BTS primarily rely for supply. Donor service, particularly in the reduction of delays, and the public perception of blood banks are seen as critical factors in maintaining a volunteer donor system. Some BTS directors contend that funding on the basis of output (used in all developed transfusion services except those of Australia, Canada, and Scotland) would improve the responsiveness of blood services to customer needs.[53]

A succession of issues in recent years led to the first substantial restructuring of the blood industry. The regulatory regime was overhauled under the Therapeutic Goods Act of 1989, which came into effect in February 1991. The previous act of 1966 did not apply to locally manufactured drugs and blood products, but the 1989 legislation brought Australia into line with regulation by the U.S. FDA and the European Medical Evaluation Authority. The tradition of quarantine, reinforced by the thalidomide experience, made Australia reluctant to accept overseas drug approvals. A campaign in 1990 by ACT-UP and other AIDS organizations to obtain rapid access to new U.S. treatments led to a committee of inquiry and reform of drug approval by the Therapeutic Goods Administration (TGA). In July 1992 publication of the TGA's Australian Code of Good Manufacturing Practice for Blood and Blood Products stimulated a considerable amount of change within the Blood Transfusion Services. For the first time they were brought under rigorous external inspection, requiring them to shift from the culture of a volunteer organization to that of a pharmaceutical manufacturer. Although the Commonwealth lacked authority to regulate the collection of whole blood not destined for plasma production, guidelines on all BTS activities were substantially changed.[54]

The Commonwealth Serum Laboratories, like other Australian statutory corporations during the late 1980s, went through a series of redefinitions of its relationship to government,[55] ending as a private corporation in 1994. CSL Ltd now supplies blood products on contract to the Commonwealth government, giving it a 10-year monopoly on fractionation; a 10-year contract with the Red Cross also formalizes previous arrangements. A critical analysis of the privatization notes that

> the Government is simultaneously one of CSL's principal suppliers, its principal customer and its regulator. Despite its commercial facade, the privatised CSL remains for most practical purposes a regulated monopoly with the rate of returned [sic] being determined by the Commonwealth Government. This means that the profitability of the company will depend on the vicissitudes of the relationship between CSL management, the Therapeutic Goods Administration (of the Commonwealth Health Department) and the Government.[56]

This judgment overlooks the facts that CSL Ltd's fractionation plant, the only one in the South Pacific and Southeast Asia, has separate commercial agreements with other countries, and that the Bioplasma division is only one of four of the company's business units.

The Auditor-General and Parliament's Joint Committee on Public Accounts were critical of several aspects of the sale of CSL. They were particularly concerned with the 147% rise in prices charged to the Commonwealth for blood products, largely attributable to previous subsidy, and the grant of 10 years of further indemnity against HIV and other infection claims. They also sought to persuade the government to establish through the Therapeutic Goods Administration a code of good manufacturing practice for blood fractionation, but were informed that international pharmaceutical regulation was adequate.[57]

CSL privatization provided the occasion for bringing together within the Commonwealth department the sections handling financial relations with CSL Ltd and the Red Cross, in proximity with the Therapeutic Goods Administration, making it possible for the first time to develop an overall Commonwealth government perspective on blood issues. The lessons of HIV compensation led the department to recognize the need for a capacity for national policy on blood, and the problem was brought to a head by disagreement among the states over screening for HTLV-1.[58] In order to legitimate the concept of a national policy, the Commonwealth department proposed to the Australian Health Ministers Council the establishment of a review of the Australian blood and blood product system, and this was conducted by consultants who had been Blewett's former Secretary for Health and First Assistant Secretary for Health Advancement.

The McKay-Wells report[59] proposed the vertical integration of blood recruitment and supply under a national Red Cross blood service. This was to be financed by triennial output-based contracts with the state governments, funded 40% by the Commonwealth, to supply an essential core of blood products free to patients, and to provide non-core products at market prices. It would be advised by a standing committee of the Australian Health Ministers Council, replacing the National Blood Transfusion Committee, and would receive Commonwealth blood-shield protection.

The McKay-Wells report was submitted to the health ministers early in 1995, together with the report of a working party on factor VIII supply[60] and a study on transmission of Creuzfeldt-Jacob disease through pituitary hormone therapy[61]; the latter demonstrated the difficulties of joint decision making among the Therapeutic Goods Administration, the Red Cross, CSL Ltd, and state governments. The McKay-Wells proposals were referred to a new Blood and Blood Products Advisory Committee, reporting to the Australian Health Ministers Advisory Committee rather than the national policy body recommended in the McKay-Wells report. There are constitutional problems raised by the latter arrangement, and constitutionality also limits the prospects for blood-shield coverage of the Red Cross, requiring uniform legislation by the states.[62]

However, the national secretary-general of the Red Cross, who had been Blewett's predecessor as Commonwealth health minister, seized on the structural proposals in the McKay-Wells report and an offer of Commonwealth funding for the first three years. He persuaded the national Red Cross board and the state BTS directors, some of them reluctant to lose their autonomy, to accept these proposals and an Australian Red Cross Blood Service came into existence at the end of 1996. The new Blood Service is responsible for coordinating the procedures of donor recruitment and selection and the distribution of blood and blood products, including those processed by CSL Ltd. Its board of management, with financial, legal, medical and Red Cross representation, replaces the National Blood Transfusion Committee and its new chief executive officer is charged with developing with the BTS directors a five-year strategic plan on blood service management, incorporating "total quality management and systems analysis." It is committed, nonetheless, to continue with voluntary, unremunerated donations, "the proven formula for the safest and most efficient blood services around the world."[63]

Conclusion

If Australia presents, by comparative standards, a case of positive responses to the challenge of blood transmission of HIV, this is due in part to the geographical and historical features that shaped its unique blood supply system and its scientific communities. Geographical isolation created a need for self-sufficiency in blood and blood products, and the absence of a substantial market meant that government funding was essential. Isolation also created an emphasis among research scientists on maintaining close international linkages with major centers in the United States and United Kingdom. These linkages produced early access to the tests that provided awareness of blood contamination, and the government's implication in blood funding created a responsibility for urgent political action once contamination was apparent. The quality of that political action depended in part on the nature of the government and the minister of the day, particularly in the choice of health promotion as an approach to preventing sexual transmission,[64] but the response in relation to blood was likely to be assured no matter what government was in office.

All of this indicates that once the signals of risk to the blood supply were read clearly in Australia, there was a capacity and a political will to respond quickly. What constituted adequate signals in 1983 and 1984 was the subject of intricate and expensive consideration in the courts. The courts generally held that the Red Cross and CSL maintained appropriate standards of action in the light of international practice; however, there were clearly differences in the reading of signals by Gordon Archer and the other BTS directors. A few voices asserted a higher standard of caution. Peter Gordon of Gordon and Slater concludes in a review of the HIV litigation,

[r]egrettably, it seems that the treatment of the AIDS epidemic by blood bankers and others entrusted with the responsibility of protecting the Australian blood supply, was tardy, unco-ordinated and compromised by self-interested pressure groups.[65]

Bryce Courtenay, Australia's most widely read author, argues in an account of his son's treatment that AHF should have been withdrawn in favor of cryoprecipitate and homosexual men excluded from donation in early 1983, in a chapter entitled "Where Pooled Blood Led to Murder by Decree and Doctors and Politicians Stood by with their Hands Firmly Clasped about their Buttocks."[66]

For signals to be read more clearly than they were would require broader social knowledge than technical expertise alone provides. The National Blood Transfusion Committee of 1983, apart from resolving widespread uncertainty about the etiology of AIDS, would have needed to know—as the venereologists did—something of the ethnography of Sydney's gay community and its U.S. links, in order to understand that the international flow of semen might undermine a hermetic blood supply. This degree of breadth would require a culture of consultation such as developed later in AIDS prevention campaigns in combining medical and community interpretations of risk.

The course of later developments, in the handling of claims for compensation and the restructuring of the blood system, was less predictable. But the proactive stance of Australian governments and their choice of the principles of the Ottawa Charter in shaping AIDS strategies made it likely that they would eventually take a course of consultation and negotiation. Those involved as plaintiffs found Australian governments dilatory and ungenerous, and Peter Gordon finds the compensation experience proof of the need for retaining intact common law rights and trial by jury[67]; a contrary view holds that confronting governments with the threat of costly and lengthy litigation subverted the common law by preventing judicial determination.[68] The scheme finally arrived at resolved a difficult set of issues in a manner that is considered exemplary by the only international comparative evaluation of HIV blood compensation.[69]

The changes to the system of blood supply and control introduced in the mid-1990s create in principle greater coherence in planning for new threats and greater accountability. What it eliminates is a cardinal virtue of federal arrangements, which allow for local initiative based on different perceptions of risk by institutions and individuals like Gordon Archer. Risk is now calculated in national cost-benefit terms, and this will work against the adoption of absolute standards of protection such as that sought by the Red Cross in seeking full security through national blood shield legislation or by the Haemophilia Foundation in seeking subsidized access to recombinant factor VIII. Discussion is already engaged concerning the need for policy concerning blood screening to be made beyond the parameters of the ARCBS.[70]

As one participant in policy making over the past two decades has observed, "the AIDS epidemic closed an age of innocence for blood banking."

NOTES

I am grateful for discussion of a first draft of this chapter by those who attended the project workshop held at Castello di Santa Maria Novella in July 1996, and for helpful comments on various drafts from Gordon Archer and Bob Beal, former directors of the Sydney and South Australia Blood Transfusion Services; Brian Candler, Mike Mossop, and Alex Proudfoot of the Commonwealth Department of Health and Family Services; Ian Gust, now of CSL Ltd; Jenny Ross of Haemophilia Foundation Australia; Glyn Davis, Margaret Duckett, Norbert Gilmore, and Julie Hamblin.

1. See J. A. Ballard, "Australia: Participation and Innovation in a Federal System," *AIDS in the Industrialized Democracies: Passions, Politics and Policies* ed. David Kirp and Ronald Bayer, (New Brunswick: Rutgers University Press, 1992); J. A. Ballard, "The Constitution of AIDS in Australia: Taking Government at a Distance Seriously," *Governing Australia: Studies in Governmentality* ed. Barry Hindess and Mitchell Dean (Melbourne: Cambridge University Press, 1998).

2. L. Stubbings, *'Look What You Started, Henry': A History of the Australian Red Cross 1914–1991* (Melbourne: Australian Red Cross Society, 1992), pp. 6–20.

3. A. H. Brogan, *Committed to Saving Lives: A History of the Commonwealth Serum Laboratories* (Melbourne: Hyland House, 1990), pp. 1–10.

4. A. H. Brogan, *Committed to Saving Lives: A History of the Commonwealth Serum Laboratories* (Melbourne: Hyland House, 1990), pp. 66–67.

5. M. L. Verso, "Fifty Years of the Red Cross Blood Transfusion Service in Victoria," *Victorian Historical Journal*, 51 (1980), pp. 218–236.

6. M. L. Verso, "Fifty Years of the Red Cross Blood Transfusion Service in Victoria," *Victorian Historical Journal*, 51 (1980), pp. 218–236; L. Stubbings, *'Look What You Started, Henry': A History of the Australian Red Cross 1914–1991* (Melbourne: Australian Red Cross Society, 1992), pp. 232–237.

7. Australian Red Cross Society to prime minister, April 1, 1977.

8. A. H. Brogan, *Committed to Saving Lives: A History of the Commonwealth Serum Laboratories* (Melbourne: Hyland House, 1990), pp. 94–98.

9. K. Beauchamp, *Red Alert: Is Regulation Working for Imported and CSL Blood Products?* (Canberra: Rupert Public Interest Movement, 1994), pp. 61–81.

10. For example, K. Beauchamp, *Red Alert: Is Regulation Working for Imported and CSL Blood Products?* (Canberra: Rupert Public Interest Movement, 1994), pp. 138–145.

11. W. Muraskin, "The Silent Epidemic: The Social, Ethical, and Medical Problems Surrounding the Fight against Hepatitis B," *Journal of Social History*, 22 (1988), pp. 277–298.

12. B. Courtenay, *April Fool's Day* (Sydney: William Heinemann, 1993).

13. *The Australian* (May 10, 1983), p. 1.

14. *Campaign* (June 1983), pp. 5, 10.

15. For example, G. Bell, "Bad Blood," *Who Weekly* (April 20, 1993) 38–41; M. Goldsmith, *Political Incorrectness: Defying the Thought Police* (Rydalmere: Stoddard and Houghton, 1996), p. 75.

16. Victoria adopted the wording "many partners," which later raised an issue in litigation for compensation.

17. K. Mutton, and I. Gust, "Acquired Immune Deficiency Syndrome," *Medical Journal of Australia*, 138 (1983) pp. 540–541.

18. D. A. Cooper, "The Acquired Immune Deficiency Syndrome: Conference Report," *Medical Journal of Australia*, 138 (1983) pp. 564–566.

19. National Health and Medical Research Council, "Acquired Immune Deficiency Syndrome (AIDS)," *Medical Journal of Australia*, 141 (1984) p. 561.

20. A. I. Adams, "AIDS and Blood Donors," *Medical Journal of Australia* 141 (1984) 558.

21. Gust later tested sera from 601 people who had tested positive to hepatitis B core antigen and found no evidence of HIV infection. He testified in the PQ case that neither HBc antibody nor T4/T8 ratio tests were appropriate surrogate tests for HIV.

22. *Daily Telegraph* November 17, 1984.

23. *The Australian*, November 17, 1984.

24. The Belgian tests, based on French antigen, proved ineffective, as did other European tests until manufacturers obtained the U.S. antigen.

25. J. Godwin et al., *Australian HIV/AIDS Legal Guide*, 2nd ed. (Sydney: Federation Press, 1993), pp. 57–60.

26. National Centre in HIV Epidemiology and Clinical Research, *HIV/AIDS and Related Diseases in Australia: Annual Surveillance Report 1997* (Sydney: NCHECR, 1997), p. 51.

27. *House of Representatives Hansard* May 22, 1985.

28. National Centre in HIV Epidemiology and Clinical Research, *An Epidemiological Assessment of the HIV Epidemic in Australia*, (Canberra: Australian Government Publishing Service, 1996), pp. 116–118.

29. Gust, in testimony to PQ case.

30. National Centre in HIV Epidemiology and Clinical Research, *An Epidemiological Assessment of the HIV Epidemic in Australia* (Canberra: Australian Government Publishing Service, 1996), p. 118.

31. A look-back program for New South Wales was introduced under Jenny Learmont, a counselor at the Sydney BTS. Records of donors dated back to January 1980 and as of September 1983, when they were computerized, could be linked to recipient records; the NSW program identified 129 cases of HIV acquired by transfusion. Learmont's program was extended nationally and her research later assisted rapid identification of hepatitis C in the blood supply back to the 1960s. She also identified an HIV-transfusion group of non-progressors, leading in 1995 to the discovery of a mutant strain of HIV. See *The Australian Magazine* (September 16, 1955), pp. 10–14.

32. P. O'Keeffe, "AIDS, Blood and Rights: A Scrutiny Role for a Senate Committee," *Legislative Studies* 2(2) (1987) 32–38; Cooney in *Senate Hansard* (May 11, 1987, June 4, 1987); Collins in *Senate Hansard* (May 25, 1988).

33. See J. Godwin, et al., *Australian HIV/AIDS Legal Guide*, 2nd ed. (Sydney: Federation Press, 1993), pp. 435–446.

34. Commonwealth of Australia, *AIDS: A Time to Care, A Time to Act: Towards a Strategy for Australians* (Canberra: Australian Government Publishing Service, 1988), pp. 189–191.

35. Personal communication, David Sinclair, Administrator of the Mark Fitzpatrick Trust, May 27, 1996.

36. *Dwan v Farquhar* 1 QR. 234 [1988].

37. *H v Royal Princess Alexandra Hospital for Children* [1990] Aust Torts Reports 80-000; see R. Plibersek, "Transfusion-Acquired AIDS: Is Anyone Legally Liable?" *Law Society Journal* 28(5) (1990), pp. 53–58.

38. 99 ALR 601, 105 ALR 53 [1991].

39. See M. P. Bastianon, "AIDS and the Blood Bank: The Argument for Strict Liability Exemption," *University of Tasmania Law Review* 11 (1992), pp. 191–205; J. Godwin, et al., *Australian HIV/AIDS Legal Guide*, 2nd ed. (Sydney: Federation Press, 1993), pp. 434–435.

40. *Sydney Morning Herald* (June 15, 1996).

41. G. Peter, "HIV Litigation in Australia," *Convention Papers, 28th Australian Legal Convention, Hobart, 28–30 September 1993* 1 (1993), pp. 187–189.

42. *PQ v Australian Red Cross Society*, 1 VLR 19 [1992].

43. Supreme Court of Victoria, February 25, 1991; appeal dismissed March 7, 1991, unreported, No 5065 of 1990.

44. See further discussion of this issue in R. S. Magnusson, "Public Interest and the Confidentiality of Blood Donor Identity in AIDS Litigation," *Australian Bar Review* 8 (1992) 226–244; J. Godwin, et al., *Australian HIV/AIDS Legal Guide*, 2nd ed. (Sydney: Federation Press, 1993), 70–72; J. Hamblin, "Identifying Blood Donors Infected with HIV," *Australian Health Law Bulletin* 1 (1993), pp. 69–70.

45. Parliament of New South Wales. Legislative Council. Standing Committee on Social Issues, *Medically Acquired H.I.V.* (1991), p. 21.

46. *PD v Australian Red Cross Society*, unreported, App Ct NSW; see J. Hamblin, "Identifying Blood Donors Infected with HIV," *Australian Health Law Bulletin* 1 (1993) pp. 69–70.

47. S. Loane, "How the Blood Bank became a Blood Bath," *Times on Sunday* (May 3, 1987), p. 13.

48. K. Kenrick, "Quality Control," *Living with AIDS: Toward the Year 2000—Report of the 3rd National Conference on AIDS* (Canberra: Australian Government Publishing Service, 1988), pp. 317–326; E. M. Dax, and T. A. Vandenbelt, "HIV Antibody Testing in Australia", *Journal of Acquired Immunodeficiency Syndromes* 6(Suppl 1) (1993), pp. S24–S28; B. R. Wylie, "Blood Transfusion in 1993," *Modern Medicine* 36 (11) (1993), pp. 89–95.

49. B. R. Wylie and R. Y. Dodd, "Protecting the Blood Supply from HIV," *Medical Journal of Australia* 165 (1996), pp. 264–265.

50. *The Australian* (August 27, 1997).

51. *Sydney Morning Herald* (May 22, 1998).

52. G. S. Whyte and B. R. Wylie, "Thanksgiving Day for the Gift of Life," *Medical Journal of Australia* 167 (1997), pp. 7–8.

53. Personal communication, Dr Gordon Whyte, Director of Victorian BTS, October 1996.

54. See D. R. M. Buckley and H. I. Starr, "Blood Banks, Plasma Derived-Therapeutics and the Therapeutic Goods Act 1989—The Commencement of Good Manufacturing Practice Auditing and the Lessons Learned," *Transfusion Transmissible Infectious Agents*, ed. Kenneth G. Kenrick, (Sydney: NSW Blood Transfusion Service, 1994), pp. 70–80.

55. A. H. Brogan, *Committed to Saving Lives: A History of the Commonwealth Serum Laboratories* (Melbourne: Hyland House, 1990).

56. C. Hamilton and J. Quiggin, *The Privatisation of CSL*, Discussion Paper 4 (Canberra: Australia Institute, 1995), p. 10.

57. Australian National Audit Office, *The Sale of CSL: Commonwealth Blood Product Funding and Regulation* (Audit Report No. 14, 1995–96), (Canberra: Australian Government Publishing Service, 1995); Australia. Parliament. Joint Committee on Public Accounts, *Review of 1995–96 Auditor-General's Reports*, (Report no. 349 of February 1997), pp. 10–21.

58. For background on the latter, see G. S. Whyte, "Is Screening of Australian Blood Donors for HTLV-1 Necessary?" *Medical Journal of Australia* 166 (1997), pp. 478–481.

59. B. McKay and R. Wells, *Commonwealth Review of Australian Blood and Blood Product System: Final Report* (1995).

60. Australian Health Ministers' Advisory Council, *Working Party on Factor VIII Supply: Report, February 1995* (Canberra: Australian Government Publishing Service, 1995).

61. M. Allars, *Inquiry into the Use of Pituitary Derived Hormones in Australia and Creutzfeldt-Jakob Disease: Report* (Canberra: Australian Government Publishing Service, 1994).

62. This had been achieved with human tissue legislation drafted by the National Law Reform Commission in the early 1980s.

63. R. Hetzel and R. Kimber, "The Australian Red Cross Blood Transfusion Service," *Medical Journal of Australia* 166 (1997), pp. 453–454.

64. J. A. Ballard, "The Constitution of AIDS in Australia: Taking Government at a Distance Seriously," *Governing Australia: Studies in Governmentality*, ed. Barry Hindess and Mitchell Dean (Melbourne: Cambridge University Press, 1998).

65. P. Gordon, "HIV Litigation in Australia" in *Convention Papers, 28th Australian Legal Convention, Hobart, 28–30 September 1993* 1 (1993) p. 186.

66. B. Courtenay, *April Fool's Day* (Sydney: William Heinemann, 1993); J. Wiltshire, "Tales of AIDS in Australia: Politics and Narrative," *Quadrant* 38 (6) (1994) 36–42, provides a detailed rebuttal.

67. P. Gordon, "HIV Litigation in Australia," *Convention Papers, 28th Australian Legal Convention, Hobart, 28–30 September 1993* 1 (1993), p. 197.

68. P. Blair, "Blood Money," *Polemic* 3(1) (1992), pp. 22–25.

69. J. Kelly, "The Liability of Blood Banks and Manufacturers of Clotting Products to Recipients of HIV-Infected Blood: A Comparison of the Law and Reaction in the United States, Canada, Great Britain, Ireland and Australia," *John Marshall Law Review* 27 (1994), pp. 465.

70. J. Kaldor, "HTLV-1 and Blood Safety: Let the Community Decide," *Medical Journal of Australia* 166 (1997), pp. 454–455.

II COMPARATIVE PERSPECTIVES ON THE POLITICS OF MEDICAL DISASTER

9 Cultural Perspectives on Blood

Dorothy Nelkin

B lood is a substance "thick with magical significance, mystical claims, pharmacological prodigies, alchemistical dreams," writes Piero Camporesi in *The Juice of Life*.[1] In earlier centuries, this substance was a daily reality, far more visible than it is today: "From birth to death, the sight and smell of blood were part of the human and social pilgrimage of each and all . . . as barbers, phlebotomists, pork butchers, midwives, brothers hospitalers opened, closed, cauterized veins."[2]

Today, in most of the countries that are represented in this volume, blood is more a virtual than a visual reality, enjoyed by audiences of grisly gangster films in abstract settings, observed by the voyeurs of televised massacres in distant lands, and managed mainly by the remote control. It is a substance, not of daily experience, but of accidents, illnesses, battles, or orgies—a substance to be avoided "in the flesh." Says Umberto Eco in his foreword to Camporesi's book, "We who use the Internet think blood of interest only to surgeons and the scholars of the new planetary pestilences."[3] Yet, he observes, there is remarkable rapport between the cultural myths of the time when blood was a daily and visible reality and the impulses of the present day.

We are just such scholars of the new planetary pestilence. So, in thinking about the responses to the devastating problem of HIV-contaminated blood products, I want to follow up Eco's observation. The realization that the blood supply had been contaminated—that private companies manufacturing blood products had been careless in their safety procedures and public regulators careless in their regulation—evoked furious responses throughout the world. In France, the scandal was compared to the Dreyfus affair, the great political trial of the Third Republic. In Japan, the scandal evoked a rage that forced public officials to make humiliating public apologies. In countries that have long tolerated corporate practices causing serious environmental pollution and occupational hazards responsible for deaths and disabilities, the public officials and private entrepreneurs involved in the distribution of contaminated blood products were publicly humiliated and severely punished. And at a time when international ideology celebrates our "global society" and the extension of international cooperation, the goal of plasma policy is national "self-sufficiency."

Why has this tragedy assumed such deep social and political significance? Why, when many risks are accepted as inevitable, is there such a visceral response to disclosures of HIV blood contamination? What accounts for variations in the responses in different societies? To illuminate these questions, it helps to consider some of the cultural and symbolic meanings that are associated with blood, and to tentatively explore their relevance to present-day impulses.

Blood is obviously an objective, biological substance; at the technical level, scientists share a set of common understandings about its physical attributes. But blood is more than a biological substance; it is also a cultural entity with complex social meanings that vary in different cultures and change over time. The social meanings placed on the body and on body parts often relate to the structure and strains of social relationships. Herbert Spencer drew a direct analogy between "the blood of the living body and the consumable and circulating commodities of the body politic."[4] Mary Douglas described the physical body as a metaphor for society—a "symbolic medium," a "visible expression of social relationships."[5] A similar assumption—that perceptions of the body reflect historical associations, political circumstances, and social relationships—will frame the analysis of this chapter on the cultural meanings of blood and their implications for controlling the safety of the blood supply.

Metaphors of blood have diverse and sometimes contradictory connotations. Blood is seen as a source of life and energy, but it is also a symbol of violence and danger. It is a metaphor for social solidarity and the connection between the individual and society, but it has also represented the biological distinctions between peoples and is linked to the politics of race and social class. Blood is a social fluid that calls for altruistic relationships, but blood plasma is an economic product that can be competitively bought and sold. Purity of blood is a clinical concept associated with physical health, but it is also a racist construct used to define ethnicity and to justify exclusion and discrimination. In its social meanings, blood can stand at once for purity and contamination, vitality and death, community and corruption, altruism and greed. With its multiple connotations and complex associations, blood is a malleable and powerful construct; the idea of tainted blood both reflects and effects social relationships, public trust, and the way people relate to authority and community.

In his classic book, *The Gift Relationship* (1971), Richard Titmuss wrote about how beliefs about blood are related to the organization of transfusion services and the safety of the blood supply.[6] Today, the problem of blood contamination has evoked what Theodore Marmor calls "the politics of scandal."[7] This politics has been partly influenced by the symbolic aspects of blood. Beliefs about blood find expression in the economics and politics of blood product distribution and regulation, the behavior of health care institutions in their efforts to assure a safe blood supply, the claims and expectations of HIV-infected individuals, and the public's perception of the nature, causes, and dangers of devastating disease.

Blood metaphors, collected from historical and contemporary sources, frequently cluster around four repeated and related themes:

> First, blood is defined as an essentialist substance, the essence of personhood, the basic life force.
>
> Second, blood—and the exchange or donation of blood—is an important symbol of community and social solidarity.
>
> Third, metaphors of blood are a means to represent the prevalence of danger and risk.
>
> Fourth, the concept of pure blood contains associations that extend well beyond the properties of a biological substance to include references to social relationships and moral as well as physical contamination.

In exploring metaphorical associations I do not wish to minimize the real tragedy of those affected by HIV-contaminated blood. Nor do I intend to provide an
exhaustive history of the beliefs, images, and myths surounding this evocative fluid.
Rather, I want to suggest that certain historical meanings associated with blood have
helped to define the tragic problem of HIV contamination, shape the systems of
blood donation, and influence the focus of responsibility and blame when safety
systems fail.

Blood as the Essentialist Substance

The cultural depiction of blood draws on the powerful essentialist images. The substance, for example, has been sacrilized and endowed with religious valorization. It
is, of course, of central importance in the eucharist doctrine of Roman Catholicism,
where bread and wine are transubstantiated into the body and blood of Christ. Here
the symbol of blood denotes the "real presence" of Christ in the church. Though
Calvin eliminated mystical practices from liturgical observance, the eucharist remains
a sensitive issue in discussions of the ecumenical movement.

An essentialist substance, blood is equated with life itself. In *The Juice of Life*,
Piero Camporesi described blood as "the seat of the soul—that invisible, elusive
principle that was deemed to ebb and flow in hiding, swelling and diffusing in the
oily liquid of life."[8] And as a life-sustaining fluid, blood in some cultures has been
associated with courage and with vital rejuvenating powers. The ancient Egyptians
bathed in blood to regain the powers of youth. Witches in the Middle Ages were
believed to drink the blood of youth as a way to keep their magical powers. And
Nicolae Ceausescu, the infamous and hypochondriacal Romanian dictator, was
suspected of harboring little boys in his castle both to brainwash them with his political ideology and to periodically draw blood from them for his own rejuvenation.[9]

In Japan, many people believe that blood type determines personal character.
More than a biological indicator, it is a "template" of identity.[10] According to Japanese folklore, a person who claims to be the heir of a deceased man drops a bit of
blood on the skeleton. If the bones absorb the blood, the relationship is established.
The Japanese press regularly publishes blood type analyses as a way to predict personality and behavior. Much like the American horoscopes, they are presumably to
be understood as partly playful, but partly serious. Magazine profiles of Japanese
political candidates include information about their blood types, dating services use
blood analysis to make matches, and mismatched blood types have been grounds for
divorce.[11] A Japanese company sells condoms that indicate blood type.[12] In Tokyo
the Blood Type Human Studies Research Institute analyzes the relationship of blood
type to personality and behavior. Perhaps this preoccupation with blood and its association with character helps to explain why Japanese persons with hemophilia (an

estimated 1800 people, 40% of whom are infected with the HIV virus) hide their condition, and, until recently, never publicly acknowledged that they have hemophilia or AIDS.

It is not only in Japan that blood is associated with behavioral characteristics and personality traits. In American popular culture, "blood" frequently appears as the word for "genes," implying that it holds meaning for the heritability of essential traits. In the American eugenics movement during the early part of this century, blood represented "stock," or "lineage," or "bloodlines."[13] The language of eugenics faded from public discourse after World War II. But today, encouraged by the highly promoted advances in genetics, the importance of heritability is again a prevalent theme in popular culture and the metaphor is still the "blood." For example, an American prime time TV film called "Tainted Blood," tells the fictional story of a pair of teenage twins who had been adopted as infants into "good" families in different parts of the country. Nevertheless they both ended up by murdering their parents as their biological mother had done. For they had inherited violent (tainted) predispositions. Criminal behavior was "in their blood."[14]

The use of blood to identify individuals has reinforced its essentialist meanings. Blood samples have served as a means of identification since the discovery of the Mendelian inheritance of blood groups in 1910. Blood-matching techniques developed at this time were understood to reveal the invisible biochemical properties that are the essence of a person and the definition of relationships. They were first applied in the 1920s to establish the relationship between parents and children, for example, in cases of infants switched at birth. Subsequently, increasingly sophisticated blood tests became a tool of investigation in cases of disputed paternity, inheritance claims, and criminal identification.

Acceptance of the use of blood for identification has varied in different countries. While accepted in the German legal system in the 1920s, the courts in the Anglo-American tradition would not admit serological evidence until much later, fearing that blood evidence would become a form of self-incrimination. In France and Italy, guided by the assumptions of the Napoleonic code, blood tests were rarely accepted. Their law codes followed the Roman principle of *pater semper incertus* (the father is always unknown). Thus, the use of blood to contest paternity challenged the "higher truth" of family unity. As a jurist explained in 1948, "Serological truth is perhaps a good thing, but the unity of the family is on a higher level."[15] Not so different was the court's decision in the 1995 trial of O.J. Simpson. The powerful scientific evidence provided by DNA analysis of Simpson's blood was, to the jury, far less important than the social issue of racism in the Los Angeles police department.[16] To scientists, blood reveals serological truth, but its social meaning is conditional on far broader social values.

Also, to scientists, blood is replenishable material. But in its social meaning, blood is more than material—it is the essence of personhood, an inviolable substance.

The taking of blood has evoked questions about individual rights. Is blood an inalienable part of the body, the property of an individual, a commodity, or a communal resource? Body parts such as a liver or kidney are regarded as inalienable, but blood as a replenishable substance is often exempt from this classification. Blood products such as factor VIII, manufactured from the blood of many persons, are generally defined as a commodity. But, in most countries, whole blood, donated by an individual, becomes a "good" or a product only when it is parted from the body, and the individual has no control of the disposition of his donated blood.[17] France, for example, imposed restrictions on "transfusions diriges" based on the assumption that an individual could not dictate the specific uses of a resource that belonged to the collectivity.[18] The practice in Holland apears to be an exception. There blood, according to de Vroom, remains "part and possession of the person who donates the blood." Blood taken for one purpose, therefore, cannot be used for another, even for research. This policy, reinforcing the individual's control over the use of blood, may have been the result of the origin of the modern blood donation system during World War II. This system developed as an underground movement to counter the routine collecting of blood from Dutch citizens for the transfusion of German troops.[19]

Conflicts between the scientific and essentialist meanings of blood underly an ongoing dispute over the Human Genome Diversity Project (HGDP). This is a project developed by scientists and several pharmaceutical and biotechnology firms to collect, store, and analyze blood taken from 25 individuals from each of 400 indigenous populations around the world.[20] The HGDP has several goals: to trace patterns of immigration, to develop a history of world populations, and to salvage the DNA of indigenous groups in remote areas that are believed to be destined for extinction. The scientists from the HGDP themselves use strikingly essentialist language when they talk about their plans to "immortalize" these populations by drawing their blood and banking it in order to preserve their DNA.

Some of the DNA collected from indigenous populations is also valued for its insight into rare genetic diseases, and its potential usefulness for the development of pharmaceutical products. Sometimes the cell lines and genes are patented. For example, researchers from the National Institutes of Health obtained a patent on the DNA from a man in New Guinea whose genes protected him from leukemia. And the Wellcome Foundation patented a cell line from an African child with a rare form of lymph cell cancer and then used the cell line to produce interferon.[21]

This explicit commercialization of blood through the patent process has been highly controversial. In 1993, the Rural Advancement Foundation International (RAFI) a non-governmental organization that conducts research and educational programs on the social impact of new technologies on rural people, received a copy of the HGDP proposal and distributed it to several indigenous organizations. To RAFI's constituency, the diversity program was a "vampire project," a pernicious form of "biopiracy."[22] They saw the project as a form of power and domination that would contribute to the further undermining of indigenous communities. They saw tampering with blood, and especially commercializing this essential fluid, as a desecration of the sacredness of the body. The negative publicity influenced the patent policy of the NIH, which eventually dropped its patent application for the New Guinea gene.

The continued scientific interest in the HGDP, however, continues to draw criticism. Indigenous groups have compared the drawing of blood to the stealing of the relics that are used in their community rituals, suggesting that blood not only has meaning as a religious substance but also plays a role in maintaining community solidarity.

Blood as a Symbol of Community

Beyond its essentialist meaning, blood — in social rituals and in the system of blood tranfusion — has come to represent community spirit, altruism, and social cohesion. Donna Shalala, Secretary of the U.S. Department of Health and Human Services, defined the blood supply as "a well spring of life, a source of security, and vivid testimony to the civic spirit that unites us as one people."[23] This communal or social meaning of blood is expressed in the common sayings that extend relationships of blood beyond the bonds of kinship: we often refer to "blood brothers" or "blood ties."

As a symbol of social solidarity, blood has been a critical substance in collective rituals. Anthropologist Mary Douglas suggests that rituals "work upon the body politic through the symbolic medium of the physical body."[24] To Douglas, blood rituals are a way that societies deal with the points of tension in their communities. Premodern societies, for example, have celebrated their salvation anxieties in rites of violence and blood. In such rites, blood was spilled in "dramatic presentation of collective mortification."[25]

Anthropologist Victor Turner described the Ndembu practice of carving the Mukula tree during circumision and childbirth rituals.[26] The tree secretes a red, blood-like gum that represents menstrual blood and the blood that accompanies the birth of a child. The ostensible purpose of the ritual is to coagulate the blood, and some of the symbolic acts in the ritual represent the desired coagulation. But the ceremony also has symbolic meaning for the community. The Mukulu tree represents both the woman's matrilineage and the principle of matriliny itself. The purpose of the ritual, according to Turner, is to make the woman accept her lot in life and thus to "celebrate and reanimate . . . tribal continuity through matriliny." Similarly, Rodney Needham, who observed blood rituals among the Penan of Borneo, suggests the association of blood with the Penan's mystical ideas about their relationships to the spiritual world. Such rituals maintain tribal continuity and community by ascribing and reinforcing the rules that govern appropriate behavior.[27]

In a contemporary analysis of blood contamination and the social meaning of "poisoned" blood, Thomas Murray, a bioethicist, describes how the gift of blood— a form of altruism—has served to bind and affirm social connectedness and community by linking the blood donor to strangers and the donation to the public good.[28] In this social context, the fears of pollution that are expressed in the responses to HIV-contaminated blood extend beyond individual risk to threaten the sense of community solidarity.

Autologous blood donation is a common way that individuals have responded to the AIDS crisis. But this growing practice has implications for the social meaning of blood donation. A common supply of available blood is frequently associated with ideas of justice and fairness. In France the blood donation system is based on an ethic of equality and national solidarity. After the Revolution, according to Jane Kramer, "the sang impur of aristocrats and priests and other degenerates of the ancien regime . . . was supposed to be the last bad blood in France."[29] The blood of every individual represented "the blood of France" and revolutionary ideals proclaimed that the people's blood be "held in common because the people were a community."[30]

Yet until World War II, the blood distribution system in France remained under the control of private physicians or hospitals, and they had their own network of paid blood donors.[31] Later, during the Second World War, the French Partisans formed a system of voluntary blood donation to help their injured troops. Volunteer donors were viewed as courageous patriots helping in the national liberation. At this time, the practice of paid donation became associated with "bad" blood taken from poor and exploited people. After the war, the voluntary system became the basis of a 1952 decree establishing public blood centers. Blood, as a symbol of equality and community in France, was to be freely donated and cost free.[32] Self-donation or "tranfusion dirige" were avoided until the risk of AIDS shattered the ideology of solidarity associated with the "people's blood."

The strength of such associations, the relationship between the ability to donate blood for the public benefit and the sense of belonging to a community, has made it difficult to exclude high-risk groups from blood donation. The concern about safety that encourages the exclusion of certain groups with a high prevalence of AIDS directly conflicts with the idea of community associated with giving blood. This fundamental dilemma was strikingly expressed in a riot of Ethiopian Jews in Israel in January 1996. They had discovered that the health authorities were secretly dumping their blood donations out of fear that, given the relatively high rate of AIDS in the Ethiopian population, their blood might be contaminated. The blood was disposed of quietly to avoid stigmatizing the donors. But to the Ethiopians, the very act of rejecting their blood became a symbol of their exclusion from the community. Thus, the incident evoked extraordinary anger and violence: "Our blood is a red as yours," proclaimed a protestor's banner.[33]

Exclusion from donation reflects accepted boundaries of community. In Japan, where blood is a symbol of national identity, blame for contamination was placed on the importation of foreign blood, especially blood from particular ethnic groups.[34] But even where blood is not a special symbol of national identity, foreign blood has been suspect, as in the United States where Haitians were excluded from the blood donation system.[35] In southern Italy, where group loyalty is strongly focused on the family rather than on the collectivity or the nation, another pattern prevails.[36] There, loyalty sentiments—within the family or among closely associated workers—have determined the pattern of blood donation; for the most part, people donate blood only to family members. The resulting shortage of available blood in Italy has required the importation of more than 75% of plasma needs.

In stark contrast, the Indian blood-banking system depends mainly on paid donations by professional blood sellers, often "pavement dwellers" who earn their livelihood through selling their blood.[37] Commercialization of blood donation is the norm. Payment for blood donation here and elsewhere is a response to shortages and the need to provide incentives to give blood. At the same time, where blood is identified as both an essentialist and a communal substance, its commercialization becomes suspect. For to place economic value on blood through the payment of blood donors threatens the value of altruism underlying its distribution.

The individualistic culture of the United States formally maintains a dual system, but paying individuals for donating whole blood is rare.[38] However, about 90% of source plasma comes from paid donors, often from prisoners or the poor.[39] Ambivalence about paying plasma donors, however, is apparent in language—Americans still talk of "donation" and "giving" even when "donors" are paid. We would scarcely be comfortable with a label of "blood vender," or a description of a "blood market." And "donations" that are based on economic interests rather than altruism tend to be devalued and stigmatized. For example, anthropologist Martin Kretzman studied the American system of blood donation as a participant observer and found that paid donors were kept waiting, pushed around, and treated as morally suspect. The staff assumed that they might be concealing information and worried that they had "bad blood." After their blood was drawn, their money was placed on the counter "in the way a prostitute might be paid after sex."[40] Donation—as the literal meaning of the word implies—is supposed to be an altruistic act.

Profitting from blood is widely considered to be aggregious and exploitative. In 1973, the Nicaraguan dictator Somoza helped to open a blood center that purchased and then exported plasma. A newspaper editor criticized Somoza for "inhuman trade in the blood of Nicaraguans." The editor was later killed and at his funeral, a riotous crowd burned the plasma center.[41] Yet, in the United States, similar practices of purchasing plasma do not evoke a public reaction. While common phrases such as "blood money" or "bloodsuckers" suggest the pejorative implications of connecting blood with money, commercial blood banks are not burned. They are, however, sometimes suspect. In 1955, an early commercial blood bank in Kansas City in 1955 was commonly referred to as the Vampire bank.[42] Turning blood into an economic product seems to violate beliefs about its importance as a public good, and economic motivations raise questions about communal values. Is it right to "break the bonds of community" through directed donations rather than maintaining a communal blood supply? The commercial interests involved in the banking of blood or the manufacturing and selling of blood products maintain a fragile credibility.

The situation in Canada is particularly revealing. There blood donation had long been a voluntary and respected humanitarian activity; about 700,000 people offered their blood annually as a "gift of life" and the Canadian Red Cross Society was a trusted institution.[43] But the ideology of altruism was disrupted when blood was used for the commercial manufacturing of blood products such as factor VIII. The highly respected Red Cross became suspect. Reflecting tensions with the United States, self-sufficiency—that is, independence fom American plasma sources—became the goal.

In the United States, the fundamental tensions over the social meaning of blood are explicit in an ongoing debate over the privatization of cord blood.[44] Placental blood can be harvested from the umbilical cord immediately after birth, and banked for the future as a substitute for bone marrow transplantation. This cord blood was once considered waste and thrown away, but the ability to freeze and store the product has turned it into a valued commercial resource. Thus, this substance has become a focus of property disputes. Who owns cord blood—the infant, the parents, or the society? Is placental blood the private property of an individual or a public resource—a common good? Private commercial interests are involved in the storage of cord blood in special private "banks." Who should be able to deposit or withdraw blood from these banks? The original plan had been to store umbilical cord blood in publicly funded blood banks. As a public resource, the material would be available for those in need of a bone marrow transplant. Cord blood is immunologically naive and matching is usually unnecessary. Moreover, any given individual is unlikely to need a transplant, so that it is an ideal communal resource. Yet companies are tracking pregnant women and urging them to privately bank their children's cord blood as a kind of insurance against future medical needs. These companies charge a one-time fee (of about $1500) to store the blood plus an annual storage charge.

The dispute over cord blood reflects broader tensions in American society over property rights, and especially over the commercialization of the body. It is further complicated by the fact that genetic information can be derived from stored blood. Even a drop of blood can be genetically analyzed to reveal a great deal about an individual's future health status and personal characteristics. Indeed, in the age of genetic diagnostics, blood is increasingly associated with the powers and dangers accruing to those with access to personal and predictive information.

Blood as a Symbol of Danger

The association of blood with power and danger is explicit in the stories and myths surrounding the violent history of colonialism. The response to the HGDP is but one example of how the taking of blood has become a metaphor for exploitation. A Guatemalan myth dwells on a practice that supposedly occurred when the Spanish Conquistadors invaded the highlands. According to the story, these pale-skinned people drained the blood of brown-skinned babies to cure their own anemia.[45]

Anthropologist Luise Whyte, collecting oral histories in Uganda, has documented similar rumors about white people who captured Africans and extracted their blood.[46] Her stories suggest that between 1918 and 1925, vampires appeared in Uganda and used needles to suck the blood of Africans. The vampires sold or drank the blood while their victims, drained of blood, collapsed. So powerful were these rumors that in the 1950s a white doctor in Kampala could not convince Ugandans to donate blood because they believed that the doctor drank the blood himself.

The vampire stories were a colonial phenomenon that disclosed anxieties about Western medical practice and experimentation. Whyte cites an informant: "When the Europeans were here . . . it was not easy to convince somebody that they were going to do research so what they did was kidnap those people." Another informant told her that Europeans came from hospitals where "people are required to donate blood for their sick relatives."[47] In 1972, a letter to the editor in a Tanzanian newspaper reported the mysterious disappearance of people whose "blood was used to treat the white man only."[48] Such rumors revived a widespread belief that "Europeans wandered around the country seeking human blood for purposes of making medicine." The taking of blood was equated with exploitation. Similar stories reappear whenever blood is collected; they circulated in the 1980s, for example, when officers from a veterinary department in Uganda collected blood in order to find out whether yellow fever was endemic to the territory.

Variations in the vampire myth have appeared in many other contexts where there are social tensions, for they serve as a way to identify the sources of danger and to place blame. They appeared, for example, in the nineteenth century blood libel stories about Jews who purportedly killed Christian boys and used their blood to make matzoh during the Passover holidays. These powerful and pernicious stories were myths of danger and they were employed to reinforce stereotypes and to justify the pogroms. They persisted until World War II.

Ideas about dangerous blood have long been used to stereotype women, especially in historical descriptions of menstruation.[49] Menstruation has been categorized in medical textbooks as a disease and associated with defilement, dirt, disorder, and danger.[50] Physicians during the Victorian age wrote of women "harboring polluted blood." One doctor described the uterus as "the sewer of all the excrements existing in the body."[51] But even contemporary physicians have referred in medical journals to menstruation as "endocrinopathy," in effect a blood disease.[52] As a source of putrefaction, menstrual blood was a symbol of danger and violence. And, related to intense emotion, it was associated with hysteria, long believed to be a characteristic woman's disease that must exclude her from occupational opportunities.

Vampire myths enjoyed a revival in the 1990s. They appeared in popular culture narratives that associated blood with violence, or with a fear of predators or "bloodsuckers" who threaten the integrity of the person. In the classic vampire myth, common in Slavic countries, the soul of a dead man quits his body to suck the blood of living persons. Then, when the grave is opened, the corpse will be fresh from the infusion of fresh blood. The story is about the power and danger of the dead. A 1992 vampire film, Bram Stoker's Dracula, conflated blood transfusion with sex—the men who gave their blood to Lucy talked about it as if it were a sexual act. In a deluge of 1990s American vampire films, including The Melrose Vampire, Vampires 90210, Bordello of Blood, and Kindred—the Embraced, blood is routinely used for spectacular effects to suggest grave danger and mortal risk. A trashy film called "Hellraiser: Blood Line" manages to associate blood with sex, violence, and also heredity. Drenched in blood, this film, specializing in torture, S & M, and decapitation—all to the tune of bloodcurdling screams—is about a man who carries demonic spirits in his blood. He inherited his uncontrollable tendency toward violence through his "bloodline."

The revival of the vampire myth has also generated a scene in the East Village of New York City where vampire fans have formed nightclubs, published magazines (the Vampire Information Exchange Newsletter), and created a form of punk music called Gothic rock. It is a kinky and trendy pastime marked by a taste of blood that may represent a defiance or a denial of AIDS. In an ad in the newsletter, one man offered "to become a donor to a female vampire."[53]

Finally, the association of blood with danger appears as well in the enormous genre of AIDS art, which is replete with bloody representations.[54] In AIDS art, the use of blood represents a source of danger, pollution, and risk. The precisionist painter, Frank Moore, for example, links AIDS with pollution by depicting beaches that are covered with the debris of syringes and the remains of impure blood.[55] Such ubiquitous images are associated with danger, but they also convey notions of blood purity. The social meaning of pure blood is complex, including references to social relationships and to moral as well as physical contamination. These associations are important to think about as we consider the variety of efforts being made to assure the purity of the blood supply.

The Social Meaning of Pure Blood

Until the seventeenth century work of William Harvey, people commonly attributed disease to bad blood. But, also, it was widely believed that the biological properties of blood varied with the socal position of the person. Nobles, for example, enjoyed superior social status because of the purity of their blood and the integrity of their bloodlines.[56]

The ascendance of a scientific world view equalized the properties of blood, which became, in effect, an exchangeable commodity. Yet the myth that races have unique blood characteristics and that these can be correlated with both physical appearance and social behavior has persisted. This was most clearly articulated in Nazi Germany where, as Anthony Synnott described it, "the ideology of blood purity spilled rivers of blood."[57] Less dramatic manifestations of the same myths appeared elsewhere. Despite the urgent need for blood during World War II and the scientific understanding of blood types, the United States Congress pressured the American Red Cross to exclude black donors from the national blood donation program. During the early years of the war, they were excluded, but later, as the need for plasma increased, the Red Cross accepted their blood, but still segregated it. Critics accused those who wanted to accept the blood of black blood donors of trying to "mongrelize" the nation.[58] Similar sentiments about the purity of Japanese blood led the Japanese to set up special brothels for the G.I. occupiers after World War II in order "to protect the purity of blood" in Japanese society.

Today, the notion of pure blood still carries associations with ideas of racial purity, social status, and, in some cases, national character. Sherry Glied has reviewed the pervasive assumption that paid blood, usually from those of lower socioeconomic status, is dangerous or likely to be impure.[59] Eric Feldman has described the beliefs of Japanese plaintiffs in the hemophilia lawsuits; they argue that paid blood was taken from "homos," blacks, and Mexicans.[60] Umberto Izzo observed that the Italian media associated paid blood with "the ghettos of large Amercian cities.[61] Blood, as suggested above, has become both an instrument for exclusion within national blood systems and an argument for the need of self-sufficiency in national blood programs.

The association of polluted blood with race in part reflects realistic concerns about the contamination of blood from high-risk groups. But its prevalence also reflects myths about race purity and the longstanding association of race categories with purity of blood. Race categories in America have long been based on ideas about "blood quanta." American Indians have been identified through "blood quantum" rulings that have required individuals to prove they have a specific percentage of Indian blood to qualify for land allotments and services. But this has also excluded them and subjected them to discrimination. So too, African Americans were identified by the "one drop of blood rule," which defined a person with even a drop of "black blood" as black. Blood became a metaphor for pedigree or ancestry in the American South, where miscegenation laws used the metaphor of "black blood" to separate the legal concept of race from skin color. The skin could lie, allowing a person to pass, but the blood represented "serological truth"; it defined and identified race.[62] Southern judges, called upon to determine the race of individuals, expressed concern about the "purity and defilement" that could result from interbreeding.[63] Thus, ideas about the purity of blood served to reinforce prevailing social biases.

Xenophobia and nationalism still pervade arguments about blood purity, as we have seen in the willingness to blame foreigners for HIV blood contamination.[64] In Japan, tainted blood became a metaphor for the mistrust of foreigners and foreign blood products.[65] In Canada, reflecting longstanding political and economic tensions, it is assumed that Canadian blood is cleaner than American blood.[66] Because the entire world had been forced to rely on plasma collected from American sources, America has been often the focus of blame. The solution, proposed in most countries is "self-sufficiency."

The use of blood metaphors in immigration debates suggest the depth of this xenophobia. Blood language is a way to express political anxieties about the threat of foreigners to national borders. Beliefs about body pollution reflect fears of social pollution, as Mary Douglas claims.[67] In the early part of the century, concerns about growing immigration in the United States were expressed in the language of blood pollution. The dangers of mixing blood and the need for purity were instrumental in the passing of restrictive immigration laws in 1926. A similar set of metaphors have reappeared today in the rhetoric of nativists. Using blood as a word for genes, they believe that "mixing blood" will lead to race suicide. In his anti-immigration book, *Alien Nation*, Peter Brimelow writes that "a link by blood" is essential to the successful functioning of a nation.[68] Brimelow and other nativists of the 1990s worry that the mixing of race groups that inevitably follows immigration is threatening the social order and the existing structure of power. Worrying about miscegenation, they draw on metaphors of blood purity that have long been invoked as a way to protect societies against foreign intrusion.[69] And they are reflected today in the tendency in many countries to place the blame on foreigners for contaminated blood.

Notions of blood purity are also invoked to maintain moral boundaries. Stories and myths of blood pervade the moral discourse about AIDS. Disputes over the rights of people infected with AIDS bring forth such myths. In 1985, for example, a decision to allow a seven-year-old child infected with AIDS to attend a public school in New York provoked a raging public dispute.[70] The debate revolved around the danger of body fluids—saliva, tears, and, especially, blood. Some parents insisted on the isolation of children with AIDS because of the danger of their blood. What would happen if an AIDS child has a nosebleed or cuts himself? Little boys, after all, fight. What if children prick themselves and exchange blood through blood brother rituals, draw blood in a fight, or get bitten by the same mosquito? During an angry public hearing—after all, a modern form of ritual—participants spelled out contamination scenarios in detail. A child with AIDS gets a nosebleed; the blood spurts onto the floor or onto another child's desk. A second child has an open wound and touches the blood. Children are usually innocents in our pantheon of images, but these scenarios turned them into monsters, wallowing in their secretions, unsocialized in sanitary behavior, and basically out of control. The stigma of AIDS as a symbol for moral as well as physical contamination evoked images of impurity, guilt, and sin even among children, and this was enhanced by its association with body fluids—with tainted blood.[71] Unclean fluids, taboo conduct, and deadly disease became connected in this discourse, reinforcing fears of physical, moral, and social danger.[72]

Similar associations appeared in response to the attempts of Ryan White—another child with AIDS—to enter the Kokomo Indiana school system. When the community's parents found that he was infected with the HIV virus, they organized a boycott of the school. Later, Ryan's photograph appeared in an Associated Press article in which he was identified as a "homophiliac (sic) who had contacted AIDS through a blood tranfusion."[73] This typographical error, conflating hemophilia and homosexuality, is a frequent malapropism that has even been heard in the context of our international meetings involving sophisticated physicians, academics, and administrators involved AIDS policy. It is an amusing slip except in the context of the stigmatization of children who test positive for the HIV virus. For they are, inevitably, morally contaminated by their "bad blood."

I have suggested in this chapter that the social meaning of pure blood has associations that extend well beyond the problem of biological contamination. Some of these associations are based on biological realities—there are certainly high-risk groups. But often they reflect social stereotypes, political tensions, or moral rigidities. "Contaminated blood" implies bad social relationships; it is a source of social and moral as well as physical illness, a cause of divisiveness and conflict, a basis for profound mistrust. The blood contamination incidents, therefore, have had an extraordinary tendency to evoke political scandals as well as to cause disease.

Analysis

In the Cold War context of 1985, a striking AIDS cartoon appeared in the Soviet newspaper, *Pravda*, just at the time of the freeze in American-Soviet relations. The artist portrayed an American general paying a sleazy-looking scientist for a test tube of AIDS-contaminated blood, presumably to be used as a weapon of biological warfare. The viruses swimming about in the test tube were tiny swastikas. The cartoon also depicted the dead, the victims of AIDS, as holocaust victims, stacked like cordwood. The Soviet cartoonist used contaminated blood to portray the United States as sadistic and degenerate. His powerful image of blood contamination associated American imperialism with Nazi fascism and dread disease.[74]

The symbolic importance of blood contamination relates to social and political strains—including the antagonisms of the Cold War, race and social class tensions, and even anxieties about our ability to contain terrorism. A revealing fictional scenario depicting possible forms of biological terrorism appeared in the *Journal of the American Medical Association.* A disgruntled supervisor of a large blood bank introduces the Ebola virus into blood products, exposing thousands of people to deadly infection.[75] Such stories suggest how the special anxieties or vulnerabilities of a society may be expressed through defining danger and attributing blame for disease. In this project, we have seen how blame for contamination has sometimes focused on race stereotypes or on foreign blood products; sometimes on regulatory incompetence and often on corporate greed. The rhetoric is replete with xenophobic references and each country has its own favorite scapegoats. Where blame is focused reflects historical or social circumstances and prevailing attitudes toward industry, medical professionals, and the regulatory bureaucracies of the state.

In American society, for example, debates over the risk of HIV-infected blood products reflect the risk debates taking place in many other arenas—over environmental threats, toxic contamination in the workplace, leaking breast implants, and harmful food additives. These quite different disputes share a common discourse of responsibility and blame, for they have revolved around a widespread belief that commercial greed would undermine responsible behavior, that government is in collusion with corporate interests, and that scientists are "hired guns." Depending on the cultural context, dangers—from environmental pollution or from blood contamination—are blamed on corporate irresponsibility, individual behavior, or social failure. (Signficantly, disasters, these days, are seldom blamed on fate or bad luck.) The specific location of responsibility and blame for blood contamination is influenced by prevailing political perceptions as well as science-based evidence.

Different actors within a country have inevitably defined the problem of contamination in different ways. This became explicit in the public testimony presented at the public hearings convened by the National Academy of Sciences, Institute of Medicine, in 1995 to examine the causes of the contamination of the clotting factor used by hemophiliacs.[76] At these hearings, representatives from the blood banking and manufacturing community talked about statistical estimates of risk, accepted standards of safety, and the risk-benefit calculations that were relevant at the time. They described the situation as a "tragic accident." To those who had been responsible for technical evaluations of blood safety, the crisis was not just a matter of the bad blood that had contaminated the clotting factor, but also the lack of public confidence and trust, and especially what they believed to be an unrealistic public expectation of zero risk. They viewed the problem of assuring a safe blood supply as manageable, to be resolved through technical and organizational solutions.

To hemophiliacs, the meaning of contaminated blood was nothing short of genocide resulting from corporate greed, and callousness, the drive for profit, and the corruption and collusion of the regulatory system. They compared factor VIII to Zyklon B, the poison gas used in the holocaust death chambers. Understandably enraged, they sported T-shirts at the public hearing depicting a "hemophilia holocaust." In his public testimony, Bob Baldwin described himself as a "hemophilia holocaust victim." "I stood in a line of death. To the left was commercially prepared clotting concentrate . . . the gas chambers. To the right was cryoprecipitate . . . working in the fields." Jonathan Botelho, representing the National Hemophilia Foundation, defined the tragedy as "a clear sign of fatal complacency in the Body Politic." It is, he said, a breakdown in the society. "The big guys kill off the little ones." The message from the hemophiliacs was their mistrust of industry, government, and the medical profession as well. "What does this tell us about the industry's view of the value of our lives and those of our families. . . . We were expendable in the face of corporate profits. . . . The alleged regulators at the FDA had abdicated their statutory responsibility to protect the safety of the nation's blood supply." It was, claimed the hemophiliacs, no less than criminal inaction. It was all a "big lie," a "slaughter for money." "Profit and spread sheets were more valuable than our lives." They called for recompense and retribution.

The participants in these public hearings expressed their beliefs in often extreme language. Yet, their views reflected the broader context of risk disputes in the United States and other countries—a context marred by mistrust of government, fear of risk, and a growing ambivalence about the value of scientific and technological progress. On the one hand, contemporary consumers and patients seek the latest technological solution to their problems, but on the other, they mistrust technology. Many people suspect that their cancers have been caused by environmental contamination, or their diseases by faulty consumer products. They often blame their illnesses on the excesses of companies driven by the profit motive—by corporate greed. They are convinced that companies and regulators are "in bed together." Disputes over risk—whether from contaminated blood, silicone breast implants, radiation, or dioxin—express profound suspicion of industry and regulatory authorities, and growing mistrust of scientific expertise.

The responses to blood contamination in many of the countries we have examined in this volume take place within this broader framework of mistrust. Though blood is more a virtual than a visible reality in modern society, concepts of blood and pollution remain embedded in the symbolic associations that have shaped our fears and guided our responses to the tragedy of AIDS from contaminated blood. How people think about blood reflects their views about the competence of their institutions, the integrity of their leaders, and the meaning of their social world.

NOTES

1. Piero Camporesi, *The Juice of Life* (New York: Continuum Publications, 1995), p. 54.
2. *Ibid.*, p. 27.
3. Umberto Eco, Foreword to Camporesi, *ibid.*
4. Cited from Herbert Spencer, *Social Statistics* (London: Chapman, 1651), pp. 323–4, in Sally Shuttleworth, "Female Circulation," *Body/Politics*, ed. Mary Jacobus, Evelyn Fox Keller, and Sally Shuttleworth (New York: Routledge, 1990), p. 58.

5. Mary Douglas, *Purity and Danger* (New York: Routledge, 1966), Introduction and Chapter 7.

6. Richard Titmuss, *The Gift Relationship* (New York: Pantheon Books, 1971).

7. Theodore Marmor, Patricia Dillon, and Stephen Scher, "Conclusion: The Comparative Politics of Contaminated Blood: From Hesitancy to Scandal," Eric Feldman and Ronald Bayer, eds., *Blood Feuds: AIDS, Blood, and the Politics of Medical Disaster* (New York: Oxford University Press, 1999).

8. Camporesi, *op. cit.*, p. 32.

9. Personal communication with Radu Popa.

10. Eric Feldman, "HIV and Blood in Japan: Transforming Private Conflict into Public Scandal," Feldman and Bayer, *op. cit.*

11. See *New York Times* (December 30, 1995); and Abigail Hayworth, "Secret Asian Love Formula," *Marie Claire* (February 1996), p. 36.

12. Advertised in *Colors*, Winter 1997.

13. Daniel Kevles, *In the Name of Eugenics* (New York: Knopf, 1985).

14. *Tainted Blood*, USA Channel, March 3, 1993.

15. See William Schneider, "Blood Group Research between the World Wars," *Yearbook of Physical Anthropology*, 1995. Schneider cites Pierre Barbier, "L'Examen du sang et le role du juge dans les proces relatif a la filiation," *Revieu Trimestrielle du Droit Civile* (1949), pp. 345–371.

16. Jeffrey Toobin, *The Run of his Life: The People v. O.J. Simpson* (New York: Random House, 1996).

17. See discussion in Ronald Bayer, "Blood and AIDS in America: Science, Politics and the Making of an Iatrogenic Catastrophe," Feldman and Bayer, *op. cit.* and Umberto Izzo, "Blood, Bureaucracy, and Law: Responding to HIV-Tainted Blood in Italy," Feldman and Bayer, *op. cit.*

18. Jane Kramer, "Bad Blood," *The New Yorker* (October 8, 1993), pp. 74–95.

19. de Vroom, personal communication.

20. L. L. Cavalli-Sforza et al., "Survey of Human Genetic Diversity: A Vanishing Opportunity for the Human Genome Diversity Project," *Genomics*, 11 (1991), pp. 490–491.

21. Andrew Kimbrell, *The Human Body Shop* (San Francisco: Harper, 1994).

22. Rural Advancement Foundation International *Communique*. See issues dated Jan/Feb 1994, Nov/Dec 1994, and May/June 1995. Also see *Cultural Survival Quarterly*, special issue, "Genes, People and Property," Summer 1996.

23. Donna Shalala, cited in a news press release by the U.S. Department of Health and Human Services, July 13, 1995.

24. Douglas, *op. cit.* p. 153.

25. *Ibid.*

26. Victor Turner, *The Forest of Symbols* (Ithaca, NY: Cornell University Press, 1967).

27. Rodney Needham, "Blood, Thunder and Mockery," *Sociologus*, 14,2 (1964) pp. 136–149.

28. Thomas Murray, "The Poisoned Gift," *A Disease of Society, Cultural and Institutional Responses to AIDS*, ed. Dorothy Nelkin, David Willis, and Scott Parris (New York: Cambridge University Press, 1991).

29. Kramer, *op. cit.*

30. *Ibid.*

31. Monika Steffen, "The Nation's Blood: Medicine, Justice, and the State in France," Feldman and Bayer, *op. cit.* Also Marie Angele Hermitte, *Le Sang et le Droit* (Paris: Edition Seuil, 1996).

32. Note that sperm donation in France is also unpaid and donors are drawn from a special pool of men with children.

33. *New York Times* (January 29, 1996) and *Nature-Medicine* 2 (March 1996) p. 260.

34. Eric Feldman, "HIV and Blood in Japan: Transforming Private Conflict into Public Scandal," Feldman and Bayer, *op. cit.*

35. Ronald Bayer, "Blood and AIDS in America: Science, Politics and the Making of an Iatrogenic Catastrophe," Feldman and Bayer, *op. cit.*

36. Umberto Izzo, "Blood, Bureaucracy and Law: Responding to the HIV-Tainted Blood in Italy," Feldman and Bayer, *op. cit.*

37. Zarin Bharucha, "AIDS and Blood in India," unpublished paper prepared for the project HIV-Contaminated Blood: Policy and Conflict.

38. The relative percentage of paid and voluntary donation keeps changing. In the 1970s, voluntary donation increased with awareness of the need for blood (see Alvin Drake, Stan Finkelstein and Harvey Sapolsky, *The American Blood Supply* [Cambridge: MIT Press, 1982]).

39. Sherry Glied, "The Circulation of Blood: AIDS, Blood and the Economics of Information," Feldman and Bayer, *op. cit.*

40. Martin J. Kretzman, "Bad Blood," *Journal of Contemporary Ethnography* 20 (January 1992), pp. 416–441.

41. Thomas Murray, "Gift of the Body and The Needs of Stangers," *Hastings Center Report*, April 1987.

42. Andrew Kimbrell, *The Human Body Shop* (San Francisco: Harper, 1994) ch. 1.

43. Norbert Gilmore and Margaret Somerville, "HIV/AIDS and the Canadian Blood System," Feldman and Bayer, *op. cit.*

44. Declan Butler, "US Company Comes Under Fire in Patent on Umbilical Cord Cells," *Nature*, 382 (July 11, 1996), p. 99.

45. Introduction to Stuart J. Youngner, Renee Fox, and Laurence O'Connell (eds), *Organ Transplantation* (Madison: The University of Wisconsin Press, 1996), p. 8.

46. Luise White, "Cars out of Place: Vampires, Technology and Labor in Eastern and Central Africa," *Representations* (Summer 1993), pp. 27–50.

47. *Ibid.*

48. *Ibid*, p. 31

49. Margaret Lock, *Encounters With Aging* (Berkeley: University of California Press, 1993).

50. *Ibid.* and Shuttleworth, *op. cit.*

51. Shuttleworth, *op. cit.*, p. 56.

52. I. H. Thorneycroft, "The Role of ERT in Prevention of Osteoporosis," *Journal of Obstetrics and Gynecology*, 160 (1989), pp. 1306–1310.

53. *New York Times*, August 10, 1996.

54. Richard Goldstein, "The Implicated and the Immune: Responses to AIDS in the Arts and Popular Culture," in D. Nelkin, D. Willis, and S. Parris, *op. cit.*

55. Frank Moore, *Eclipse* (1992), at Sperone Westwater Gallery in New York City.

56. Davydd Greenwood, *The Taming of Evolution* (Ithaca, NY: Cornell University Press, 1984), ch. 4.

57. Anthony Synnott, *The Body Social* (New York: Routledge, 1993), p. 32.

58. Spencer Love, *One Blood* (Chapel Hill: University of North Carolina Press, 1996).

59. Glied, *op. cit.*

60. Feldman, *op. cit.*

61. Izzo, *op. cit.*

62. Eva Saks, "Representing Miscegenation Law," *Raritan*, (Fall 1988), pp. 29–41.

63. Kenneth L. Karst, "Myths of Identity," *UCLA Law Review*, 43 (December 1995), pp. 263ff.

64. David Wolff, "Blood Without Borders," unpublished paper prepared for the project HIV-Contaminated Blood: Policy and Conflict.

65. Feldman *op. cit.*

66. Norbert Gilmore, personal communication.

67. Douglas, *op. cit.*

68. Peter Brimelow, *Alien Nation* (New York: Random House, 1995).

69. For documentation of this language, see Dorothy Nelkin and Mark Michaels, "Biological Categories and Border Controls," *International Journal of Sociology and Social Policy*, 18 (1998), pp. 33–62.

70. For an analysis of this dispute, see Dorothy Nelkin and Stephen Hilgartner, "Disputed Dimensions of Risk: A Public School Controversy over AIDS, *The Milbank Quarterly*, 64, Suppl 1 (1986), pp. 118–142.

71. For discussion of stigmatization, see Norbert Gilmore and Margaret Somerville, "Stigmatization, Scapegoating and Discrimination in Sexually Transmitted Diseases," *Social Science Medicine*, 39, 9 (1994), pp. 1339–1358.

72. Sander Gilman, *Death and Representation: Images of Illness from Madness to AIDS* (Ithaca, NY: Cornell University Press, 1988).

73. *Ithaca Journal* (May 1, 1986).

74. J. Seale, "AIDS Virus Infection: A Soviet View of its Origin," *Journal of the Royal Society of Medicine*, 79 (1986), pp. 494–495.

75. Joan Stephenson, "Confronting a Biological Armageddon," *JAMA*, 296 (August 7, 1996) p. 349.

76. National Academy of Sciences, Institute of Medicine, *HIV and the Blood Supply* (National Academy Press, 1995). As a member of the IOM Commission, this author was present at these public hearings.

10 The Politics of Blood

Hemophilia Activism in the AIDS Crisis

David Kirp

Ideas, once called into being and rooted in important social groups, have a life of their own.

Eugene Genovese, *Roll, Jordan, Roll:*
The World the Slaves Made (1974)

The "Zap" at the Bayer Plant

On a warm afternoon in the autumn of 1996, a limousine pulled up at the gates of the Bayer AG plant in Berkeley, California.[1] A handful of young men piled out of the car, megaphones to the ready. "We are here to take your name away!" they shouted. "I.G. Farben, I.G. Farben, Zyklon B, Zyklon B"—an unsubtle reference to the lethal gas manufactured by the German pharmaceutical house and used to devastating effect in the Holocaust—"4000 dead, 4000 dead, 4000 dead." A cameraman recorded the scene, hoping to persuade local TV stations to air this "great source tape."

"Demo by limo," these demonstrators—"the wrecking crew . . . the Northern California boys in the band," as they called themselves—exulted in their Internet posting.[2] "How much more newsworthy can a story be?" Abruptly, however, the tone of the posting shifted and the demonstrators stood revealed as desperately sick, if still defiant, young men. "We might not be able to walk, but we can still demo!"

During the late 1980s and early 1990s, AIDS activists launched similar "zaps" against drug companies. Those demonstrators were mainly gay men, members of ACT-UP, expert practitioners in dramaturgical activism.[3] The object of their animus was the alleged profiteering by pharmaceutical companies that put AZT and other drugs in the HIV arsenal out of the reach of many people with AIDS. By 1996, ACT-UP, with its "Silence=Death" insignia, had disappeared from public view. The demonstration at the Bayer plant borrowed from the ACT-UP script, but there the similarity ended.[4] What united this new generation of activists wasn't their sexual orientation but a clotting deficiency in their blood. These men were hemophilia sufferers, and the *j'accuse* they directed at the pharmaceutical house was deadly serious.

Bayer is one of five U.S.-based companies that manufactures the blood-clotting products, factor VIII and factor IX concentrate, upon which people with hemophilia rely to live "normal" lives.[5] Because blood contaminated with HIV was used in preparing these concentrates, the hemophiliac population in the United States was decimated—these are the "4000 dead" to whom the demonstrators refer. And because many nations have depended on the United States to supply blood products to their hemophiliacs (in the 1980s, 60% of the world's plasma supply was collected in the United States), the deadly consequences of HIV contamination have been felt worldwide.[6]

A tragic accident, the pharmaceutical houses called it,[7] and a generation earlier, there would have been few dissenters from that judgment. But thalidomide,

Chernobyl, Agent Orange, Three Mile Island, Bhopal, Love Canal, mad cow disease—places and things that represent narratives of blame, not chronicles of inevitability—have made the public less inclined to accept fate rather than fault as an explanation for the horrific. Now a disaster of the scope of hemophilia AIDS invariably sparks a search for cause and culprit. The progression is so familiar as to appear lockstep, from naming the event to blaming and then to claiming. Injuries become comprehended as grievances, which are then formalized as disputes.[8]

So too with hemophilia and AIDS: the victims ultimately regarded what happened as no accident but rather as the inevitable result of decisions driven by corporate greed. Just as drug companies were complicit in the Holocaust of half a century ago, at the Bayer plant and other public forums they stood accused of another holocaust: hemophilia genocide. [9]

The Mobilization of a Social Interest Group

Beginning in the mid-1980s, as the deadly effects of HIV-contaminated blood products became widely apparent, hemophilia sufferers mobilized in countries as politically and socially diverse as Australia, Japan, Germany, and the United States.[10] They transformed themselves from a loosely linked group of patients whose health was paternalistically managed by medical professionals and pharmaceutical houses into an insurgent movement—a social interest group with an identity, an animus, and a strategy. How this astonishing mobilization happened, and with what consequences for both hemophilia sufferers and AIDS policy, is the focus of this chapter.

This flurry of activity flies in the face of the conventional wisdom, which holds that persuading people to take collective action is very hard work. People are not natural joiners. They do not readily form new associations with the aim of influencing public policy, even when they share hopes or grievances. When they do come together, their involvement is often as evanescent as a day-long strike to protest proposed cuts in French social welfare programs or the 1995 "Million Man March" on Washington. "Homo civicus," as Robert Dahl observes in *Who Governs?*, his landmark account of political behavior, "is not, by nature, a political animal."[11] In *The Logic of Collective Action*,[12] a classic in economic literature, Mancur Olson contends that the rationally self-interested individual, homo economicus, will not participate in organized activities intended to secure some collective good, because the costs of such involvement outweigh whatever benefits he will receive. Only in extraordinary circumstances, Olson concludes, do people shift away from "hopeless submission . . . to an aroused readiness."[13]

If organization is hard work generally, disease is an especially unpromising starting point from which to launch a social movement. "All people are potential patients, but as long as they are healthy they usually are not concerned about hospitals, doctors, and drugs" — or disease-based organizations.[14] When they do become sick, they regard that circumstance as a personal and private matter. A diagnosis is less obviously the basis for constructing an identity than an affliction from which the sufferer devoutly wishes to recover.

Moreover, because many illnesses carry social stigmas, patients' talk is often filled with self-denigration, attributions of bad genes or ill-considered lives.[15] Better health is conventionally understood as depending not on the actions of one's fellow sufferers but rather on one's own willingness and capacity to comply with expert medical advice. (In this regard, the medical language is revealing: When a treatment does not work the patient is said to have "failed the treatment," not vice versa.) This emphasis on individualism undercuts the usual rationale for collective action, that joint activity is needed for a mutually desired end.

Patients with a chronic disease like kidney failure or hemophilia aren't quite so unorganizable, for they already possess some shared social capital.[16] Their persisting health problems make them aware of the need for a particular type of care — dialysis for those with kidney failure, the regular and reliable supply of blood products for people with hemophilia — and in seeking this care they come into contact with fellow sufferers. There has historically been a role for organizations like hemophilia foundations that claim to look after the interests of patients with chronic diseases. But AIDS evoked both a radically different world view and a different kind of collective action. Like other social movements, its members were "claiming collectively the right to realize their own identity: the possibility of disposing of their personal creativity, their affective life, and their biological and interpersonal existence."[17]

Among the scores of hemophilia rights groups that sprang up across the globe, there are significant differences, and these are rooted in varying political and social histories. Australia and Canada have a robust tradition of interest group organization, for example, whereas France and Japan do not. The role of the public health system also varies from place to place — it is stronger in Germany than Italy — and so does the capacity of the legal system to furnish substantial relief.[18] Hemophilia organizations in some countries have operated like traditional interest groups, concentrating on pressuring government for favorable action; elsewhere the emphasis has been on the self-reflexive construction of an identity that is the hallmark of new social movements.[19] Many of the hemophilia groups have engaged in both insider politics and identity formation. [20]

Such variation is to be expected. What is unusual, and so noteworthy, are the cross-national similarities.[21] All these groups adhere to the core belief that a regime of incompetents and evil- doers, not a tragic accident, caused the deaths, worldwide, of more than half of those with severe or moderate hemophilia. Their anger has been directed at multiple targets: at the pharmaceutical firms that manufactured the deadly product; at governments, for their failure to deliver timely warning of the danger; at the doctors, who misled them; even at their own organizations, despised by the newly mobilized for having minimized the risk of exposure to HIV. In country after country, they have demanded and obtained compensation from drug companies and governments.[22] The movement has forced the creation of public tribunals, seeking and winning apologies for wrong-doing, or pressed its agenda in the courts, securing criminal verdicts against wrongdoers.

The emergence of a social interest group—and, concomitantly, a politics of identity—among hemophilia sufferers invites a platoon of questions. How did this transformation come about? Why did activists define themselves as they did, as innocent victims entitled to recompense? How were polities in so many nations prompted to revisit their conception of hemophilia sufferers and respond so sympathetically to their claims? How did people with hemophilia relate to the gay-led AIDS movement?[23] And what does the emergence of a hemophilia movement imply, not only for policy making about AIDS or the blood supply but also for any health policy issue whose implications intersect with the politics of identity—consequences that after the fact can be perceived as tragic or, so very differently, as genocidal?

Hemophiliacs and Gay Men: The "Odd Couple" of AIDS

During the early years of the AIDS epidemic, hemophilia sufferers and gay men were the two hardest-hit groups in the population.[24] Even though on the face of it they have little in common (aside from the fact that both are all-male), their social histories are intertwined. Joined in stigma, they mobilized very differently in the face of AIDS.

Both gay men and hemophilia sufferers have habitually been regarded as less than normal, tainted by bad blood or deviant behavior.[25] Indeed, the differences between them have sometimes been blurred. Before factor VIII concentrate enabled them to live close to normal lives, many young hemophiliacs, frail and effeminate in manner, were derided as "hemo-homos."[26] Derogatory judgments also found their way into the intimate precincts of the family, as parents blamed themselves for having passed along a defect, whether through genetic inheritance (bad genes) or environmental influence (overprotective mothers and distant fathers producing homosexuals, in the classic psychoanalytic account). Homosexuals and hemophilia sufferers responded by internalizing the shame of their circumstance, living closeted lives, concealing or camouflaging the significance of their condition.

Liberation came to hemophiliacs and homosexuals at almost exactly the same time, at the end of the 1960s. But liberation took entirely different forms. For hemophiliacs, factor VIII was the medical miracle, the "magic bullet" that promised to make their individual lives close to normal.[27] For gays, liberation began with a political event—the unprecedented refusal of homosexuals, gathered on a sultry evening in the summer of 1969 at a New York City bar called the Stonewall, to submit to a police roust.[28] Their defiance sparked emulation in cities across the United States and in scores of nations.[29] "Come out, come out!" became the rallying cry of a new movement, shame and secrecy upended by pride in gay identity.

Unsurprisingly, liberation meant very different things for these two groups. Hemophiliacs and gay men had distinct aspirations, differed in their inclination to construct a social movement, and held opposing attitudes toward the professionals who regulated their lives. During the 1970s, none of this mattered much, as newly liberated gays and hemophiliacs lived in separate universes. With the advent of AIDS, however, these differences proved consequential.

People with hemophilia simply wanted to be rid of their condition, to live lives as close to normal as medically possible.[30] Because normality was understood in medical terms, their liberation wasn't accompanied by organization building. On the contrary: with factor VIII readily available, hemophiliacs saw themselves as having less need for solidarity. Hemophilia associations had been organized a generation earlier, but these were tiny groups, often little more than letterhead organizations that teetered on the edge of bankruptcy.

People with hemophilia saw nothing problematic about the lack of solidarity. They implicitly trusted their caregivers, the physicians, and the pharmaceutical establishment, who had brought normality within reach. Even in the mid-1980s, many continued to believe the pharmaceutical companies' assurances that factor VIII concentrate was basically safe. They clung to the belief that they were safe from AIDS because the virus killed only homosexual men.[31] Not until the terrible impact on their community was too plain to deny did people with hemophilia begin turning to collective action.[32]

Normality for gays, by contrast, was not a medical construct but a controversial cultural idea. After Stonewall, some homosexuals did (and do) aspire to be offered a "place at the table."[33] Others joined forces with emergent social movements in coalitions of the newly liberated. Still others—the "nelly queens" of an older generation, the self-proclaimed "queers" of today—devised an alternative identity for themselves.[34]

Until the epochal events at Stonewall, homosexuals were not organized because of their well-founded fears about the consequences of public exposure. It soon became evident, however, that if the goals of gay liberation were going to be achieved, individual gestures were insufficient. Collective action was required. During the 1970s, gay groups of varying ideological stripes formed under the banner of this new social movement. The emergence of a "gay pride" movement began in the United States, then was adapted elsewhere by homosexuals who now had the reason, the opportunity, and the wish to come together.

Not every homosexual got involved in movement building. Some remained closeted for fear of exposure. Others behaved as free riders, declining to participate in these social interest groups even as they benefited from the movement's accomplishments. Still, at the outset of the AIDS epidemic there was a pool of homosexuals, trained in politics and organizing, prepared to take up the AIDS cause.[35] Even as some of these insurgent groups focused on questions of identity, making their presence felt by blockading the New York Stock Exchange or marking sidewalks with "Silence=Death" insignias, others sought to influence the policy debates. They insisted that national governments treat AIDS as a public priority[36] and pressed for a role for homosexuals in devising and implementating AIDS policy.[37]

The narrative of gay-dominated AIDS organizations was mostly borrowed from gay liberation. AIDS was a disease against which war had to be waged, not a moral judgment. Although doctors and scientists were essential allies in this fight, they had to be prodded to act less cautiously than was their custom, and also had to overcome homosexuals' long-standing suspicions.[38]

This history of distrust encouraged considerable initiative-taking by gays with AIDS. In the United States, gay-led AIDS groups pushed for quicker access to promising treatments and went abroad to obtain drugs that weren't legally available at home.[39] Stingy governments, foot-dragging bureaucrats, and money-driven drug companies: these were the enemies in the gay AIDS narrative. Gays infected by the disease rejected the labels of AIDS victim, AIDS sufferer, or AIDS patient, because such terminology implied passivity and helplessness, traits that were inconsistent with the group's self-composed identity. "People with AIDS" or "people living with AIDS" were the proper signifiers for people determined to shape their own fates.[40]

For gays and hemophilia sufferers alike, AIDS marked the end of a brief chapter of personal liberation. The first cases of what would become known as AIDS were identified in 1981: that was less than a generation after Stonewall, less than a decade after factor VIII concentrate became widely available.

Hemophiliacs, Gays, and the Blood Supply

Almost from the outset of the AIDS epidemic, and well before HIV was identified as the responsible agent, scientists speculated that one likely way this disease could be spread was through blood. Because the earliest cases had been reported in gay men, it was proposed that to reduce this risk of blood-borne contagion, homosexuals be prevented from donating blood. As the head of AIDS activities at the U.S. Centers for Disease Control argued, "people are dying. The medical problem is more important than the civil rights issue."[41]

Gay-run AIDS groups and the professional-dominated hemophilia organizations initially resisted such restrictions. For different reasons, each downplayed the risks of an AIDS-tainted blood supply.[42]

Gay groups feared that excluding homosexuals as blood donors would define them as outcasts. Gay men would be singled out as responsible not only for their own deaths but also, through the vector of blood, for the deaths of "innocents." Such a construction of the nascent epidemic would undermine gays' standing in society and threaten their own liberation, so recently and imperfectly won.

The priority of the hemophilia associations was to assure the continued availability of factor VIII concentrate. Hemophilia sufferers would accept the risk of blood contamination, presumably minuscule, the head of the Danish Hemophilia Society contended, in exchange for the benefits of access to this blood product. In taking that position (identical to the stance adopted in the 1970s, when factor VIII was contaminated with hepatitis B), the hemophilia professionals had the support of their patients. Many hemophiliacs were strongly resistant to switching from factor VIII concentrate back to cryoprecipitate, for such reasons as convenience, cost, denial of risk, and unwillingness to give up the freedom that concentrate provided.[43]

The split between gays and hemophiliacs became plain in 1982, when the first three cases of an AIDS-related pneumonia were reported among hemophilia sufferers. Hemophilia organizations joined with public health officials to push for the exclusion of men who reported having had sex with men from the blood donor pool. While in some countries, gay AIDS groups accepted this change in policy, elsewhere, as in the United States, they were furious. "The concern of the National Hemophilia Foundation has been the safety of the blood products upon which the survival of hemophiliacs is based," the National Gay Task Force observed. "But to single out any segment of our society is divisive and dangerous. . . . Pitting victim against victim will serve only to divert attention from the vital medical and ethical concerns that lie at the heart of this crisis."[44]

This feared assault on gays never came to pass, and the policy of barring anyone who acknowledges having engaged in a homosexual act since 1978 was maintained, even after the development of a test to detect HIV antibodies. The issue has recently resurfaced in the United States and the Netherlands, where homosexuals who have tested HIV-negative for many years have requested that they be permitted to donate blood as an act of social solidarity. In the United States, neither public officials nor gay medical groups have sided with these would-be donors, but the manager of the Dutch Central Laboratory for Blood Transfusion Services has lent his support to this request. Meanwhile, tensions persist between gay and hemophilia groups, rooted in conflicting visions of a just AIDS policy as well as different strategies for mobilization.

From Acquiescence to Activism

If a new social movement is going to take off, "passionate issue engagement" is essential.[45] "[P]eople must collectively define their situations as unjust and subject to change through group action. . . . Shifting political conditions supply the necessary 'cognitive cues' capable of triggering the process of cognitive liberation while existent organizations afford insurgents the stable group-settings within which that process is most likely to occur."[46] In short, members of these groups must agree on their collective identity.[47] Among hemophiliacs, such a process of identity formation began in the mid-1980s.

Central to this transformation of consciousness is the construction of a narrative, an account of how things are that is both persuasive to watchful outsiders and true to members' sense of themselves.[48] Such a narrative "assigns meaning to, and interprets, relevant events and conditions in ways that are intended to mobilize potential adherents and constituents, to garner bystander support, and to demobilize antagonists."[49] It gives voice to the deep concerns of those in the group—belonging and exclusion, agency and powerlessness, grievance and response—and so provides the membership with "moral capital."[50] It values the authenticity of constituents' experience over the claims of expertise, which are perceived as elitist and dependency-promoting. The narrative comes replete with heroes and villains, horror stories and war stories, ideological truths and (because it is an organizing tool) the anticipation of happy endings. It is the statement of a calling, a mission. In place of a politics of give-and-take is the purity of a politics of struggle, as everything that matters becomes a matter of justice.[51]

As the toll of blood-linked AIDS deaths mounted, both among people exposed to the virus through transfusions as well as hemophiliacs, levels of anger also rose. Whether this anger became a precursor to collective action—whether naming and blaming led to framing—depended on whether or not these individuals were able to mobilize. Hemophiliacs organized. Transfusees, though similarly afflicted, did not.

People infected while receiving HIV-contaminated transfusions were widely diffused among the population. They represented a near-random sampling of their nation's citizenry, with no history of being oppressed by their condition and no organization to which they could turn. In this respect, they were much like those characters, beloved by playwrights and novelists, who at some fateful moment chance to be on the bridge at San Luis Rey, or taking a cruise on the "Ship of Fools." The fact that these individuals shared an AIDS diagnosis and an animus against blood banks wasn't reason enough for them to come together.

With a handful of exceptions (notably an Australian group, TRAIDS—Transfusion-based AIDS), this category of AIDS patients has not organized. Instead, they have gone to court, not as a group but singly, arguing that the hospital or blood bank that supplied them with tainted blood should be held liable. Those cases have thrust upon judges and juries the familiar task of assigning legal responsibility. Some cases have resulted in monetary awards (of varying amounts), and others have ended in dismissals, a range of outcomes that mirrors the individualization of grievances.

Hemophiliacs, unlike transfusees, were organized. But the institutions that spoke for them were effectively led by medical professionals, with whom the blood-processing companies were "shamelessly aligned."[52] Association officials, themselves doctors, routinely had contractual ties to and hence a financial stake in pharmaceutical houses. The plasma derivative industry routinely made grants to these associations, underwriting youth camps, periodicals, and conferences. Such links had been unquestioned in the small world of hemophilia because during the era of "golden boys (doctors)" and "golden patients,"[53] no conflict was perceived among the parties at interest.[54] This web of mutual dependencies prompted hemophilia associations to be hypercautious in their initial responses to the AIDS epidemic, anxious not to give offense to their corporate backers.

Commenting on the 1983 decision of a drug company to withdraw a batch of factor VIII concentrate, the U.S. National Hemophilia Foundation (NHF) declared: "It is not the role of the NHF to judge the appropriateness of corporate decisions made by individual pharmaceutical companies. . . . . [such corporate decisions] *should not* cause anxiety or changes in treatment programs." Some months later, the NHF reaffirmed that "the life and health of hemophiliacs depends upon the appropriate use of blood product [as prescribed by their physicians]."[55] Nor was the organization willing at this crucial period to push for heat-treated factor VIII, citing cost as the reason for its reluctance to act.[56]

The consequences of financial dependence were even more obvious at the international level. Since its launching in 1963, the World Federation of Hemophilia had relied on the pharmaceutical firms to underwrite its activities. In 1980, federation founder Frank Schnabel (who earlier had formed the Canadian Hemophilia Society) used the bully pulpit of the *WHF Bulletin* to praise Cutter Laboratories for its financial contributions, unsubtly chiding other "benefiting companies" for "hav[ing] failed to participate in the funding . . . in effect, enjoying a free ride. . . . Will the other members of industry match Cutter's contribution . . . ?"[57] Although the WHF insisted that it was autonomous, so tight were these linkages, so substantial the dependency of the medical specialists on their pharmaceutical patrons, that the federation forbade as unseemly any criticism of the drug companies until its 1994 conference.[58]

Beginning in the mid-1980s, hemophilia activists changed this pattern. In country after country, they either took control of their organizations, shattering the familiar arrangements, or split off to form new organizations.[59]

The French Hemophilia Association had adopted a policy of quiet diplomacy concerning AIDS. In 1987, when the blood scandal that would eventually threaten the government was breaking in that country, the organization made quiet over-tures to the health ministry, justifying this backdoor approach by its concern "not to have hemophiliacs talked about" and its reluctance "to accuse either doctors or the State." Barely a year later, however, a newly launched splinter group, the Asso-ciation of Poly-Transfused Persons, brought claims against the blood banks — and against the Association as well — for failing to assist hemophiliacs in lodging their grievances. "The prospect of jail," said the organization's leader, "tends to cure bureaucratic amnesia."[60]

In the United States, the Committee of 10,000 was launched in 1991 by hemo-philiacs who rejected the posture of the established organization, the National Hemo-philia Foundation.[61] The Committee's report, "The Trail of AIDS in the Hemophilia Community," based on documents turned over during litigation, was offered as "evi-dence that demands a verdict."[62] On the West Coast, another newly formed group, the Hemophilia/HIV Peer Association, took an even more aggressive stance.

The Turin branch of the Italian Hemophilia Foundation broke off from the par-ent organization in 1987, complaining about its timidity. A year later, a new and more activist-minded group, the Association of Poly-Transfused Persons, based in Turin, was started. In Denmark, the Netherlands, and Canada, among other countries, leader-ship of hemophilia associations passed into activists' hands.

With these shifts in leadership came a new policy direction. In the early years of the epidemic, hemophilia organizations had regarded AIDS as a tragedy for which no one was at fault. This new generation of activists constructed a narrative in which blame was pivotal. The companies that manufactured factor VIII should have known earlier in the epidemic that they were likely producing an AIDS-tainted product. Government officials should have stepped in more quickly, to protect them more vigorously. Their own doctors should have informed them of the true character of the risk they were running in relying on a blood product that, because it was drawn from so many donors, was so vulnerable to contamination.[63]

These newly energized groups adopted tactics that, if commonplace for other social movements, were anathema to hemophilia traditionalists — demonstrations, revelations of damaged lives, confrontations. In the Netherlands, a country long noted for its consensual style of decision making,[64] a 1983 debate over the blood supply became known as "Bloody Sunday" because of its acrimonious tone. In Denmark, doctors and hemophiliacs split in 1985 over the propriety of a more public and con-frontationist strategy.[65] The fact that the chairman of the Danish society's medical committee was a blood products manufacturer became a point of contention; no longer was there a perceived identity of interest between the pharmaceutical houses and the hemophiliacs. The Canadian Hemophilia Society, in the words of its presi-dent, started "crying scandal" on behalf of self-styled "victims," as hemophilia suffer-ers publicized their plight and called for an official investigation into the use of HIV-contaminated blood products. In Italy, the insurgent organization shattered the norms of privacy when it publicized stories of individual hemophilia sufferers on TV in order to stir public sympathy.[66] HIV-infected hemophiliacs in Denmark ignored the request of the Hemophilia Society that they not publicize their situation, and told their stories on television.

Among the 33 member nations of the World Hemophilia Federation, including countries such as Greece, Brazil, and Hungary, which had only modest public health systems, the major demand was that hemophiliacs with AIDS (or their families, in case of death) be financially compensated by the government and/or by the pharmaceutical companies that distributed contaminated blood products. The federation supported these efforts, even as it tiptoed through the social minefield of guilt and innocence. In a memo to its member nations, it noted with exquisite delicacy that "the public has to be convinced that hemophiliacs are *particularly eligible* for compensation, especially with respect to psychic and social aspects."[67] A few months later, the federation urged that governments recognize "the *uniquely tragic position* of people with haemophilia who have become HIV-seropositive through the use of medically indicated blood products."[68]

Initially, government and industry were unresponsive to this demand. Pharmaceutical firms denied any responsibility for the tragedy. Governments were loath to provide compensation, which carried the implication of blameworthy conduct and so might set a precedent for other AIDS-infected groups to lodge claims for their members. Support was eventually provided, though, once governments and drug companies found a way to do so while still saving face and avoiding the appearance of setting precedent. Financial help was accompanied by denials that payments were related to fault.

Public officials in France and Germany likened their compensation efforts to aid that they had previously provided after a health system breakdown — as for children who suffered the consequences of thalidomide or innoculation with a bad batch of polio vaccine — or in the wake of a natural disaster like a fire or flood. Canadian officials were willing to provide "humanitarian assistance" — a form of relief that didn't acknowledge blame — mainly because the government, wounded by criticism leveled against it at the International Conference on AIDS in Montreal, "couldn't afford the [political] consequences of a spate of lawsuits."[69] In Japan, monetary awards were proffered as the sweetener ("candy and a whip," in the Japanese phrase) in a 1987 law that otherwise rejected the concerns of hemophilia groups.[70] In Australia, assistance was referred to as no-fault compensation; in Britain, shades of Richard Titmuss, it was proffered as a "gift."[71]

The behavior of pharmaceutical houses was much the same. Even where they have set aside funds for hemophiliacs with AIDS — these firms have acknowledged wrongdoing only when extraordinary pressure has been brought to bear. Instead, settlement offers have been made to dispose of a troublesome situation at the least cost to their public image. Although the precise amounts of assistance widely vary (in several countries, Australia, Japan, France, Germany, and Canada among them, the payments have been substantially increased over time), payments are typically less than what a person who proved that his life had been shortened by the negligent or willful conduct of a drug company could hope to win through litigation.

"J'accuse"

As new information surfaced in the late 1980s and early 1990s about what was known about AIDS and tainted blood, when, and by whom, the narrative of the hemophilia movement became even more permeated with accusation. Pharmaceutical houses were charged with deliberately putting hemophiliacs' lives at risk by knowingly distributing tainted batches of factor VIII. Even after tests that could detect HIV antibodies in blood became available, the new revelations suggested that companies had failed to use them, for periods ranging from months to years, because doing so would have required them to destroy existing stocks. These firms also opted, mainly for economic reasons, not to switch to heat-treated factor VIII, a process that kills the AIDS virus, until their supply of the non-heat-treated product had been used up.[72] For their part, public health officials were charged with acting in criminal concert with the pharmaceutical houses. An accusatory finger was pointed at the United States, the leading supplier of factor VIII, as peddling death.[73]

In constructing this narrative of blame, hemophilia groups looked for tutelage across national borders. The World Hemophilia Federation's newsletter informed member country associations about what was happening elsewhere, and informal networks also swapped information. The advent of the Internet has been a godsend. Several hemophilia web sites offer a mix of personal accounts and policy discussion, creating a virtual movement in tandem with organizations on the ground.[74]

The drumbeat of betrayal and evil-doing reverberated around the industrial world. A "genocide" was occurring, the newly formed U.S. Hemophilia/HIV Peer Association declared in 1991, because of the "commercially driven practices of certain large pharmaceutical corporations." Those firms had failed to counter the earlier threat of hepatitis B." Had they done so, "they would have prevented the transmission of HIV." Moreover, "with the exception of persons who were transfused with contaminated blood, only our community has been brought down by AIDS precisely because we followed the advice of our doctors." The National Hemophilia Foundation was condemned in equally pungent language. Its sins, like those of the drug companies, began before the advent of AIDS, with its failure "to sound an alarm" about hepatitis B. When AIDS appeared, the foundation stuck with its head-in-the-sand approach: "[T]he NHF . . . advised hemophiliacs not to be alarmed and not to change their treatment methods. . . . That remained the advice we were given . . . into 1985. . . . In effect we were told by NHF to use [clotting factor] just as though there were no danger of AIDS." Such reassurances amounted to acts of betrayal. "We—the alienated—do not identify with the hemophilia institutions. After all the debacle of the 80s, we do not need an organization that cozies up to the corporate decision makers. . . . We need an organization that demands—not in lip service but for real—that every person who needs it gets the safest factor available and that is affordable."[75]

At the NHF's 1992 convention, protesters wearing death masks confronted "the corporate mass murderers." A "shame list" of physicians was posted, which included all the leaders in hemophilia treatment. A year later, hearings conducted by a committee of the Institute of Medicine, convened at the behest of several U.S. senators and the Secretary of the Department of Health and Human Services, became the setting for a drama of grief and rage. Those who spoke demanded justice, defined as apologies and compensation from the government[76] and the pharmaceutical houses. As one mother of two hemophiliac sons, dead of AIDS at age 36, declared: "Today we demand justice and shout to the world and to this committee, 'How did you let this happen to us? Why did you do nothing to prevent this?'"

The NHF refused to go along with the demand for compensation. Such a strategy, the organization argued, would be dangerously socially divisive—"an ideological throwback to Elizabethan Poor Laws, with notions of 'deserved' and undeserved populations." The new cadre of activists had no time for such ethical niceties. Compensation was demanded not only as financial relief but also as vindication, "a partial payment for wrongs that had been done."[77]

Across the nations, social interest groups sounded variations on this cry for justice. In France, which had a long tradition of venerating its blood donors, scandals over tainted batches of factor VIII and whole blood being used for financial reasons despite knowledge of their likely impurity led to an alliance of "'rebellious' hemophiliacs, career-motivated journalists, and lawyers interested in the case." So angry were the hemophilia sufferers that at the criminal trial of health officials, police were fearful that infected syringes would be thrown at the accused. Some high officials were jailed and others disgraced.[78]

Hemophiliacs in Australia, who from the outset of the AIDS epidemic had been asked to advise the government on policy, were not interested in apologies. However, they did want more financial support than had initially been offered.[79]

Although the strategy of the hemophilia movement in Japan was shaped by lawyer-advocates, the campaign reached far beyond the courtroom. When the Friends of Hemophilia Association announced in 1990 that it was suing the government and five drug companies, "[p]laintiffs were organized into several associations . . . modeled on Japanese citizens' movements of the 1970s. These organizations published newsletters, held symposia, and appeared in the media at every opportunity. . . .

Emphasizing the importance . . . of mobilizing a large citizens' movement, an attorney . . . stated, 'I think that we have learned on other occasions that rights will not be bestowed from above if we are silent.'"[80] Mass demonstrations were led by a charismatic teenager who went public as "a victim of the drug-induced disaster." On World AIDS Day in 1995, 1400 students demonstrated at Waseda University. Two weeks later, rallies were held in eight cities across the nation, while 2000 demonstrators massed at Tokyo's Ministry of Health and Welfare.

This vigorous public campaign, a rarity in Japan, forced drug company executives and health officials to rethink their earlier dismissal of the hemophiliacs' demands. A few months earlier, Green Cross, the primary supplier of blood products in Japan, had patronizingly said that "[w]e feel pity for the patients rather than being sorry for them." In 1996, amid a widening scandal, the company's director reversed field. When, during a meeting with spokesmen for the hemophilia group, his initial gesture of apology was rejected as superficial, he "got down on his hands and knees, and bowed so deeply that his forehead touched the floor. That was the defining moment of the conflict; a display of physical and psychological vulnerability."[81] One high-ranking Japanese government official has been sentenced to prison for his role in the blood products scandal, and officials at companies that manufacture blood products stand accused of falsifying data.[82]

Hemophilia organizations in the Netherlands initially cooperated with some seven hundred professional health care and welfare groups to develop a common strategy, an "AIDS platform"; however, this coalition collapsed early in the 1990s. The Dutch Hemophilia Society first sought an independent investigation into the origins of AIDS-tainted blood, and later filed a formal complaint against the medical authorities. In 1993, the ombudsman who investigated that complaint issued a report faulting officials for acting too slowly in failing to ban unsafe blood products and not increasing the supply of heat-treated factor VIII.

In Canada, 90 people who participated in blood policy-making and disseminating have been the focus of a several years'-long investigation by a government-appointed Commission of Inquiry. Some fifty thousand pages of testimony have been gathered, at a cost of $14 million (Canadian). Testifying before the Commission in 1996, hemophilia rights advocates argued that what had happened in Canada was as outrageous as the events in France, and anticipated a report that would result in criminal charges against the miscreants.

Activists in Germany criticized the German Hemophilia Association for failing to inform hemophiliacs about the risks of contracting AIDS until the mid-1980s. A quick financial settlement led to what health officials termed the "pacification" of the opposition, but the issue flared again in 1992 when UB Plasma, a German pharmaceutical company, was found to have used blood and plasma untested for HIV antibodies.[83]

Around the globe, as hemophiliacs looked back in anger, few nations have been free from recrimination. Even Switzerland—home of the International Red Cross, widely regarded as having set the gold standard for purity of the blood supply—had its own tainted blood scandal, its own *j'accuse*.

Innocent Victims—and Everyone Else

New social interest groups need to differentiate themselves in order to survive.[84] Antagonisms emerge in the competition for scarce resources, financial and otherwise. Narratives magnify differences and sharpen boundaries among movement organizations. Although the most familiar targets of social movements are repressive governments[85] and malevolent corporations, other interest groups may also become the foci of animus: we–they distinctions begin to get made. Concerning AIDS, hemophiliac groups came to speak of their "innocence" not only in the context of wrongdoing by government and blood product suppliers but also in contrast with the "guilt" of others, gay men and drug users, who carried the virus.

The worldwide campaign provided hemophiliacs who had been largely isolated from one another with a common identity and a common cause. Nowhere, however, have hemophilia sufferers formed mass-based activist groups like ACT-UP. Although the leadership changed—now it is fellow hemophiliacs, not doctors, who speak for them—levels of active participation in the movement have remained generally low. Zaps like the event at the Berkeley Bayer plant, and demonstrations where people with hemophilia were joined by others who took up their cause, as happened in Japan, have been rarities.[86]

Nor did the hemophilia movement form strategic alliances with gay-dominated AIDS groups. For hemophiliacs, the psychic wounds from the old schoolyard insult, hemo-homo, played a part in keeping the two groups separate. Some hemophilia activists, "obsessed with not having a link made between homosexuality and hemophilia," practiced "homophobia-phobia."[87] There was also a residue of distrust from conflicts early in the epidemic over whether homsexuals should be prevented from donating blood, as well as bitterness on the part of hemophilia organizations at gay groups that had seemingly ignored their plight. "Many homosexuals didn't want a public link made between the blood disorder and the 'gay plague,'"[88] because they remained fearful of being blamed for the deaths of hemophilia sufferers.

Gay and hemophilia groups have often skirmished. The president of the Danish National Organization for Gays and Lesbians complained in a 1985 newspaper interview that hemophiliacs were getting too much attention. In France, hemophilia association leaders relied on homophobic fears to justify maintaining a separation between hemophiliac and gay-led AIDS groups. Because all hemophilia sufferers are men, the spokesmen contended, the fact of their joining forces with gay groups could be read as suggesting that hemophiliacs were themselves homosexual. Hemophilia activists in Canada chastised the government for having acquired blood products from "a San Francisco centre with many gay donors."[89] Depending on the audience, such a charge could be heard as a straightforward commentary about unsound public health practice or as a suggestion that homosexuality itself was a menace to health. The Italian Hemophilia Association demanded hospitalization for hemophiliacs with AIDS separate from other terminally ill AIDS patients. Although the Association's stated intention was to secure treatment from "familiar" doctors, the result was to secure distinctly better accommodations for these "innocents." In Germany, after hemophiliacs infected with HIV were financially compensated, gay activists made a similar claim on the public fisc for their constituents, but received no support in their efforts from the hemophilia movement.

Underlying these skirmishes were basic differences in the aspirations, indeed the identity, of gay and hemophilia AIDS groups. With the exception of Germany, special compensation for gay AIDS patients was nowhere contemplated. Equal treatment was the goal—health benefits, drug treatments, disability insurance; the very things heterosexuals would receive under similar circumstances. Early in the epidemic, gay spokesmen invidiously contrasted the government's neglect of "their" disease, AIDS, with the prompt official response to epidemics that threatened the mainstream population, notably Legionnaires' disease in the United States and Toxic Syndrome in Spain.[90] Nor did gay organizations focus on identifying and punishing the culpable parties. At the outset of the epidemic, rumors swirled that AIDS represented a CIA plot to kill off homosexuals, but that claim was quickly dismissed as paranoid. Although Randy Shilts' international best seller *And the Band Played On* focused on "Patient Zero," a "Typhoid Mary" for AIDS, the idea that one person was responsible for the epidemic drew no support.

Gay men have regarded AIDS as a disease, not a conspiracy, and the gay AIDS narrative has emphasized empowerment, not victimhood. Participation in making and carrying out policy has been regarded as important as an expressive act, and also as a way to press for better AIDS treatment, a vaccine, and a cure. Some activists even developed expertise in the scientific underpinnings of the discourse in order to participate effectively in forums usually reserved for scientists.

Hemophilia groups took a very different approach. Well before the AIDS epidemic, a treatment system geared specifically for their needs was in place in many countries, the great achievement of the old-line organizations. Although AIDS meant new types of care were required, the movement didn't have to concentrate on obtaining specialized care. What's surprising, however, is that these organizations displayed little interest in AIDS science, the development of an AIDS vaccine, or a cure for the disease, even though that would help people with hemophilia. Instead, their demands have been expressed in terms of financial settlements and gestures of contrition.

The political strategy of the hemophilia movement has also depended on its distinguishing itself from other groups, relying on political and media allies from outside the realm of AIDS. In country after country, the narrative was much the same: a tiny minority, born with a medical condition that it sought to overcome with the help of modern science, is betrayed by the very forces that it regarded as its saviors. That story line plays irresistibly on the appeal of personality and the presence of a villain.

Politicians allied themselves with the hemophiliacs' cause for an assortment of reasons. In Japan, an ambitious health minister seized upon grievances over tainted blood products to clean house in his bureaucracy, in the process boosting his own career. In the United States, hemophilia sufferers formed alliances with the political right, as politicians openly hostile to gay rights concerns have been the prime backers of federal legislation that would benefit hemophiliacs with AIDS.

In France, the hemophilia movement joined forces for a time with the ultra-rightist National Front Party. To the National Front, which ran a hemophiliac with AIDS as a parliamentary candidate, the hemophiliac sufferers' plight illustrated the menace posed by foreigners and gays. "[T]here were posters on walls all over France—they were traced to the [National Front] Party's printer—which featured a torch with a flame of letters that spelled out 'Socialisme, Immigration, Delinquance, Affairisme,' for SIDA, the French acronym for AIDS."[91] This coalition angered other AIDS activists because National Front sponsorship divided people with AIDS into the innocent and the guilty. The popular press played up this division, featuring stories about "beautiful dying children, grieving parents, chilly villains and a disease of dark, carnal origin corrupting innocent French blood." Hemophilia activists saw the National Front as giving their cause new visibility at a time when no other politicians were paying attention. Once hemophiliacs' grievances were incorporated into the mainstream agenda, the movement severed its ties with the rightists.[92]

The international success of the hemophilia rights movement has been remarkable. In less than a decade, compensation has been awarded to people with hemophilia in almost every nation where it has been sought—66 countries as of December 1996, according to the World Hemophilia Federation. Apologies have been made to those infected with AIDS by government officials and blood product manufacturers. Tighter controls have been placed on the suppliers of blood and blood products, including the various Red Cross organizations. Widespread investigations have been launched, and criminal prosecutions pressed. In these triumphs, the movement may have sown the seeds of its own demise.

W(h)ither Activism?

The last chapter of the saga of AIDS, hemophilia, and bad blood—an account not only of how hemophiliacs themselves will fare, but also of how health policy generally will be affected—remains unwritten.

"Hi all and what can we do?": That question was posted on the Internet by an American hemophiliac named C. Williams in November 1996, on the eve of the settlement of the drug company litigation. "I am speaking about the need to become seen by the mainstream population. Without resorting to violence, what can we do to once again become a topic of disucssion in the press . . . to be seen not as trouble-makers but as people who will Not Go Away."

"The world needs to know the contempt these folks have for their best customers." (In the United States, the annual cost of blood products is more than a hundred thousand dollars per patient.) But the possibilities for effective movement action are limited—"Some kind of Factor strike? A long-term occupation or sit-down of some sort?" Williams ends his message on a note at once brave and fearful. "Hang in there fellow screw-ees. We shall not be screwed again (I hope not, anyway)."[93]

The hemophilia rights movement has been a hybrid of several familiar types of organization. Like the civil rights movement, it is identity-based. Like the animal rights movement, it is morally driven, its moral imagery centered on injustice. Like anti-war movements, it has an ideological element, opposition to corporate greed and its deadly consequence. It shares the concern of traditional interest groups, like labor and seniors' organizations, in getting more benefits for its membership.

Even as social interest groups come and go, political and societal structures carry on. But the residue of a movement's efforts, the taste left in the mouth, affects how officials react to claims voiced by the next wave of insurgent organizations. It also influences how policy is made and politics is conducted even in the absence of direct pressure. The practice of AIDS science, for example, continues to bear the imprint of ACT-UP–type activism,[94] even as the conduct of health policy generally has been affected by public responses to AIDS. In these ways, the impact of social movements can outlast their organizational life.

If a social interest group is to survive for more than a season, it must devise a language and structure fit for permanence. Charisma has to be routinized, the hardest stage in the life cycle of any organization.[95] Groups such as ACT-UP, which nurture themselves on a diet of high-pitched outrage, implode because they can't sustain the requisite level of fury. Old-line civil rights, farmer, and labor organizations degenerate into the very kind of hierarchical entity, unresponsive to constituents' concerns, that their organizers once sought to unhorse.[96]

The future of the hemophilia rights movement is as uncertain as C. Williams' Internet posting suggests. Blood-related controversies continue to break out, most recently in Ireland, yet the movement's activities have slowed. Having achieved much of what it set out to do, the social interest group has only the power of solidarity—or the possibility of a new threat to the purity of the blood supply—upon which to base its appeal.[97] Thus far, its message hasn't reached beyond AIDS and the blood supply, and as a French AIDS activist points out, "when you negotiate the price of your death, you don't do anything for your treatment."[98] Moreover, despite all the criticisms that people with hemophilia have leveled against their physicians, their continuing dependency on those physicians limits the potential for mobilization.

Tellingly, membership in hemophilia organizations declined once before—during the 1970s, with the availability of factor VIII, the supposed magic bullet that people with hemophilia believed negated the need for solidarity.[99] That faith was mistaken, of course, but if appeals to solidarity and fearfulness remain insufficient, this movement will have exhausted itself in the battle over AIDS-tainted blood.[100]

That scenario invites reappraisal not only of the politics of blood but also of political decision making in other arenas dominated by social interest groups like the hemophilia groups. What happens when health organizing intersects with identity organizing, as is more and more the case? When groups succeed in mobilizing an active constitutency and influencing a vulnerable state, they have the power to democratize decision making, opening up processes controlled by elites to broader scrutiny.[101] That is all to the good. But this conception of politics also carries troubling implications.

Social interest groups tend to focus on the grievances of a narrowly defined group. That is the surest way to provide coherence, to gain and maintain a membership, to construct a story with which the group's members can identify. In a world where such organizations hold sway, the public interest comes to be defined as representing the aggregation of group grievances. Meanwhile, claims of comparable moral or social importance go ignored for want of a group to press them.

In the context of AIDS, gays and hemophiliacs operated differently. Homosexuals were well organized before the epidemic, but widely disliked. They faced a hostile media and a phobic polity from which they needed to extract support for life-prolonging care and treatment. People with hemophilia, although lacking a history of organizing, were already hooked into a system of specialized care.[102] They were also able to marshall public and media sympathy, while turning apparent scandals into the tools of group mobilization. Although homosexuals have had to depend on doctors and drug companies for progress in fighting AIDS, hemophiliacs confronted a medical-pharmaceutical establishment on which they had been, and would continue to be, dependent for lifetime specialist care.

Hemophiliacs used their comparative advantage in ways that shaped—distorted—public responses to the epidemic. In France, the annual budget for indemnifying hemophiliacs is more than twice the budget for AIDS prevention and many times the budget for AIDS research.[103] In the United States, individuals exposed to

HIV through blood transfusions will not benefit from pending federal legislation that provides compensation—but only for hemophilia sufferers. Nor were the blood-transfusion AIDS victims invited to appear before the U.S. commission that reviewed the operation of the blood supply system, for that commission's mandate was expressly limited to hemophilia. In these instances, differential treatment of people with AIDS cannot be explained by pointing to the merits of their respective claims.

When social interest groups carry their agenda into the public arena, they often play the game of divide-and-conquer. Gay AIDS organizers focused on the needs of the gay community, while ignoring intravenous drug users, who in most countries are less organized and several rungs farther down the social acceptance scale. Hemophilia groups have done the same thing. In describing themselves as "innocent victims," they invited hostility toward gays and intravenous drug users, who could not so readily occupy the moral high ground. The argument that help should be predicated on a judgment of innocence also made it easier for public officials to focus on socially favored groups, hemophiliacs and children, while devoting less attention to the vast majority of AIDS cases, which are not blood-linked.

If the manufacture of symbols and sympathies is rapidly becoming a staple of political campaigns, the reliance on poster-children to carry the weight of argument in the AIDS domain—Kimberly Bergalis in the United States, allegedly infected with HIV by an irresponsible gay dentist; the charismatic adolescent who has personified the hemophile movement in Japan—is still noteworthy. Uniquely in American annals, the two major pieces of AIDS legislation are both named for hemophiliac child-martyrs. Federal funding for AIDS care is provided under the Ryan White Act, named for an adolescent whose battle for social acceptance made him a celebrity in the AIDS wars. The hemophilia compensation measure (introduced in Congress but not yet passed) is known as the Ricky Ray Act, after another boy whose fame derived from his struggle against hemophilia, AIDS, and bigotry.

Stories have a legitimate place in policy discourse because they bring abstract-sounding problems to vivid life. If such emotion-laden strategies assume pride of place in "democratized" policy conversations, however, analytically driven approaches will be pushed to the margins, because cost-benefit analyses are no match for the personification of outrage.[104] Public officials will also be less inclined to make the hard, and potentially tragic, choices that public health frequently demands.[105] What public servant is willing to make the kinds of swift, sure judgments that risk being labeled as "Blood Britta," the Danish health minister who, it was claimed, "wants dead bodies on her table"[106]? Who wants to be called "the Mengele of the Hemophilia AIDS Holocaust," as was said of an American doctor whose professional life had been devoted to the care of hemophilia sufferers?[107]

The successes of the hemophilia movement have brought help for people who needed it, and that is an undoubted social benefit. Yet in another kind of society—one less committed to the justice of Elizabethan Poor Laws, more inclined to shared social responsibility—the fact that a person is seriously ill would be reason enough to deliver such help. Moral tests would not be imposed before assistance was forthcoming.

The prevailing calculus of support, which invites distinctions between the deserving and the undeserving in delivering help, also signals prudent public health officials how to respond to the next health crisis, and the one after that. Consider blood policy. One current debate has to do with the need to introduce expensive antigen screening. Another focuses on whether blood that has the potential to carry Creutzfeldt-Jakob disease should be recalled, and recipients of such blood informed, even though there is no evidence that this disease can be transmitted by blood, because there is no way to prove the absence of risk.[108] In such instances—as well as a raft of public health decisions far beyond the domain of blood—the lesson from AIDS is that it is politically astute to promote zero risk for groups that command popular support, even at costs that would not withstand cost/benefit scrutiny,[109] while ignoring risks that will never be captured in vivid policy dramas.

What is politically astute, of course, doesn't always make for wise practice. The selective hyper-caution of such an approach to health policy could vastly increase the cost of care, even as it keeps off the market products and practices of potentially great benefit that fail to satisfy impossible tests of risklessness. Ironically, this may be the major legacy of the politics of blood that has emerged in the era of AIDS.

NOTES

A caveat: Although this chapter draws on case studies of 13 nations, the limited comparability of data across those case studies means that, of necessity, the cross-national analysis is suggestive. A full-blown comparative study of the hemophilia rights movement remains to be done.

1. Ronald Bayer, Eric Feldman, the organizers of the project for which this chapter was written, as well as Erik Albaek, John Ballard, Steven Epstein, Joshua Gamson, Sherry Glied, Dorothy Nelkin and Umberto Izzo, offered insightful critiques of a draft version.

2. Postings can be found at Hemophilia-Support@Web-Depot.COM; the World Wide Web site is http://ww.web-depot.com/hemophilia.

3. See Joshua Gamson, "Must Identity Movements Self-Destruct? A Queer Dilemma," *Social Problems*, 42 (1995) pp. 390–407.

4. Similar demonstrations were held each week during the fall of 1996. FAX zaps, which tied up the company's FAX machines, were part of the demonstration.

5. The cost of factor VIII and factor IX is prohibitive in third world and some second world nations; in those countries, other methods of replenishing the blood clotting factor are used. See C. Nuchprayoon, "AIDS and Blood in Thailand," unpublished paper prepared for the project HIV-Contaminated Blood: Policy and Conflict.

6. In 1975, the World Health Organization had recommended that nations be self-sufficient in blood and blood products. Though that recommendation is not without its problematic aspects, it does minimize the risk of worldwide contamination; had it been followed, many fewer hemophilia sufferers would have contracted AIDS.

7. Philip Bobbitt and Guido Calabrese, *Tragic Choices* (New York: Norton, 1978).

8. William Felstiner, Richard Abel, and Austin Sarat, "The Emergence and Transformation of Disputes: Naming, Blaming, Claiming . . . ," *Law and Society Review*, 15 (1980–81), pp. 3–4.

9. On the uses of the Holocaust in social movements, see Arlene Stein, "Mobilizing Memories: The Holocaust as a Symbolic Resource for Social Movements." Unpublished paper, 1996.

10. On many AIDS-related matters, from the recognition of the epidemic to the development of effective treatments, the United States was first; not so, however, with respect to hemophilia activism. Ronald Bayer and David L. Kirp, "The United States: At the Center of the Storm," *AIDS in the Industrialized Democracies: Passions, Politics and Policies* ed. David L. Kirp and Ronald Bayer (New Brunswick, NJ: Rutgers University Press, 1992), pp.7–49.

11. Robert Dahl, *Who Governs?* (New Haven, CT: Yale University Press, 1961), p. 225.

12. Mancur Olson, *The Logic of Collective Action* (Cambridge, MA: Harvard University Press, 1965). See also Anthony Downs, *An Economic Theory of Democracy* (New York: Harper, 1957).

13. Doug McAdam, *Political Process and the Development of Black Insurgency, 1930–1970* (Chicago: University of Chicago Press, 1984), p. 34.

14. Piet Hagen, *Blood: Gift or Merchandise?* (New York: Alan R. Liss, 1982), p. 53.

15. See Erving Goffman, *Stigma* (Englewood Cliffs, NJ: Prentice Hall, 1963); Susan Sontag, *Illness as Metaphor* (New York: Farrar Straus and Giroux, 1978); Susan Sontag, *AIDS and its Metaphors* (New York: Farrar Straus and Giroux 1987); James Jones, *Bad Blood* (New York: Free Press, 1992). The welfare rights movement, which briefly flourished in the United States in the 1970s, had to overcome a similar sense of shame, and a desire for secrecy, on the part of welfare recipients. See Piven and Cloward.

16. Robert Putnam, *Making Democracy Work: Civic Traditions in Italy* (Princeton, NJ: Princeton University Press, 1993). See also Robert Bellah, Richard Madsen, William Sullivan, Ann Swidler, and Steven Tipton, *Habits of the Heart* (Berkeley, CA: University of California Press, 1985).

17. Alberto Melucci, "The New Social Movements: A Theoretical Approach." *Social Science Information*, 19 (1991) pp. 199–226 at p. 218.

18. Robert Kagan, "Adversarial Legalism," *Journal of Public Policy and Managment*, 10 (1991), p. 3.

19. Joshua Gamson, "Silence, Death and the Invisible Enemy: AIDS Activism and Social Movement 'Newness,'" *Social Problems*, 42 (1989), pp. 390–407.

20. See Enrique Larana, Hank Johnston and Joseph Gusfield, eds, *New Social Movements: From Ideology to Identity* (Philadelphia: Temple University Press, 1994); Aldon Morris and Carol McClurg Mueller, eds., *Frontiers in Social Movement Theory* (New Haven: Yale University Press, 1992); Craig Calhoun, *Social Theory and the Politics of Identity* (New York: Blackwell, 1994); Sidney Verba, Kay Lehman Schlozman, and Henry E. Brady, *Voice and Equality* (Cambridge: Harvard University Press, 1995); David Knoke, "Associations and Interest Groups, *Annual Review of Sociology*, 12 (1986) pp. 8–9; Jack Walker, "Survey Research and Membership in Voluntary Associations," *American Journal of Political Science*, 32 (1988), pp. 908–928; Bonnie Erickson and T. A. Nosanchuk, "How an Apolitical Association Politicizes," *Canadian Review of Sociology and Anthropology*, 27 (1990), pp. 206–219. The focus on distinction-making may reflect the narcissism of small differences, from which disciplines are not immune.

21. Bert Klandermans and Sidney Tarrow, "Mobilization into Social Movements: Synthesizing European and American Approaches," *International Social Movement Research*, 1 (1988), pp. 1–38.

22. For a summary of how nations responded, see the newsletters published by the HIV Financial Assistance Committee (formerly the Committee on Compensation) of the World Hemophilia Federation.

23. For a discussion of gay activism as a trans-national phenomenon, see Kirp and Bayer at pp. 368–9, 375.

24. Two other groups were also perceived as disproportionately affected by HIV: intravenous drug users and, in the United States, Haitians. In some countries, such as the Netherlands, drug users mobilized; elsewhere, as in the United States, they remained outside the policy debates. Haitians in the United States did organize, and successfully pressured the government to remove them from the list of especially vulnerable groups. See Ronald Bayer, *Private Acts, Social Consequences: AIDS and the Politics of Public Health* (New Brunswick, NJ: Rutgers University Press, 1991).

25. On blood and social taint, see Mary Douglas, *Purity and Danger* (London: Routledge, 1979).

26. Andre Picard, *The Gift of Death: Confronting Canada's Tainted-Blood Tragedy* (Toronto: Harper-Collins, 1995). The not-infrequent slip, "homophiliac," reiterates the confusion.

27. Compare Allan Brandt, *No Magic Bullet* (New York: Oxford University Press, 1987).

28. Martin Duberman, *Stonewall* (New York: Dutton, 1993).

29. See, for example, Dennis Altman, *Homosexual: Oppression and Liberation* (Sydney, AU: Angus and Robertson, 1972); Dennis Altman, "The Emergence of Gay Identity in the USA and Australia," *Politics in the Future: The Role of Social Movements* ed. Christine Jennet and Randal Stewart, (Melbourne: McMillan, 1989).

30. In this desire for normality, hemophiliacs differ from many hearing-impaired people, who in the past generation have formed a social movement premised on the belief that there is a distinct (and perhaps distinctly better) deaf culture, and who resist assimilation of the hearing-impaired into the hearing world.

31. Picard, *op. cit*. p. 160.

32. In this respect, Denmark is the exception. In 1974, the Hemophilia Society—which had been founded just five years earlier—shifted from being a society for hemophiliacs to a society of hemophiliacs, with the medical members forming a medical committee. Even there, when AIDS struck, hemophiliacs had no experience in dealing with the health policy system.

33. Bruce Bawer, *A Place at the Table* (New York: Poseidon, 1993).

34. Gamson (1995), *op. cit.*

35. In Italy, the absence of overt state hostility impeded the organization of gays. See Umberto Izzo, "Blood, Bureaucracy and Law: Responding to HIV-Tainted Blood in Italy," Eric Feldman and Ronald Bayer, eds., *Blood Feuds: AIDS, Blood, and the Politics of Medical Disaster* (New York: Oxford University Press, 1999).

36. In the United States, despite statements from the Secretary of Health and Human Services that AIDS was the nation's "number one health priority," the administration remained loath to act. Not until 1987 did President Reagan even say the word "AIDS." In Europe and Japan, AIDS was widely regarded as an American issue.

37. This pattern holds true for the eleven nations whose AIDS policy history is recounted in Kirp and Bayer, *op. cit.*

38. Many gay men regarded doctors as ignorant of their special health needs, if not overtly hostile, and there were good reasons for such suspicions. Medical journals ran highly judgmental accounts of homosexuals' diseases, written by doctors who based their homophobic generalizations on an atypically promiscuous sample of gay patients. When gay men sought psychological treatment, they often got "cures" instead. Not until 1973 did the American Psychiatric Association, whose standards influence therapeutic practice worldwide, ceased to label homosexuality as an illness. Ronald Bayer, *Homosexuality and American Psychiatry* (New York: Basic Books, 1981).

39. Steven Epstein, Impure Science: AIDS, Activism and the Politics of Knowledge (Berkeley: University of California Press, 1996).

40. See, generally, Kirp and Bayer, *op. cit.*; Randy Shilts, *And the Band Played On* (New York: St. Martins, 1987); Sandra Panem, *The AIDS Bureaucracy* (Cambridge, MA: Harvard University Press, 1988); Dennis Altman, *AIDS in the Mind of America* (Garden City, NY: Anchor Books, 1986); Charles Perrow and Mauro Guillen, *The AIDS Disaster: The Failure of Organizations in New York and the Nation* (New Haven, CT: Yale University Press, 1990); Rolf Rosenbrock, *AIDS Kann Schneller Besiegt Werden (AIDS Can Be Treated Faster)* (Hamburg: VSA-Verlag, 1986); M Frings, ed., *Dimensionen einer Krankheit (Dimensions of a Disease)* (Reinbek: Rowohlt Verlag, 1986); Wilson Tuckey, "The Politics of AIDS" in Department of Community Services and Health, *Living with AIDS* (Canberra: Australian Government Publishing Service, 1988); Ricardo Lorenzo and Hector Anibitarte, *AIDS: A Burning Topic* (Madrid: Editorial Revolucion, 1987); Oscar Guasch, *The Pink Society*, unpublished Ph.D. dissertation (University of Barcelona School of Public Health, 1990); Peter Aggleton, *AIDS: Individual, Cutural and Policy Dimensions* (London: Falmer Press, 1990); Simon Watney, *Policing Desire* (Minneapolis: University of Minnesota Press, 1987); Eric Fee and Daniel Fox, eds., *AIDS: The Burdens of History* (Berkeley, CA: University of California Press, 1988).

41. Ronald Bayer, "Blood and AIDS in America: Science, Politics and the Making of an Iatrogenic Catastrophe," Feldman and Bayer, *op. cit.*

42. Blood banks were also resistant. They depended on their reputation as providers of a product that was symbolic of life itself. Concern about the purity of the blood supply, they feared, would cause panic. Moreover, in such a climate of fear, some people who required transfusions as part of an appropriate medical procedure would reject the procedure, against advice, in order to protect themselves from the possibility of contracting AIDS through contaminated blood, thus putting themselves at greater risk. The blood banks were also fearful that patients would insist on using only their own previously collected blood or else blood drawn from a pool of known donors, a practice that called into question a key tenet of the blood system, its universality. Stories about possible contamination of the blood supply even threatened to reduce donations from people who believed that donating put them at risk for contracting AIDS. In response, blood banks emphasized the safety of the system, initially rejecting even the possibility of risk, later minimizing it, insisting that the odds of AIDS contamination were higher than being struck by a falling satellite. On the social significance of blood, see Richard Titmuss, *The Gift Relationship* (New York: Random House, 1971).

43. *Ibid.*, p. 203.

44. Bayer, Feldman and Bayer, *op. cit.*

45. Verba et al. *op. cit.*, pp. 398–415.

46. McAdam *op. cit.*, p. 51.

47. Alberto Melucci, "The Process of Collective Identity," in Hank Johnston and Bert Klandermans.

48. Sociologists, who once used the language of esprit de corps to describe this phenomenon, Herbert Blumer, "Collective Behavior," *An Outline of the Principles of Sociology* ed. Robert Park (New York: Barnes and Noble, 1939) pp. 68–121, now speak of a "culturally appropriate frame." Hank Johnston and Bert Klandermans, eds., *Social Movements and Culture* (Minneapolis: University of Minnesota Press, 1993). See also Johnson, Larana, and Gusfield; Gitlin. Compare Paul Sabatier and Susan McLaughlin, "Belief Congruence Between Interest Group Leaders and Members: An Empirical Analysis of Three Theories and a Suggested Synthesis," *Policy Sciences*, 6 (1990), pp. 301–342.

49. David Snow and Robert Benford, "Ideology, Frame Resonance, and Participant Mobilization," *International Social Movement Research* 1 (1985) 197–217, p 198. See also David Snow, E. Burke Rochford, Jr., Steven Worden, and Robert Benford, "Frame Aligment Processes: Micromobilization and Movement Participation. *American Sociological Review*, 51 (1986) 464–481; David Snow and Robert Benford, "Master Frames and Cycles of Protest," in Morris and Mueller, pp. 133–155.

50. Paul Gilroy, *The Black Atlantic: Modernity and Double Consciousness* (London: Verson, 1993).

51. William Gamson, Bruce Fireman, and Steven Rytina, *Encounters with Unjust Authority* (Homewood, IL: Dorsey, 1982).

52. Picard, p. 162.

53. Laura Resnick, "The Hemophilia Movement in the United States," unpublished Ph.D. dissertation, (School of Public Health, Columbia University, 1994).

54. See, generally, Elliot Friedson, *Professional Dominance: The Social Structure of Medical Care* (New York: Allerton, 1970).

55. Bayer, Feldman and Bayer, *op. cit.*

56. Resnick, *op. cit.* p. 220.

57. Hagan, *op. cit.* p. 54.

58. E-mail from John Ballard to David Kirp, November 15, 1996.

59. See the country case studies in Feldman and Bayer, *op. cit.*

60. Picard, p. 200.

61. The organization's founder joined ACT UP–Boston when he first became politicized around AIDS issues Though by his account he was often the only heterosexual in the room, he found the situation far preferable than trying to get anywhere with the Hemophilia Foundation. E-mail from Steven Epstein to David Kirp, September 24, 1996. On the history of the American hemophilia movement, see generally Resnick.

62. The Committee of 10,000 would later take the lead in negotiating the settlement with the pharmaceutical companies.

63. These hemophilia sufferers saw themselves as innocent victims, who bore no responsibility for their fate. Complexities and inconvenient truths were ignored in this narrative.

For one thing, because of the long latency period of AIDS, some exposure to AIDS was essentially unavoidable. It's estimated that as many as 40% of hemophilia sufferers with HIV were infected prior to 1981, before this strange new disease had emerged, and in the year between the first reported cases among gay men and the first reported cases of blood-borne transmission. Also, and far more controversially, the desire of many people with hemophilia to live normal lives at almost any cost may have inclined some of them to minimize the risks of reliance on a product that, while possibly contaminated, was otherwise so beneficial. In this respect, those who were exposed to AIDS through blood transfusions and newborns born with the disease due to intrauterine transfer of the virus could make a different moral claim.

The distinction is advanced not to patrol the lines between guilt and innocence, victim and perpetrator in the AIDS realm, but for quite the opposite reason: to suggest the problematics of such a view.

64. Simon Schama, *An Embarrassment of Riches* (Cambridge: Harvard University Press, 1975).

65. E-mail from Erik Albaek to David Kirp, November 5, 1996.

66. E-mail from Umberto Izzo to David Kirp, October 28, 1996.

67. World Federation of Hemophilia, "Memo to National Member Organizations," March 16, 1989 (italics added)

68. World Federation of Hemophilia, Memo to National Member Organizations, May 3, 1989 (italics added).

69. Picard, *op. cit.* p. 168.

70. Eric Feldman, "HIV and Blood in Japan: Transforming Private Conflict into Public Scandal," Feldman and Bayer, *op. cit.*

71. Rosemary Taylor, "AIDS and Blood in Great Britain," an unpublished paper prepared for the project HIV-Contaminated Blood: Policy and Conflict; and John Ballard, "HIV-Contaminated Blood and Australian Policy: The Limits of Success," Feldman and Bayer, *op. cit.*

72. Another contributing fact was disagreement over the efficacy of heat-treated factor VIII concentrate.

73. One exception was Australia, which was self-sufficient in blood products as well as blood.

74. Hemophilia organizations are listed on the Web at http://planetmaggie.pcchcs. saic.com/hepcontacts.html. See also Hemophilia-Support@Web-Depot.COM, with a separate site for anonymous postings.

75. Bayer, Feldman and Bayer, *op. cit.*

76. The Ricky Ray Relief Act, which would provide compensation to hemophiliacs, is pending in Congress.

77. Bayer, Feldman and Bayer, *op. cit.*

78. Monika Steffan "The Nation's Blood: Medicine, Justice, and the State in France," Feldman and Bayer, *op. cit.* Jane Kramer, "Bad Blood," *New Yorker* (October 11, 1993), pp. 74–95.

79. Ballard, *op. cit.*

80. Feldman, *op. cit.*

81. *Ibid.*

82. For all the finger-pointing at the United States, an American subsidiary of Green Cross, Alpha Therapeutics, contends that it warned the parent Japanese company of the dangers of unheated products in 1982, but that its warnings weren't heeded.

83. Stephan Dressler, "Blood 'Scandal' and AIDS in Germany," Feldman and Bayer, *op. cit.* A criminal investigation against former health ministers, for their alleged misdeeds in the mid-1980s, resulted in a 1996 decision not to bring charges. "German Ministers Clear in German AIDS 'Bad-Blood' Scandal." *Reuters*, October 29, 1996.

84. See Myra Ferree and Beth Hess, *Controversy and Coalition: The New Feminist Movement* (New York: Twayne, 1994); Carol Mueller, "The Organizational Basis of Conflict in Contemporary Feminism," in Myra Ferree and Patricia Martin, eds., *Feminist Organizations: Harvest of the New Women's Movement* (Philadelphia: Temple University Press, 1994), pp. 263–275.

85. This is particularly true of radical political movements. See Donatella della Porta and Sidney Tarrow, "Unwanted Children: Political Violence and the Cycle of Protest in

Italy, 1966–1973." *European Journal of Political Research* 14 (1990), pp. 607–632; Donatella della Porta, ed., *Social Movements and Violence: Participation in Underground Organizations* (Greenwich, CT: JAI Press, 1992).

86. The likeliest explanation for this relatively low level of participation is a tragic one: the very high proportion of hemophiliacs who had already been infected by HIV at the outset of the epidemic, whose energies have been focused on simply keeping themselves alive.

87. Picard, *op. cit.* p. 81. See also Resnick, *op. cit.* p. 199. Ironically, as Picard notes, several of those leaders were in fact closeted homosexuals.

88. *Ibid.*, p. 160.

89. *Canada Financial Post* (December 10, 1996), p. 2.

90. Jesus de Miguel and David L. Kirp, "Spain: An Epidemic of Denial," *op. cit.* pp. 166–185.

91. Steffen, *op. cit.*

92. In the United States, the case of Kimberly Bergalis, the young woman purportedly infected by her (gay) dentist, was similarly seized upon for gay-bashing purposes by right-wing politicians.

93. "CWilliams"<charwill@aneas.net>

94. Steven Epstein, *Impure Science* (Berkeley CA: University of California Press, 1996).

95. See, for example, Anne Costain, *Inviting Women's Rebellion* (Baltimore: Johns Hopkins Press, 1992).

96. See Frances Piven and Richard Cloward, *Poor People's Movements* (New York: Vintage Books, 1979).

97. Some countries now clean blood plasma with a detergent solvent, which is seen as more effective than heat treatment in killing viruses such as HIV.

The development, by pharmaceutical houses, of substitutes for human blood—spurred by the advent of AIDS—promises to greatly reduce, if not eliminate, the risk of contamination from viruses such as HIV. "These products are likely to end up being the largest-selling products in the pharmaceutical industry" within a decade, says the editor of the Medical Technology Stock Letter. Richard Jacobsen, "USA: Advances Rekindle Blood Substitute Debate" *Reuters* November 24, 1996.

98. "The [French] Socialists . . . say their mistake was not paying off the hemophiliacs quickly, and 'solving the problem' that way." Kramer, p. 93.

99. During the 1970s, the NHF was in or near bankruptcy on several occasions. Resnick, *op. cit.* p. 168.

100. In the United States, as of November 25, 1996, a Reuters wire story notes that 90% of AIDS-infected hemophiliacs had approved a $640 million settlment with four drug companies, Bayer AG, Baxter International, Armour Pharmaeuticals, and Alpha Therapeutic Corporation, a division of Japan's Green Cross Some 800 suits were still pending.

101. In France, as an outgrowth of the blood scandal, the law concerning legal proceedings against cabinet ministers was changed to enable a citizen to make a claim against a member of government for decisions taken in office, rather than having to depend on political majorities in Parliament to act. Steffan, *op. cit.*

102. In the United States, which relies more than other industrial democracies on the market to furnish care, hemophiliacs have had access to publicly supported treatment centers since the passage of federal legislation in 1975 Resnick, p. 131.

103. Kramer, *op. cit.*

104. The point is not that benefit-cost analyses are entirely devoid of their own ideological content; the differences among persuasive techniques are matters of degree, not kind. See Deborah Stone, *Policy Paradox* (New York: Norton, 1997).

105. The heroes of public health are those who act decisively, to do the greatest good for the greatest number, without concern for political consequences. Dr. Rieux, the central figure in Camus' *The Plague*, is viewed as heroic because of the swift sureness of the measures he proposed to contain the plague in the Algerian city of Oran. Had Rieux been wrong in his scientific judgment, mistaken in urging quarantine, he'd be indistinguishable from the National Front activists in France, who sounded the cry of alarm, or from Lyndon LaRouche, the public health *bete noir* of AIDS in the United States. (Albert Camus, *The Plague* [New York: Random House, 1948].)

106. Eric Albaek, "Denmark: The Political 'Pink Triangle,'" in Kirp and Bayer *op. cit.*, p. 306; Eric Albaek, "The Never-Ending Story? The Political and Legal Controversies over HIV and the Blood Supply in Denmark," Feldman and Bayer, *op. cit.*

107. Bayer, Feldman and Bayer, *op. cit.*

108. The former president of the National Hemophilia Population raises the same concern. "If it turns out twenty years from now that DNA products have a presently unknown side effect, will we then be demanding compensation. We have consistently argued that for a small population such as those with hemophilia, if we wait for new products until they can be fully tested on thousands of people, no new drugs will be marketed."

109. One Canadian physician, who has informed recipients of CJD-contaminated blood, declared: "The risk as far as I am concerned is zero. . . . We knew this would be alarming for families but we felt it was our responsibility to tell them." Norbert Gilmore and Margaret Somerville, "From Trust to Trajedy: HIV/AIDS and the Canadian Blood System," Feldman and Bayer, *op. cit.*

11 The Circulation of the Blood
AIDS, Blood, and the Economics of Information

Sherry Glied

The story of HIV and blood systems can be usefully divided into three eras: pre-1982, 1982–1985, and post-1985. The institutional structures of the blood systems in the 10 developed countries studied in the project from which this volume emerged were quite similar in the pre-1982 period. None of these systems implemented decisive measures for improving the quality of blood before 1985 (other than very limited efforts at donor exclusion), yet none failed to implement HIV testing and heat treatment by 1986. They differed mainly in the pace of implementing screening and heat treatment in the brief 1985–1986 period.

Prior to 1982, these 10 countries developed similar institutional structures of blood collection and distribution that solved a common problem of asymmetric information about the quality of blood. Although this structure may have been optimal for dealing with the information problem presented by the principal threats to blood quality prior to 1982, the blood supply in each country became contaminated by HIV in 1982–1985. In every large developed country (population greater than 1 million) in Europe, Australia, and North America, people developed AIDS as a consequence of the transfusion of blood or blood products. My analysis will address why this happened and why all the national systems in our study failed to respond effectively over the 1982–1985 period, a failure that had particularly adverse consequences in countries with relatively high rates of non-transfusion-related AIDS. Finally, I will examine the response of these national systems in the aftermath of the development of an HIV test in 1985.

The Blood Supply Before 1982: Hepatitis and Asymmetric Information

From the Second World War until 1982, the infectious disease problem that occupied the energies of blood bankers, regulators, and policy analysts around the world was the transmission of hepatitis B through blood transfusion. Hepatitis is a disease that developed in the nineteenth century entirely as a consequence of the transfer of human blood and blood components from one person to another (initially because of vaccination using human source vaccines). After a brief latency period (of about 60 days), infection with hepatitis B leads to a serious and sometimes persistent illness. People who have had this illness remain carriers and can continue to transmit hepatitis to those who are given transfusions of their blood. In the 1960s, hepatitis B was a very significant problem. Reliable tests for detecting antibodies in the blood did not exist. As many as 1 in 150 individuals over 40 in the United States who received transfusions died of hepatitis-related causes.[1] In Japan, a hepatitis-infected transfusion endangered the health of U.S. Ambassador Edwin Reischauer.[2]

The medical problem that is hepatitis can be translated into economics as a problem of asymmetric information. This economic problem has two dimensions. First, from the perspective of a blood collector, the quality of the blood that courses through the veins of a potential donor cannot be fully known. A blood donor may know that he has had hepatitis, but the blood collector does not. Second, from the perspective of a patient or physician, the characteristics of the donor who provided a unit of blood to a collector, characteristics that may be correlated with the risk of hepatitis, cannot be ascertained. A blood collector may know that she has collected a particular unit on skid row, but the patient and physician, who see only the blood and not the donor, do not. The collection and distribution of blood need to be organized in a way that responds to these two closely related informational asymmetries.

A considerable economic literature exists about this type of asymmetric information problem. Much of that literature addresses the question of how to design "revelation mechanisms"—ways to get people to disclose the private information that they have. The organization of the blood system in the pre-1982 period provided such a revelation mechanism.

Blood collection systems typically relied on three institutional mechanisms to ensure product quality. First, blood donors did not receive cash payments for giving blood. Even the United States stopped using paid donors for whole blood transfusion by 1980. Second, blood collection systems did not, on the whole, profit from the sale of blood. Third, government regulatory authorities enforced standards and oversaw the operation of the system. As Table 11-1 suggests, there were strikingly few differences among the developed countries we are studying along these dimensions of institutional structure. Germany, alone among them, collected a small amount of blood from donors who were paid cash, but this commercial blood collection ap-

Table 11-1. Organization of the blood system in selected countries

	Payment to Whole Blood Donors	*Organization of Blood Banks*
Australia	All voluntary	Nonprofit monopoly
Canada	All voluntary	Nonprofit monopoly
Denmark	All voluntary	Nonprofit monopoly
France	All voluntary	Nonprofit monopoly
Germany	Mainly voluntary	Mainly nonprofit
Italy	All voluntary	Nonprofit regional monopolies
Japan	All voluntary	Nonprofit monopoly
Netherlands	All voluntary	Nonprofit monopoly
United Kingdom	All voluntary	No-cost monopoly
United States	All voluntary	Nonprofit, mainly regional, monopolies
India	Mixed	Mixed
Thailand	All nonpaid	Nonprofit monopoly
Zimbabwe	All voluntary	Nonprofit monopoly

Source: Papers prepared for the project HIV Contaminated Blood: Policy and Conflict, presented at the Costello di Santa Maria Novella, Fiano, Italy July 1996.

pears to have had little effect on the overall organization and performance of their system.

The similarity in the structure of national blood systems in the pre-1982 period was, to some extent, due to the work of Richard Titmuss, whose book *The Gift Relationship* (1971) drew international attention to the problem of hepatitis-infected blood and called for reliance on voluntary donors.[1-4] The institutional solution prescribed by Titmuss was a remarkably successful solution to the problem of hepatitis. In combination with an imperfect test for hepatitis B, the use of voluntary donation led to significant declines in rates of hepatitis B worldwide, so that by 1980 they were at apparently "acceptable" levels.

Each of the component parts of the pre-1982 blood system worked to ensure the quality of the blood. The central element was the use of voluntary (rather than paid or replacement) donation. Why should volunteered blood be of higher quality than paid blood? There are two possible reasons. First, the *behavior* of voluntary donors can solve one problem of asymmetric information. As Kenneth Arrow noted in his comments on Titmuss, "Since no adequate test has yet been devised for the presence of hepatitis in the blood, its detection depends essentially on the willingness of the donor to state correctly whether or not he is suffering from the disease."[5] Alternatively, the quality of blood may depend not on the behavior of donors, but on their *characteristics*.[6,7] The blood-related characteristics of voluntary donors may be better than those of paid donors.

The argument from behavior suggests that volunteer blood is better because volunteers are altruists who are giving, in Titmuss' words, a gift. We give gifts to help people, not to harm them. In economic terms, blood donors have private information about their health status. Those who donate voluntarily reveal information that they are healthy. "Giving" is a simple information-revelation mechanism. This hypothesis is formalized in several economic models.[8,9]

The argument that volunteer blood is safer than paid blood because of the characteristics of volunteer donors is more prosaic. Paid donors are, on average, of lower socioeconomic status than volunteer donors. Higher income people would demand a higher dollar price for donating blood than lower income people do because their time and convenience is worth more to them.

The relationship between socioeconomic status and health is well established. Poor people have higher rates of morbidity, particularly infectious morbidity, than higher income people do. In addition, prostitutes, drug addicts, and alcoholics, groups at high risk for infectious diseases that can be transmitted by blood, are also poor. Paid blood is poor blood precisely because it is drawn from poor people. As the plaintiffs in a Japanese case suggested, paid blood comes from "homos," blacks, and Mexicans, and was collected in a "despondent" atmosphere.[2] The Italian media characterized paid blood as coming from "the ghettos of large American cities."[4] In England, paid donors were viewed as members of "down and out groups."[10]

Offering a higher price for blood donation might encourage people of high socioeconomic status to donate.[6,11,12] This policy would also, however, encourage more poor people to donate, and blood-collecting organizations would have to develop a method for screening potential donors based on socioeconomic status. Such methods are difficult to implement, particularly for whole blood, for which a minimum of two months must pass between donations. Titmuss noted of paid donors that "Many are said to give fictitious names and addresses . . . and to traffic in black markets of social security cards, 'rented' for 25 cents or so to serve as identity cards at blood banks."[1] Volunteer donation appears to be a relatively effective way to screen out of the blood donation pool persons of low socioeconomic status. Volunteer blood drives can choose where they want to establish collection facilities. Typically, they choose university campuses and the offices of large firms. They do not generally locate in poverty-stricken areas or near skid row. Today, the U.S. blood donor pool is of considerably higher socioeconomic status than the average nondonor and this is true in other countries as well.[13,14] The striking exception to this pattern is France, where blood was collected on the streets of Paris and in prisons.[15]

In practice, the behavioral and socioeconomic benefits of voluntary donation work together. Voluntary donation is a good way to elicit information both about disease risk and about socioeconomic status. It is an economically efficient way of solving the information asymmetries inherent in the hepatitis problem. In addition, as Titmuss noted, voluntary donation provides important noneconomic benefits. Under national voluntary donation systems, citizens become literal blood brothers. Voluntary blood donation allows donors to express their national solidarity. To Titmuss, and many other writers, these social benefits were as important a consequence of the voluntary system as any efficiency improvements.

The second institutional component that helped ensure the quality of blood systems was the organizational structure of blood collection. In most countries, blood banking is a monopoly—at either the national, regional, or local level. In the United States, about 95% of not-for-profit blood banks face no competition in their local markets, although some large cities do have competing blood banks.[16] Competition in blood banking is generally deplored. As one writer notes, systems with competition are "susceptible to entrepreneurial activities which, in their worst forms, can dangerously pollute the blood supply."[17] Even where multiple blood banks exist in a region, explicit rules and implicit norms discourage them from competing.[12]

Furthermore, blood banks typically operate on a not-for-profit basis and do not charge more than the cost of transfusing blood. In some cases, (e.g., the United Kingdom), blood banks do not receive *any* payment from end users (hospitals) for the sale of their blood. The ethic of voluntarism is explicitly extended from the donor-collector relationship to the collector-physician relationship. Blood banks do not earn a profit in part because volunteer donors would object to others profiting from their gift. In the United States, local blood banks do sell blood to hospitals (usually at the cost of collection), but they also receive subsidies from local organizations that give them a price advantage in selling to local markets.[16]

As a result of this organizational structure, there is little advantage (and quite possibly a net disadvantage) for a blood bank to collect more blood than is needed within a region and transfer it to an out-of-region facility (within that country). Unlike other producers, blood bankers reap little financial reward when the demand for their product rises (within limits). The lack of interbank competition, the non-profit structure of blood banks, and the low or nonexistent payments bankers receive for blood make economic sense in the context of voluntary blood banking. They reduce blood bank incentives to "cheat" by recruiting more donors from lower socioeconomic status populations.[18] Increasing the size of the donor pool is ordinarily not in the interest of either blood users or of blood bankers.

In addition to voluntary donation and not-for-profit noncompeting blood collection, each country also imposed regulation on its blood system. Regulators mandated conformity with a set of national rules regarding the testing and treatment of blood. These rules were designed to protect consumers from undesirable changes in the actions of blood-collecting institutions.

The regulatory principle governing blood favors maintenance of the status quo in the face of a potentially dangerous threat or costly improvement. The Japanese health regulatory system, for example, is designed to "avoid drug-induced tragedies."[2] England's efforts to protect its residents from such tragedies make it "the land of the extended clinical trial."[10] Similarly, the U.S. FDA requires evidence of both safety and efficacy before approving a new product for sale on the market.

The status quo–oriented regulatory structure conforms to that suggested by recent studies of individual behavior under uncertainty. People exhibit aversion to losses relative to the status quo, but are less responsive to the prospect of gains, leading individuals, as well as regulatory institutions, to stick with what is known.[19,20,21] A regulatory system that generated national conformity in adherence to blood safety standards, and enshrined the status quo in the face of uncertainty, was the final element in the institutional structure of the pre-1982 era.

AIDS: A New Problem for an Old Paradigm

For a brief period in the late 1970s, the blood transfusion and blood products systems of all 10 developed countries studied here appeared safe and effective. They regularly provided whole blood or AHF of high quality to their populations; hemophiliacs were able to home-transfuse using AHF; and ever-improving tests for hepatitis B promised to free recipients from the dangers of that disease. The last great threat to blood product safety, the collection of plasma in poor Latin American and Caribbean countries, had largely ended by the late 1970s. These systems, though appropriately designed to cope with the circumstances of the late 1970s, failed to protect blood and blood product recipients from HIV in the early 1980s.

In the early years of the epidemic, donors, blood bankers, and physicians were all unsure of how HIV was transmitted, the duration of its latency, how effective donor screening would be, how effective surrogate testing would be, and whether heat treatment would neutralize HIV or undesirably modify AHF. Even where some information was available, such as information about the characteristics of people with AIDS, this information was not sufficient for anyone (donor, blood bank, physician, or blood recipient) to identify individual carriers of the virus. These are problems of *incomplete* information, not problems of *asymmetric* information. Institutional structures designed to address problems of asymmetric information had no particular advantage (and were, quite possibly, at a disadvantage) in addressing these problems of incomplete information.

Uninformed Donors

In many countries, a slow response to the threat of AIDS in the blood was predicated on a false syllogism: blood from paid donors is unsafe; our blood supply excludes paid donors; hence our blood is safe.[22,23] The relative safety of voluntary blood compared to paid blood had been established in the period when hepatitis B was the main problem facing the blood system.

Hepatitis differed from AIDS, however, in some important respects. People who contract hepatitis develop symptoms within 60 days. After becoming ill, the blood of those who recover (the vast majority) continues to transmit infection for the rest of the donor's life. The period of danger with respect to hepatitis is mainly the period *after* an episode of illness. Blood banks that screened for hepatitis could ask donors whether they had ever had hepatitis (just as they asked donors whether they have had other illnesses) and exclude blood from donors who had actually had the disease (although, even in this case, some infected people do not recognize they have had hepatitis).

Unlike hepatitis, HIV was infectious for 7 to 10 years before a donor developed symptoms. Until an HIV test was developed, most prospective donors, however altruistic, did not know that they harbored the virus. Asking prospective donors whether they had AIDS symptoms screened out very few infected donors. Unlike the hepatitis case, blood bank screening had to focus on risk behaviors associated with infection, not with infection itself.

The principal strategy blood systems used before the HIV test was developed to reduce the risk of infection was to encourage donor self-exclusion. Informing people about the risks of certain behaviors and allowing them to defer donation was a way to make use of the altruism-based strengths of voluntary donation in the context of AIDS. Asking about risk behaviors—especially socially stigmatized behavior—was, however, not something that came naturally to blood banks or donors.

Nonetheless, giving prospective donors an opportunity to self-exclude by informing them of risks helped reduce the risk of transmission somewhat everywhere, and more in some countries than in others. The proportion of the donor pool in large U.S. cities that consisted of young men decreased after voluntary self-exclusion was introduced.[24] Making donors legally responsible for the quality of their donated blood, as in Australia and Canada, had much more substantial effects. The rate of infection among donors in Australia dropped by a factor of 50 after legal sanctions were introduced. Nonetheless, even in Australia, infected donors continued to contribute.[25] It is likely that the success of donor self-exclusion was related to the degree to which AIDS risk behaviors were viewed as socially stigmatized in each country.

The Limits of Altruism

The transmission of HIV through blood in the era of self-exclusion casts doubt on whether altruism alone is sufficient to guarantee blood safety. Knowledge of HIV risk factors was widespread among risk groups (particularly gay men) before 1984. Yet, in most countries, evidence suggests that people with risk factors continued to give blood voluntarily despite the possibility that they might cause harm to the recipients of their gifts. In every country under study, evidence of HIV infection in the blood supply in 1985 suggests that at least a few people with some risk factors did continue to donate. In many countries, the rate of infections in donations dropped precipitously after testing was officially introduced. It is quite clear that many of those who donated infected blood were aware of their risk of disease. In France, the rate of infection among new donors dropped by a factor of ten once testing of samples was implemented (and by a factor of nearly 12 among regular donors).[15] In Germany, the rate dropped by a factor of fourteen.[26] In Montreal, the rate dropped from 0.2% when donors did not know that samples were being screened to 0.05% when screening was official.[27] To the extent that some people donated blood after 1985 in order to be tested for HIV, these figures understate the extent of blood donation by HIV-infected individuals who knew they had risk factors before 1985.

Pure individual altruism was not enough, even in Titmuss's day, to generate an adequate supply of blood. Blood donation became a cozy experience, featuring friendly, kind volunteer organizers, coffee, sandwiches, cookies, confidential STD tests, and time off work; and in Germany, $20 to $40 for time and effort.[26,28] Most importantly, in many countries, through advertising campaigns, company drives, and the identification of blood donation with national history, blood donation was turned into a symbol of social solidarity. Blood donation became an opportunity for individuals to visibly participate in the larger society and to bask in the approbation of the community. But once participating in a blood drive became a sign of belonging, not participating became a sign of exclusion. To be unfit for blood donation, like being unfit for the draft, became a stigmatizing condition. Indeed, before the emergence of AIDS, exponents of the gift philosophy strongly opposed the idea of choosing donors based on their outward characteristics. A critic in 1976 suggested that we should be "actively concerned that the whole range of people in this society have an opportunity to give blood."[29]

The HIV epidemic destroyed the confluence between the efficiency benefits of the voluntary system and its desirable ethical consequences. Socially stigmatized groups resisted efforts at wholesale exclusion and demanded the right to give blood, even when such donations might reduce the quality of the blood supply. Groups who had been the object of other discrimination protested that exclusion from blood donation further stigmatized them. These groups included gay men, Haitians, and even communities with high HIV seroprevalence rates.[3,30] As Bayer notes, the U.S. Office of Technology Assessment decried advocates of surrogate testing because of their failure to consider the psychic costs to donors.[3] In France, blood collecting organizations failed to stop blood drives in prisons because they felt that limiting inmate opportunities to donate blood would reduce their social reintegration.[15]

Once a gift is motivated by something other than pure altruism, whether cash or other benefits, there is less reason to believe that it will be in the best interest of the recipient. The connection between blood donation and social solidarity, like the connection between blood donation and any other reward, monetary or otherwise, reduces the potency of the argument that altruism alone will lead donors to screen themselves. Volunteer donation is better than paid donation in eliciting private information about health risks. But it is far from secure as long as potential donors have other reasons for giving blood.

AIDS and Socioeconomic Status

Voluntary donation had also helped improve the quality of blood in the era of hepatitis by making it easier to choose donors according to their socioeconomic status. But the protective effects of high socioeconomic status were less important in the early days of the HIV epidemic.

In the early 1980s, HIV initially appeared among groups of relatively higher socioeconomic status than the groups among which other infectious diseases appeared (in both developed countries and in Africa). Over time, like other diseases, AIDS spread into poorer populations, while more educated groups were quicker to learn of and take precautions against further exposure. The socioeconomic status argument suggests that voluntary donors will be safer when a disease is well established and thus concentrated among the disadvantaged, but that the use of voluntary donors will not protect the supply from a newly discovered disease that strikes both the relatively affluent and the poor.

The blood system did not take many steps to protect blood in the early 1980s. The principle step taken, voluntary self-exclusion, operated entirely in the context of the existing blood collection system. More effective means of protection were, however, available. Two types of alternative strategies could have been used. By early 1982, the epidemiology of the AIDS epidemic in developed countries was well established. In every country, cases were concentrated among gay men and intravenous drug users in selected major metropolitan areas. Exploiting these epidemiological variations could have generated a substantially safer blood supply. Furthermore, by 1983, a relationship between HIV and various surrogate markers had been established and heat-treated blood products were available (indeed, such products were available even earlier in Germany).[31] Use of surrogate tests could have reduced the transmission of HIV in the United States (and the amount of HIV in plasma products) by as much as 80%.[32] Yet until a laboratory test for HIV was developed in 1984–1985, no country took strong and effective steps to reduce transmission through blood or blood products. Such steps may not have been cost-beneficial in countries that had low rates of AIDS and that relied entirely on locally collected blood and blood products. But this combination of conditions does not describe any of the countries in the group under study.

Epidemiological Responses

In its early years, AIDS was a remarkably tightly concentrated disease. Between 1978 and 1985, half of all reported cases in the *world* had occurred among residents of three metropolitan areas in the United States. (Note, however, that in 1985, reporting encompassed only North and South America, Europe, and Oceania. Many AIDS cases had already occurred in Africa and some had occurred in Asia, but these cases were not included in reports at that time.)[33] In Paris, the AIDS rate through 1985 was over 40 times as high as that in the rest of France. In Copenhagen, the rate was 18 times that in the rest of Denmark. In Milan, the rate was 20 times as high as in the rest of Italy. In Amsterdam, the rate was 45 times as high as in the rest of the Netherlands.

These variations in overall rates translated, almost one for one, into variations in blood transfusion case rates. A very good predictor of the number of AIDS blood transfusion cases in any country (or, in the United States, any state) is the number of non-blood-related cases in that country (or state). The strong relationship between all cases and blood cases suggests that information about infection rates by region (and also by sex) was readily available.

A strategy of targeting lower-risk regions and populations as a source of cleaner blood would have been valuable. Such a strategy, at the regional level, was pursued (to some extent) in Australia, and is an important component of efforts in many developing countries.[28,34] Data from within the United States suggests that increasing the use of blood from safer regions (and simultaneously decreasing the use of blood collected from men in high-prevalence regions) could have substantially reduced infections. The prevalence of HIV in the blood supply of Los Angeles was 10 times as high as the prevalence in Tulsa, Oklahoma, or Portland, Oregon.[12] One simple strategy every country could have used would have been to reduce collections in epidemic epicenters.

In principle, cross-border trade in blood would also have had beneficial consequences. France could have reduced its rate of transfusion infections by increasing the use of blood from neighboring Germany or Holland, where the AIDS case rate was half as high. Canada would have benefited from using blood from the United Kingdom, where the AIDS case rate was one third as high.

The exception that proves the rule here is the case of New York City. New York City has a relatively high donor rate, but it also contains many tertiary hospitals and uses a lot of blood. In 1973, the Red Cross in New York began purchasing "Euroblood" from blood banks in Switzerland and the Netherlands to make up for this deficiency in supply.[35] Euroblood provided a cheaper source of higher quality blood than could be obtained from expanding collection efforts in New York City itself. In consequence of the importation of Euroblood, the rate of transfusion-associated HIV in New York State is substantially lower (by half) than would be predicted on the basis of the number of other cases alone.[36]

Why wasn't information about differences in regional and national risk levels exploited more effectively? It was not impossible. Although it would have required considerable expenditures to motivate more donors to give blood in low-risk areas, particularly if the blood was intended for export to other countries, donation rates in most areas are sufficiently low that increasing donations substantially was certainly technically possible.

The institutional structure that contributed to high blood quality before 1982, however, impeded an effective response to this information about the HIV epidemic. Competition over quality among countries was very strongly discouraged by the World Health Organization and the International Red Cross, which strongly recommended national self-sufficiency in blood. Competition over quality among local blood suppliers within countries was often infeasible and always discouraged both by custom and by pricing practices. High-quality-blood collectors did not "sell" their products in low-quality markets and crowd out poor-quality local supply. Under the prevailing structure of the voluntary blood system in the early 1980s, quality could only be improved if blood bankers in high-prevalence areas voluntarily reduced their collections (through much more systematic screening, for example), or if regulators or central blood banking authorities demanded that they do so. But in this highly segmented, heavily regulated market, better screening would only create local shortages and raise the cost of collection.

Surrogate Testing and Heat Treatment

There were other steps that blood bankers and their regulators could have taken to reduce the risk of infection in the 1982–1985 period. Surrogate tests for hepatitis B surface antigen and for T cell counts were available for testing whole blood. By 1981, heat-treated AHF was available for sale in Germany. By 1983, the FDA approved the first American heat-treated AHF product.

Surrogate testing and heat treatment would have been costly (as would the epidemiology-based steps described above). German heat-treated AHF was 10 times as costly as the non-heat-treated product.[3] American heat-treated AHF was about 20% more costly than untreated product.[37] The surrogate test for hepatitis B core antigen cost $5 per unit of blood.[32] Furthermore, these steps also had significant indirect costs. Advocates of surrogate testing argued that as many as 80% of those with AIDS tested positive for hepatitis B core antigen, suggesting that the test was relatively sensitive. Roughly 5% of blood donors, however, tested positive for hepatitis B core antigen and most of them were probably not infected with HIV, so the test was not at all specific.[32] Collecting and disposing of blood from donors who tested positive for hepatitis B, and recruiting replacement donors, would impose further costs on blood banks.

Any of these steps would have imposed costs with certainty in exchange for highly uncertain benefits. Before the HIV test was developed, there was no way for anyone—blood collector or consumer—to know whether surrogate testing would greatly improve the quality of blood or whether heat treatment would kill the AIDS virus. In fact, although heat treatment successfully cleaned AHF of hepatitis B virus (that is the reason it was developed), early forms of heat treatment did not kill the non-A, non-B hepatitis virus and were not fully effective in killing HIV.[38] Indeed, heat-treating AHF could even have increased the risk of infection because if less potent heat-treated AHF were substituted for ordinary AHF, dosages would have to increase, increasing both monetary costs and, because more product would be used, the number of donor exposures.[39]

The regulatory structure that had helped ensure the quality of blood before 1982 imposed barriers to actions with unknown consequences. Regulators in all the countries under study required firm evidence of safety and efficacy before accepting a new product. In consequence, in the United States, heat-treated AHF was approved for use as a treatment for hemophilia before 1985 only because heat treatment prevented the spread of hepatitis B, an outcome that could be proved given the tests then available.[40] Testing the T-cell level in donated blood, as the Stanford blood bank did, provided no information about diseases other than AIDS, and testing for hepatitis B core antigen provided information that was of little value unless the presence of the antigen was also correlated with the presence of the virus causing AIDS. With firm evidence that the tests were costly, but no compelling direct evidence that they were valuable, regulators were loath to mandate their general use.

Even without governmental authority, blood banks could voluntarily have chosen to do surrogate testing. Regulators in the United States, however, prohibited bankers and manufacturers from suggesting that the tests were markers for the agent causing AIDS, complying with their mandate to prohibit false advertising. The evidence from the heat treatment experience suggests that regulators in other countries would have behaved like those in the United States with respect to the use of surrogate tests. Furthermore, in countries where the price of blood was set by regulators, approval would have been required to recoup the additional costs incurred through surrogate testing.

Heat-treated AHF could not be sold in most countries without regulatory approval of its safety. Although some countries permitted the sale of heat-treated product because there was evidence that it reduced transmission of hepatitis, they did not permit the product to be advertised as safer with respect to AIDS. As late as October 1984, the National Hemophilia Foundation in the United States recommended the use of heat-treated products "with the understanding that the protection against AIDS is yet to be proven."[3] No one claimed in 1983 that heat treatment stopped the spread of HIV, because there was no test for HIV. Similarly, in 1989, the use of HIV antigen screening for blood had not yet been proved, and the FDA licensed test kit was "not labelled for intended use as a blood screen."[41]

This conservative regulatory stance limited the interest and ability of nongovernmental authorities to take independent steps to clean the blood supply. Even in a market system, unless blood bankers and manufacturers could communicate the quality advantages of these steps, they could not pass along the additional cost of testing or heat treatment to customers. If they tried to sell tested or treated product at higher prices, no one would buy it. They could certainly not hope to gain market share over potential competitors through quality competition if they could not communicate quality differences.

Liability Standards

Economic analysts who wrote in response to Titmuss focused on the role of the liability regime in assuring quality. Kessel and Havighurst, for example, advocated the imposition of strict liability—on physicians and blood banks, respectively.[6,7] Under such a regime, a blood bank or manufacturer would be legally responsible for damages even if the banker or manufacturer had taken all feasible precautions. Despite the efforts of these scholars, physicians and blood bankers are not, in general, held liable for the quality of blood that they supply. Many lawsuits, in multiple countries, have held physicians and blood bankers liable for negligence in the aftermath of the

AIDS epidemic, but even these lawsuits did not impose standards of strict liability.[42] Under negligence standards, blood bankers typically only had to conform with industry practice and did not have to take all the potential costs of their actions into account.

In principle, strict liability rules could have encouraged blood bankers to take costly steps immediately (such as pursuing epidemiological strategies or implementing surrogate testing) in order to reduce the costs associated with illness occurring later. In practice, however, the nature of the HIV would likely have limited the effectiveness of strict liability in altering the behavior of these actors with respect to transfusion-related AIDS. The uncertainty surrounding the success of measures to reduce the risk of HIV, the long and variable delay between infection and the development of disease, the high rate of death from unrelated causes in the transfused population, the difficulty of identifying the source of infected blood in multiply-transfused patients, and the difficulty of proving that HIV was not contracted in some other manner make this a poor case for the prophylactic operation of liability rules.[43] Although the negligence standard did not encourage blood bankers to incur costs in anticipation of future liability savings, it is far from clear that any liability rule in 1983 would have led blood banks or product manufacturers to behave very differently.

As Table 11-1 indicates, the developed countries hit by the HIV epidemic in the early 1980s had very similar institutional structures. Thus it is hard to say from a comparative study of these countries whether an alternative configuration would have led to a better outcome. Within these countries, however, the behavior of two very distinct groups—for-profit AHF producers and individual patients and hemophiliacs—provide some indication of how different institutional structures might have responded to the epidemic.

AHF Producers

The quality of most products is assured not by laws or special institutional structures but by market forces. Quality can be generated by markets if purchasers can discern the quality of a product either before or after purchasing it. Markets generate quality through the development of reputations or brand names. Firms invest in brand names so that consumers distinguish their product from those of other suppliers and associate it with a particular level of quality. Reducing quality below that level will diminish the firm's brand name and will not be in the firm's interest if it expects to continue in business.

Not-for-profit organizations can also generate brand names and compete over quality. But the carefully constructed anti-competitive design of the blood system provided no reason for local blood banks to do so. American for-profit AHF producers, competing over brand names, were virtually the only blood suppliers who sought to use regional collection strategies and improve screening during this period.

In 1982, AHF producers stopped accepting blood from San Francisco, New York City, and Los Angeles.[11] They acted more quickly than U.S. not-for-profit blood banks (and those in other countries) in requiring donor screening (and pushed not-for-profit blood banks who relied on volunteer blood and sold plasma to them to implement such screening). Plasma producers required prospective donors to undergo physical tests and to sign statements certifying that they did not belong to known risk groups.[11] By 1986, a WHO official noted "The large experience in the USA shows that there is *no* difference between the frequency with which individuals are identified with antibody to the AIDS virus in the commercial plasmapheresis setting compared to the voluntary blood donor setting. If anything, the frequency of antibody in commercial plasmapheresis is *lower* than in voluntary blood donors" (emphasis in original).[44] Pharmaceutical manufacturers also took some other steps to improve product quality. For example, they produced some product in 1982 from plasma collected exclusively from female donors in the United States.[45]

There were limits to these strategies, however. The WHO official was comparing American voluntary and paid blood donors at a time when the United States had AIDS rates five times as high as the next highest European country. Although U.S. paid donation rates may not have been substantially different from U.S. voluntary donation rates, they were not markedly safe. U.S. plasma manufacturers did not, however, turn to other countries to get cleaner plasma, perhaps because there simply was no other plasma to use. In 1983, the U.S. plasmapheresis industry supplied 70% to 90% of the world supply of plasma.[46] In 1987, of the 14 million liters of plasma collected for fractionation use in the world, 8 million were collected through plasmapheresis in the United States. In total, over 90% of plasma collected through plasmapheresis came from paid U.S. donors.[47] Few voluntary systems were able to produce enough plasma to generate AHF concentrate for local use, let alone for export. Self-sufficiency in plasma production typically meant the use of cryoprecipitate, rather than concentrate (which could be administered at home and was preferred by hemophiliacs). In this period many countries were establishing local fractionation plants to produce AHF concentrate (and albumin), but most relied on American source plasma as input into their local production.[27,48] The ban on paid plasma collection in most other countries meant that most countries were not self-sufficient in AHF and were forced to rely on plasma collected from American donors, who, because of the epidemiology of HIV, almost certainly had higher rates of infection than paid donors elsewhere would have.

While isolated not-for-profit plasma producers in other countries took steps to improve the safety of their plasma supply, these measures never diffused, even within these countries. For example, in Australia, one region (Melbourne) began sending female-only plasma for fractionation.[28] Similarly, one Canadian province (Nova Scotia) produced concentrate from local plasma only. Unlike the for-profit pharmaceutical manufacturers who felt compelled to improve quality and keep up with their competitors, other blood bankers did not face competition from these local efforts.

Pharmaceutical companies were certainly less altruistic than not-for-profit blood banks. The market in which they operated, however, closely corresponds to that implied by the brand name theory described above. Manufacturers had well-developed brand names, faced substantial competition, and sold their product to a defined market of repeat consumers.[45] Blood product manufacturers depended on their customers and feared their competitors. They recognized that their competitors could, and would, point out differences in the safety of products. The fact that consumers did respond to brand names was one of the motivations of French and Japanese regulators who withheld initial approval of U.S.-produced heat-treated plasma.

Patients, Physicians, and the Demand for Blood and Blood Products: 1982–1985

Without the ability to inform patients and users, there was little incentive for blood bankers and product manufacturers to take costly steps to reduce transmission risk. The lack of information about these alternatives also reduced consumer demand for these steps. But the lack of safer alternatives did not close off all options for patients. The final step that could be taken in the face of evidence that AIDS could be transmitted through the blood supply was simply to reduce the use of blood and blood products. This step required the least information — only the knowledge that blood and blood products were less safe than they had been. Furthermore, it could be taken at the most decentralized level — by individual physicians and patients (who could decline surgery) and by hemophiliacs.

Evidence from blood systems around the world suggests that there were substantial possibilities for reducing the use of allogeneic blood without incurring significant costs. In the United States in 1985, an estimated 20% to 25% of red blood cell use was unnecessary, as were an estimated 95% of plasma transfusions.[49] In a comparison across European hospitals, the percentage of patients with bypass graft surgery who received a blood transfusion (allogeneic or autologous) ranged between 17% and 100%.[50] The decision to transfuse blood apparently depends on the art as well as the science of medicine. Not surprisingly, then, rates of use of blood responded to the epidemic, in the United States and elsewhere. In San Francisco, where AIDS was particularly concentrated, allogeneic whole blood use declined 14% between 1982 and 1984. Blood use grew more slowly than it had previously in other areas of the country, but only declined in high AIDS regions, so these declines are likely to have been related to the newly perceived risk of HIV infection.[51] In France, rates of "inappropriate" blood use declined 30% to 50%.[15] In Canada, 34% of patients surveyed in 1984 said that they would avoid transfusion to reduce the risk of HIV infection.[27]

Interest in alternatives to allogeneic blood, particularly autologous donation, grew in many countries.[52] Private blood banks arose in the United Kingdom, Australia, and the United States. Rates of autologous donation in the United States rose rapidly in the early years of the epidemic, again mainly in areas where AIDS was concentrated.[53,54] In other countries, regulatory authorities initially resisted the introduction of autologous donation, which is somewhat more costly than the use of allogeneic blood, but by 1990, autologous donation was an option in most developed countries.

The nature of the response to AIDS in the blood product market was quite different. Blood product use also varies substantially. In Austria, type A hemophiliacs typically received doses of 16,000 International Units of AHF per year. In neighboring Germany, doses averaged 80,000 IUs per year.[55] Considerable variation in use patterns also exists within certain countries.[56] Rates of infection among hemophiliacs are correlated with rates of use of fractionated product.

Confronted with the risk of AIDS, hemophiliacs could reduce the use of AHF or substitute cryoprecipitate made from the blood of a small number of donors. This type of change was recommended by many advisory bodies. Yet hemophilia treatment changed little in the 1982–1985 period. The rate of use of concentrate increased over the period, rather than declining.[27,56,57]

Hemophiliacs, unlike physicians and potential blood transfusion recipients, were limited in their ability to act independently. In most countries, their access to alternative treatment products was mediated by the health insurance and regulatory systems. In Japan, for example, cryoprecipitate was only available in limited quantities. German hemophiliacs could obtain heat-treated AHF only if they were not infected with hepatitis B. In Denmark, only products on a government formulary could be freely prescribed by physicians. But even where options were available, relatively little change occurred. Hemophiliacs had grown accustomed to the use of concentrate products. They had accepted the serious risk of hepatitis from the use of AHF and apparently treated the risk of AIDS as similar. In this stance, they were encouraged by their doctors and by hemophiliac associations that also strove to maintain the status quo. Although some hemophilia doctors and individual hemophiliacs did change their practices, there was no wholesale switch to cryoprecipitate anywhere.

The differences between demand changes in the whole blood sector and among hemophiliacs are consistent with the literature on economic behavior under uncertainty. First, blood transfusion users and hemophiliacs differed substantially in the nature of the status quo that they faced. Patients faced no risk of transfusion until the possibility of surgery arose. AIDS presented them with a new, highly publicized risk that compounded the existing dangers of undergoing surgery. It was in the interest of patients and of surgeons, who wanted to perform operations, to reduce patient risks, and the perceptions of these risks as much as possible. By contrast, HIV seemed to be less of a new risk for hemophiliacs (at least from the perspective of their physicians and advocacy organizations). They had grown accustomed to the use of blood products that carried significant dangers of infectious diseases and appear to have assimilated HIV to their prior experience with hepatitis.

Second, blood transfusion users and hemophiliacs differed in the kind of protection that was offered to them. Autologous donation, or the avoidance of transfusion altogether, allowed surgery patients to reduce the new risk of transfusion-associated disease to zero. For hemophiliacs, alternative products, including small-pool cryoprecipitate, could reduce transfusion risks, but they could not reduce the risks to zero. The economic literature on choice under uncertainty indicates that "certainty premiums" exist. People value products that are *completely* safe much more highly than those that are merely safer than alternatives.[19]

Complete Information

The role of loss aversion and the status quo bias in regulatory behavior becomes obvious in the regulatory reversals that occurred in each country after 1985. In April and June 1984, researchers in France and the United States identified the human immunodeficiency virus.[12] Development of a laboratory test for the identification of the virus proceeded rapidly. By late 1984, it had become possible to identify the virus in standard laboratory settings. In March 1985, one laboratory was licensed for the test in the United States. The market for testing was competitive, and the test was available at relatively low cost.[58] The development of the test had three immediate effects on the information available to generate a response to the transmission of HIV through the blood. First, it became possible to test blood for HIV and to ascertain whether a unit of blood was infected. Second, it became possible to know whether heat treatment and other efforts (including voluntary self-exclusion) were effective in preventing transmission. Finally, it became possible to identify cases of HIV transmission through the blood without waiting the 7 to 10 years until AIDS became apparent. These three developments together led to a sea change in the response to the transmission of HIV.

In the countries under study, it became instantly apparent that voluntary self-exclusion and similar efforts had not protected the blood supply from HIV. Testing revealed that some local donors were seropositive and also demonstrated that large numbers of hemophiliacs and at least a few transfusion recipients had received blood and blood products that were tainted with the virus. In Montreal a seroprevalence survey made the front page of the local paper. In Denmark, the discovery of a single case of transfusion-transmitted AIDS from a Danish blood donor was enough to change government policy on testing. In August 1985, the Japanese identified the first domestically transmitted blood case and began HIV testing. The test also made it possible to address this dismaying information without radically altering the institutional characteristics that had produced a safe blood supply in the 1970s.

As Table 11-2 shows, countries moved very rapidly in taking advantage of this information. In each country, the regulatory component of the blood system dramatically upgraded standards and reduced risks. Differences in the regulatory structure of these various countries do appear to have affected the pace of change within the brief 1985–1986 period. Trebilcock, Howse, and Daniels, in their study of the response of eight countries to the epidemic, examine the role of regulatory design in the timing of the implementation of efforts to reduce transmission, particularly HIV testing and heat treatment.[37] They conclude that regulatory institutions that were centralized and divorced from the collection and distribution of blood and blood products responded more rapidly than decentralized structures and institutions that were responsible for both regulating blood and collecting it.

These differences in response time, however, were a matter of months. In most countries, once a risk of transmission in that country had been established, the test was quickly implemented nationwide. Testing was mandated even in countries where low HIV prevalence suggested that it made little sense from a cost-effectiveness standpoint. In the United States in 1986, the cost per life saved from testing blood was over $10,000 per year.[59] In countries with much lower HIV prevalence, the cost per life saved was proportionally higher. Countries that had only gradually adopted testing for hepatitis B and hepatitis B core antigen jumped on the HIV testing bandwagon.

Table 11-2. Timing of HIV testing and heat treatment

	HIV (ELISA) Testing of Blood Supply Mandated	Heat Treatment of Factor Concentrate Mandated
Australia	May 1985	January 1985
Canada	November 1985	July 1985
Denmark	January 1986	October 1985
France	August 1985	October 1985
Germany	October 1985	Never mandated, but no reimbursement for untreated products
Italy	March 1985	July 1985
Japan	November 1986	October 1985/February 1986
United Kingdom	October 1985	June 1985
United States	March 1985	October 1984
India	1987/1989	N.A.
Thailand	1987/1989	N.A.
Zimbabwe	July 1985	N.A.

Source: Australia, Canada, France, Germany, United Kingdom, United States from Trebilcock, M., Howse, H., and Daniels, R., "Do Institutions Matter? A Comparative Pathology of the HIV-Infected Blood Tragedy 82 *Virginia Law Review* (1996), pp. 1407–1492. Other countries, data on file.

Similarly, by late 1984, studies in various countries had shown that heat-treated AHF was (relatively) effective in preventing transmission of the virus. In combination with information that showed that local donors were infected (or that American AHF was infected), this information convinced every country to switch from untreated to heat-treated products. No country had mandated the use of these products in December 1984; all of these countries mandated heat treatment by December 1985.

The Aftermath

AIDS was not hepatitis. The introduction of a new disease destabilized an existing institutional framework and led to profound changes in the way that regulators and the public viewed blood and blood-collecting institutions.

In the wake of media coverage and governmental or quasi-governmental investigations in most countries since 1985, the stance of blood regulators around the world has changed. The pre-1985 status quo of a basically safe blood supply was overturned in favor of the view that the blood supply is fundamentally at risk. Regulatory precautions have been tightened and new tests have been implemented, even where risks seem relatively small. Efforts to reduce blood use and to recycle blood during operations, as well as efforts to derive synthetic alternatives to human blood, further reduce the role of the traditional blood service.

The treatment of hemophilia, too, has changed. All AHF must be heat-treated and methods of heat treatment are constantly being improved. New methods are much more costly and plasma-demanding than earlier methods. Shortages of the new products have led some writers to complain that quality standards are being set too high.[39]

These developments in the blood transfusion and AHF markets suggest that the system has now restabilized. New tests have been introduced and blood is, once again, "safe." But AIDS has left cracks that the tests only paper over. The new regulatory stance, which places a much higher premium on blood safety, requires blood banks to perform many more tests and exclude many more potential donors. False (as well as true) positive rates on these newly standard screening tests pose a threat to the voluntary blood banking system. The pool of donors who qualify for donation shrinks (more than proportionately, because the tests are not perfectly specific) with each successive quality enhancement. This narrower pool of donors must be encouraged to make more repeat donations. More encouragement means more incentives, and more incentives, as I argue above, means less altruism and less true "voluntarism."

At the same time, better recruitment efforts, more tests, and more heat treatment raise the costs of blood and blood products during an era of worldwide health care cost containment. Pressure to control costs encourages competition and, perhaps, reduces compliance with cost-increasing regulations, further undermining the pre-1982 institutional structure. Blood is safer than it ever was, but the blood system is under much greater strain.

Most people who were infected with HIV through blood were infected before 1985, many much earlier. The HIV test was highly effective in reducing the risk beginning in 1985. Before 1982, no one was aware of the risk of AIDS and no action could be taken. But in the middle period, between 1982 and 1985, available information was put to very little use. It is important to focus on that period because the kind of information available between 1982 and 1985 is the kind of information most likely to become available rapidly if a new disease appears in the blood system.

Information available between 1982 and 1985 was epidemiological (not causal) and incomplete (not scientifically validated). Before 1985, patterns of association between disease and individual characteristics and between disease and blood characteristics appeared, but they could not be proved. The problem facing the blood supply was how to deal with such uncertain information. In general, the response everywhere was very cautious. Regulators were reluctant to mandate measures of uncertain efficacy and considerable monetary and human cost—or to devolve responsibility for evaluating this information to consumers of blood and blood products who might, or might not, have behaved differently. Of course, this status quo–favoring regulatory stance is not unique to the regulation of the blood supply in the face of AIDS. For example, activists seeking regulatory approval for drugs for the treatment of AIDS have argued that the long delays typically needed to clearly prove safety and efficacy are inappropriate in the case of a deadly disease and assert that patients deserve the opportunity to assess the risks and benefits of treatment for themselves.

The regulatory system governing blood in each country, like many aspects of the voluntary blood collection system itself, was designed to maintain quality within a static environment. It existed in a world in which population health only changed in a positive direction. In such an environment, a regulatory structure that adopts change only very cautiously makes sense. A change in the blood supply that turns out to raise costs without improving quality, or, more seriously, a change that reduces quality, is unacceptable. In retrospect, however, these principles may have been inappropriate for addressing a situation in which the status quo could change radically.

In an environment of rapid change, it becomes much more important to make use of scraps of information, even if they are incomplete. Allowing producers to make more product quality claims that patients and physicians can respond to is likely to make use of partial information faster. In turn, the use of such information can provide data to regulatory authorities as they decide what actions to take. Allowing blood collectors to compete and establish local brand names can encourage them to reveal quality-enhancing information.

Empowering patients, physicians, and producers, however, raises as many troubling questions as it solves. Errors of action may be easily as serious as errors of inaction, and the theory of loss aversion suggests that people value such errors very highly. Giving patients choices in this way raises important equity issues. If patients themselves can choose whether to use costly heat-treated products, blood that has been surrogate tested, plasma collected from women only, or their own banked blood, who is to pay the incremental costs? Such choices undermine equity standards and undermine the notions of social solidarity central to voluntary blood systems.

Furthermore, our new sense of a dynamic status quo may be mistaken. At every point in time, most diseases are old diseases, and donor characteristics can be readily correlated with disease risk. The voluntary, nonprofit, noncompetitive institutional structure is a very effective way of exploiting information in a static environment and we would give up that efficiency if we chose a more market-oriented approach.

NOTES

1. R. M. Titmuss, *The Gift Relationship: From Human Blood to Social Policy* (New York: Pantheon Books, 1971), p. 115.

2. E. Feldman, "HIV and Blood in Japan: Transforming Private Conflict into Public Scandal," Eric Feldman and Ronald Bayer, eds., *Blood Feuds: AIDS, Blood, and the Politics of Disaster* (New York: Oxford University Press, 1999).

3. R. Bayer, "Blood and AIDS in America: Science, Politics and the Making of an Iatrogenic Disaster," Feldman and Bayer, *op. cit.*

4. U. Izzo, "Blood, Bureaucracy and Law: Responding to HIV-Tainted Blood in Italy," Feldman and Bayer, *op. cit.*

5. K. Arrow, "Gifts and Exchanges," *Philosophy and Public Affairs*, 1 (1972), pp. 343–362, p. 346.

6. R. A. Kessel, "Transfused Blood, Serum Hepatitis, and the Coase Theorem," *Journal of Law and Economics*, 17(2) (1975), pp. 265–89.

7. C. Havighurst, "Legal Responses to the Problem of Poor Quality Blood," *Blood Policy: Issues and Alternatives*, ed. David B. Johnson, (Washington, D.C.: American Enterprise Institute, 1976), pp. 21–37.

8. J. Haltiwanger and M. Waldman, "The Role of Altruism in Economic Interaction," *Journal of Economic Behavior and Organizations*, 21(2) (1993), pp. 1–15.

9. H. Stewart, "Rationality and the Market for Human Blood," *Journal of Economic Behavior and Organization*, 19(2) (1992), pp. 125–143.

10. R. Taylor, "AIDS and Blood in Great Britain," an unpublished paper prepared for the project HIV-Contaminated Blood: Policy and Conflict.

11. R. D. Eckert and E. L. Wallace, *Securing a Safer Blood Supply: Two Views* (Washington: American Enterprise Institute, 1985).

12. R. D. Eckert, "The AIDS Blood-Transfusion Cases: A Legal and Economic Analysis of Liability," *San Diego Law Review*, 29 (1992), pp. 203–298.

13. National Research Council, Committee on AIDS Research and the Behavioral, Social, and Statistical Sciences, *AIDS: the Second Decade* (Washington: National Academy Press, 1990).

14. E. Albaek, "The Never-Ending Story: The Political and Legal Controversies over HIV and the Blood Supply in Denmark," Feldman and Bayer, *op. cit.*

15. M. Steffen, "The Nation's Blood: Medicine, Justice, and the State in France," Feldman and Bayer, *op. cit.*

16. P. Jacobs, R. P. Wilder, "Pricing Behavior of Non-Profit Agencies: The Case of Blood Products," *Journal of Health Economics*, 3(1) (1984), pp. 49–61.

17. A. Britten, F. Etzel, C. Carman, C. Smit Sibinga, "Supply and Need of Factor VIII Concentrates," *Haematologia* 16(1–4) (1983), pp. 109–20.

18. K. C. Fraundorf, "Competition in Blood Banking," *Public Policy* 23(2) (1975), pp. 219–40.

19. W. K. Viscusi, W. Magat, and J. Huber "Consumer Rationality in the Face of Multiple Health Risks," *Rand Journal of Economics* (1987), pp. 465–479.

20. A. Tversky and D. Kahneman, "Loss Aversion in Riskless Choice: A Reference-Dependent Model," *Quarterly Journal of Economics*, 106(4) (1991), pp. 1039–61.

21. D. Kahneman, J. L. Knetsch, and R. H. Thaler, "The Endowment Effect, Loss Aversion, and Status Quo Bias: Anomalies," *Journal of Economic Perspectives*, 5(1) (1991), pp. 193–206.

22. G. N. Russell, S. Peterson, S. J. Harper, and M. A. Fox, "Homologous Blood Use and Conservation Techniques for Cardiac Surgery in the United Kingdom," *British Medical Journal*, 297(6660) (1988), pp. 1390–1.

23. J. Kramer, "Bad Blood," *The New Yorker*, 69 (October 11, 1993), pp. 74–80.

24. J. R. Bove, "Measures other than Laboratory Testing to Exclude Donors who are at Increased Risk of Transmitting the AIDS Virus: the USA Experience," *AIDS: The Safety of Blood and Blood Products*, ed. J. C. Petricciani, I. D. Gust, P. A. Hoppe, and H. W. Krijnen (Chichester: John Wiley [WHO], 1987), pp. 125–130.

25. R. W. Beal, "Measures Other than Laboratory Testing to Exclude Donors Who Are at Increased Risk of Transmitting the AIDS Virus: Exclusion of High Risk Donors," ch. 14 in *AIDS: The Safety of Blood and Blood Products*, ed J. C. Petricciani, I. D. Gust, P. A. Hoppe, and H. W. Krijnen (Chichester: John Wiley [WHO], 1987), pp. 131–133.

26. S. Dressler, "Blood 'Scandal' and AIDS in Germany," Feldman and Bayer, *op. cit.*

27. N. Gilmore and M. Somerville, "From Trust to Tragedy: HIV/AIDS and the Canadian Blood System," Feldman and Bayer, *op. cit.*

28. J. Ballard, "HIV-Contaminated Blood and Australian Policy: The Limits of Success," Feldman and Bayer, *op. cit.*

29. M. Reddin, "Commentary," *Blood Policy: Issues and Alternatives*, ed. David B. Johnson (Washington: American Enterprise Institute, 1976) 59–62.

30. Commission of Inquiry into the Blood System in Canada. *Interim Report*. Ottawa: Canada Communication Group, 1995.

31. W. A. Check, "Preventing AIDS Transmission: Should Blood Donors Be Screened?" *JAMA*, 249(5) (1983), pp. 567–570.

32. S. A. Galel, J. D. Lifson, and E. G. Engleman, "Prevention of AIDS Transmission through Screening of the Blood Supply," *Annual Review of Immunology*, 13 (1995), pp. 201–227.

33. J. B. Brunet and R. A. Ancelle, "The International Occurrence of the Acquired Immunodeficiency Syndrome," *Annals of Internal Medicine*, 103(5) (1985), pp. 670–4.

34. D. Mvere, "AIDS and Blood in Zimbabwe," an unpublished paper prepared for the project HIV Contaminated Blood: Policy and Conflict.

35. A. Kellner, "The Need for Reform," *Blood Policy: Issues and Alternatives*, ed. David B. Johnson (Washington: American Enterprise Institute, 1976a), pp. 137–144.

36. R. M. Selik, J. W. Ward, and J. W. Buehler, "Demographic Differences in Cumulative Incidence Rates of Transfusion-associated Acquired Immunodeficiency Syndrome," *American Journal of Epidemiology*, 15;140(2) (1994), pp. 105–12.

37. M. Trebilcock, R. Howse, and R. Daniels, "Do Institutions Matter? A Comparative Pathology of the HIV-Infected Blood Tragedy," *University of Virginia Law Review*, 82 (1996), pp. 1407–1485.

38. B. T. Colvin, M. Ainsworth, S. J. Machin, I. J. Mackie, J. K. Smith, L. Winkelman, and M. E. Haddon, "Heat-treated NHS Factor VIII Concentrate in the United Kingdom—a preliminary study," *Clinical and Laboratory Haematology*, 8(2) (1986), pp. 85–92.

39. G. F. Pierce, J. M. Lusher, A. P. Brownstein, J. C. Goldsmith, and C. M. Kessler, "The Use of Purified Clotting Factor Concentrates in Hemophilia. Influence of Viral Safety, Cost, and Supply on Therapy," *JAMA*, 261(23) (1989), pp. 3434–8.

40. H. M. Meyer, Jr., "Food and Drug Administration Responses to the Challenges of AIDS," *Public Health Reports*, 98(4) (1983), pp. 320–323.

41. D. N. Mendelson and S. G. Sandler, "A Model for Estimating Incremental Benefits and Costs of Testing Donated Blood for Human Immunodeficiency Virus Antigen (HIV-Ag)," *Transfusion*, 30(1) (1990), pp. 73–75.

42. J. M. Kern and B. B. Croy, "A Review of Transfusion-Associated AIDS Litigation: 1984 through 1993." *Transfusion*, 34(6) (1994), pp. 484–91.

43. D. Dewees, D. Duff, and M. Trebilcock, *Exploring the Domain of Accident Law: Taking the Facts Seriously* (Oxford: Oxford University Press, 1996).

44. J. C. Petricciani, *AIDS: The Safety of Blood and Blood Products*, ed. J. C. Petricciani, I. D. Gust, P. A. Hoppe, and H. W. Krijnen (Chichester: John Wiley [WHO], 1987), p. 334.

45. Institute of Medicine, *HIV and the Blood Supply An Analysis of Crisis Decision-making* ed. Lauren B. Leveton et al. (Washington, D.C.: National Academy of Sciences, 1995).

46. J. L. Tullis, "Current Plasmapheresis Practice in the United States," *La Ricerca in Clinica e in Laboratorio*, 13(1) (1983), pp. 11–19.

47. J. Leikola, "Plasma Procurement World-Wide," *Beitrage zur Infusionstherapie* 24 (1989), pp. 69–73.

48. P. M. Mannucci, "Availability of Plasma Fractions for Therapeutic Use in Italy," *La Ricerca in Clinica e in Laboratorio*, 13(1) (1983), pp. 1–4.

49. U.S. Congress, Office of Technology Assessment, *Blood Policy and Technology* (Washington, D.C.: Government Printing Office, 1985).

50. Sanguis Study Group, "Use of Blood Products for Elective Surgery in 43 European Hospitals," *Transfusion Medicine*, 4 (1994), pp. 251–268.

51. D. M. Surgenor, E. L. Wallace, S. G. Hale, and M. W. Gilpatrick, "Changing Patterns of Blood Transfusion in Four Sets of U.S. Hospitals, 1980 to 1985," *Transfusion*, 28(6) (1988), pp. 513–518.

52. H. Hambley, "Revised Guidelines on Preoperative Autologous Blood Donation," *British Medical Journal*, 307(6918) (1993), pp. 1510.

53. D. M. Surgenor, E. L. Wallace, S. H. Hao, and R. H. Chapman, " Collection and Transfusion of Blood in the U.S., 1982–1988," *New England Journal of Medicine*, 322 (23) (1990), pp. 1646–1649.

54. E. L. Wallace, D. M. Surgenor, H. S. Hao, J. An, R. H. Chapman, and W. H. Churchill, "Collection and Transfusion of Blood and Blood Components in the United States, 1989," *Transfusion*, 33(2) (1993), pp. 139–44.

55. A. Britten, F. Etzel, C. Carman, C. Smit Sibinga, "Supply and Need of Factor VIII Concentrates," *Haematologia*, 16(1–4) (1983), pp. 109–20.

56. F. Rodeghiero, "Treatment of Hemophilia," *La Ricerca in Clinica e in Laboratorio*, 15(4) (1985), pp. 289–303.

57. S. Mayes, H. A. Handford, D. Szczucki, and J. H. Schaefer, "Blood Product Use by Hemophiliacs in Relation to AIDS Risk Awareness and Patient Variables," *Psychosomatics*, 35(4) (1994), pp. 354–360.

58. M. M. Heckler, "The Challenge of the Acquired Immunodeficiency Syndrome," *Annals of Internal Medicine*, 103 (1985), pp. 655–656.

59. R. S. Eisenstaedt and T. E. Getzen, "Screening Blood Donors for Human Immunodeficiency Virus Antibody: Cost-Benefit Analysis," *American Journal of Public Health*, 78(4) (1988), pp. 450–4.

Conclusion

The Comparative Politics of Contaminated Blood

From Hesitancy to Scandal

Theodore R. Marmor,
Patricia A. Dillon,
and Stephen Scher

The story of blood and AIDS is one of genuine tragedy, as the case studies in this book powerfully reveal. By the time scientific and regulatory authorities understood the sources of infection from contaminated blood, thousands of blood transfusion recipients and a substantial proportion of hemophiliacs in advanced industrial nations had already been infected with HIV. The period from 1981 to 1985 was one of uneven but profound change: from hesitancy to understanding, and from skepticism to heat treatment of blood products. It was a period of coping with confusion, of conflicting organizational priorities, and of variously channeled demands for what seemed like costly preventive actions. After these actions were taken—by the mid-1980s—the source of controversy shifted, first to restitution and later to retribution. From initial offers of victim compensation to full-scale reviews of official (mis)conduct and professional (mis)judgments, the stories have involved everything from tawdry commercialism to high scandal, from substantial punishment to diffuse regret.

The patterns of the post-1985 responses to the tragedy of HIV-contaminated blood are far more varied than the initial reactions. The central puzzle this concluding chapter addresses is what accounts—in probabilistic terms—for both the similarities in the initial reactions and for the variations that emerge thereafter. The chapter proceeds in three parts. The first sets the stage by sketching the assumptive world regarding blood products and hemophilia that was largely taken for granted at the outset of the 1980s. Our contention is that those widely shared assumptions help to account for much of the hesitancy in responding to signs of contaminated blood in the early 1980s. The second part sets out to portray what in retrospect appears to be the compressed differences in national responses to contaminated blood in the 1982–85 period. This interpretation is suggested in the introduction to this volume, illustrated in the case studies, and only briefly argued here.[1] The third and most extensive part explores the variation in national responses that began to take shape in the mid-1980s.

The variations from country to country in the post-1985 period fall into three broad categories: high, moderate, and low-intensity scandal politics. Despite its limitations, this categorization was helpful in analyzing and understanding the particular mix of institutional arrangements, cultural beliefs, and feelings of bitterness and betrayal that account for the variation the case studies reveal. In a larger context, these different national responses provide a lens through which to view the capacity of each country's institutions to assess and respond to risk under conditions of uncertainty. This is a complicated, cross-national story, however, and comparative analysis can play only a partial role in illuminating why and how such a tragedy took place and what followed from it. Nonetheless, the recurrent themes in this story—which lies at the intersection of science and policy—are hardly restricted to the AIDS crisis or to the distribution and use of blood and blood products for medical purposes.

Institutional Legacies and the Tragedy of Contaminated Blood

It is worth repeating that in 1981, after the report of the sentinel cases of *Pneumocystis carinii* pneumonia in Los Angeles,[2] and in 1982, after AIDS was reported in a patient with hemophilia,[3] the nature of this new syndrome was unclear. HIV had not been isolated. The latency period and rate of progression to AIDS were unknown. The dominant scientific and regulatory actors, uncertain about the scientific features of this new threat, and lacking clear direction within their own institutions,[4] fell back on their familiar understandings about blood safety and the risks to health in dealing with new blood-related threats. As a result, one cannot understand the unfolding tragedy of infected blood without first taking into account the institutional and belief legacy concerning blood and blood products, the regulation thereof, and responses to hepatitis B in the 1970s.

The entry of HIV into the blood supply in the late 1970s took place at a time of extraordinary technological attainment and rising expectations in the community of hemophiliacs and their specialist physicians. The development of blood products that promised to reduce spontaneous bleeding—the wonder of factor VIII—meant that young men with hemophilia, who had faced limited mobility, crippling pain, disability, and early death[5] from intracranial and joint bleeding, could suddenly look forward to normal family life and strenuous sports. Moreover, the life expectancy for hemophiliacs was rising sharply, to 60 years by 1980.[6-8] These dramatic improvements required pharmaceutical preparations that were expensive and dependent on a large, reliable supply of blood plasma. Paralleling these developments, blood banks, donor groups, and the Red Cross directed their attention toward ensuring the availability of blood products and to maintaining a blood supply that was adequate and reliable. These factors set the stage for what the introduction to this volume describes as the "iatrogenic tragedy" of blood and AIDS.

Although the reader may already be familiar with the beliefs associated with maintaining an adequate, reliable, and safe blood supply, a brief summary here will prove helpful. While a commercially driven, pharmaceutically based system was central to the production of clotting factors for hemophiliacs, the institutional framework for whole blood was based on voluntarism. Commercial blood was presumed less safe than blood drawn from voluntary sources. Because the stability of the blood supply in a voluntary system depended on willing donors, appeals to altruism and reassurances about safety had become standard procedures. Some risks—like that of hepatitis B—came to be regarded as "acceptable" and manageable for hemophiliacs, most of whom were known to have been already exposed. When balanced against the blessings of the new blood products, the threat of hepatitis B seemed remote to both blood professionals and patients. As earlier chapters have shown, the emphasis was on increasing the supply and availability of "convenience products."

This assumptive world, tragically, would prove disastrous for both hemophiliacs and blood transfusion recipients. Altruism was no safeguard against the HIV infection. Nor would assumptions about "acceptable risks" hold true for the deadly HIV virus. The gap between institutional claims about blood and blood products, on the one hand, and the realities of practice, on the other, would later shape the politics of retribution. The extent to which transfusion recipients and hemophiliacs had depended on trusted medical and political elites would contribute greatly to the sense of betrayal and the search for the guilty in the aftermath of the tragedy of HIV-contaminated blood.

The Pattern of Hesitancy, 1982–85

Despite differences in financing and institutional arrangements in the countries under study, broadly similar patterns emerged in their initial, hesitant response to the emergence of AIDS among transfusion recipients and hemophiliacs. First, physicians underestimated the extent to which those exposed to potentially contaminated blood would suffer irreparable injury. Second was the importance everywhere of blood-community elites in setting policy, with the role of other interest groups more varied. Third was delay at critical points because of difficulties in balancing industrial policy and goals against uncertain scientific information. Fourth was the reluctance to screen donors, because such efforts might have undercut public perceptions of a safe blood supply and potentially stigmatized high-risk groups. Last was the marginal political position of the hemophiliac population, a patient group that had not yet developed a political identity, and the absence of political identity among those who shared nothing but the fact that they had been patients in need of blood transfusions.

In country after country, the tragedy of underestimating the risk of the deadly new virus had a profound impact. Just as they had previously accepted the trade-off between hepatitis infection and the benefits to hemophiliacs of reduced disability, the major institutional actors were reluctant to disrupt the supply of blood and blood products by measures that promised but could not assure a measure of security against AIDS. (Although, ironically, those who feared that AIDS might spread like hepatitis were the first to sound the tocsin.) Perceptions about risk were also influenced by a common reluctance to take on the cost of screening and, later, heat treatment, and by beliefs about the groups first infected with AIDS. Because it was "the American disease" and a disease of homosexuals, drug users, and Haitians, familiar national policies were thought adequate to protect hemophiliacs. These perceptions of risk, coupled with the patterns discussed above, bred resistance to safety measures that would have protected the blood supply and, consequently, hemophiliacs in the 1982–85 period. The results of this common pattern of hesitancy would turn out to be tragic.

A common pattern does not, of course, mean an identical one. There surely were variations in the timing of heat treatment, of taking untreated blood out of distribution, and of excluding high-risk groups from blood donation.[9] And small differences—even of months—in the introduction of safety measures had deadly consequences. Nonetheless, by 1986, the nations under study had broadly similar policies. The differences among nations that would emerge in response to these policies were much greater, ranging from scandal to quiet adjustment, from punishing attacks on public officials to what was largely business as usual.

Varieties of Scandal in the Aftermath of Undeniable Tragedy

In contrast to the hesitancy and relatively narrow range of institutional responses to the appearance of HIV, the aftermath of actual infection exhibited considerable cross-national variation.[10] Each country under study in this volume experienced some elements of a blood scandal, and there were important similarities in their experiences. Most obvious was the emergence of organizations of hemophiliacs and their growing independence from (and anger at) former allies in medicine. There was a common sense of violation of deeply held social beliefs about responsible medical practice. Among other similarities were the limited role played by transfusion recipients and a pattern of initially settling for compensation in the 1980s. In the 1990s, the search for guilty parties became widespread. That search included extensive use of the media, more frequent reliance on the courts, and the demonstration of greater political influence by hemophiliacs than their numbers alone would have predicted. These common elements were nonetheless shaped by organizational and cultural differences, channeled through distinctive legal and political institutions. In the end, the results were very different.

Accounting for the variation among countries does not require a taxonomy of scandal itself, but some conceptual preliminaries are called for. First of all, measuring the intensity of scandal is not the same as measuring wrongdoing. Scandal is by accepted usage a public matter. It is not the world of closed meetings but rather the exposure of wrongdoing at such meetings. Even when wrongdoing becomes known, the intensity of the scandal it prompts need not be proportionate to the wrongdoing. Second, policy scandals typically involve the disclosure not of wrongdoing (or alleged wrongdoing) in general, but wrongdoing of particular kinds: the abuse of institutional power or the violation of some important community norm. Third, exposing scandalous conduct does not, in itself, generate a scandal. Whether a scandal emerges in any particular case depends in large part upon the degree to which those disclosing or investigating the wrongdoing are successful in capturing and maintaining public attention as the investigation and disclosures continue. Fourth, scandals generally, though not necessarily, lead to adverse consequences for the wrongdoers. Typical outcomes include criminal punishment, civil liability, loss of office or position, and damage to one's reputation. Fifth, unless scandals are very quickly contained, they tend to cast a broad net of wrongdoing and wrongdoers. Just how broad depends on how the issues are framed, on the intensity of the scandal, and on how long the public's interest is sustained. These factors will depend, in turn, not just on the social, political, and legal setting in each country, but also upon the precise role that the protagonists — in our case, hemophiliacs — come to define for themselves and how aggressively and effectively they act in pursuit of their goals.

Central to the development of the blood scandals was the transformation of hemophiliacs into a cohesive group with a core identity and political goals. What is remarkable is that this transformation — a very difficult one, as David Kirp has noted[11] — took place at all. Prior to the advent of AHF products, hemophiliacs had often suffered in isolation while they coped, as best they could, with their disease. Then, thanks to AHF products, they had come to lead mainstream lives. Though no longer in isolation and no longer suffering, they had little incentive to band together around their disease for political purposes. After exposure to HIV, they were forced into their private worlds again, to face the personal calamities of physical deterioration, financial ruin, the disease or death of family members, and even violence from frightened neighbors. Even so, despite their previously apolitical history and the personal desperation and private nightmares that resulted from being infected with HIV, hemophiliacs banded together, found identity in a group, and mobilized into social movements.

Once organized, the social movements of hemophiliacs generated the conflicts — and ultimately the scandals — we see in each of the countries we have studied. The intensity of each scandal lies on a continuum having three broad categories: high scandal, moderate scandal, and low scandal. Any such grouping of countries will necessarily be imperfect; each country has a distinctive configuration of government, health care arrangements, and political culture. The categories nonetheless are helpful in analyzing how industrial democracies confronted the tragedy of transmitting HIV through blood and blood products.

Instances of High Scandal

Canada, France, and Japan, among the nations discussed in this volume, experienced the most prolonged and bitter public debate about wrongdoing in connection with HIV infection through contaminated blood and blood products. They all punished major figures and made substantial changes in their institutional arrangements for the supply and regulation of blood. Their scandals, in short, demonstrated intensity, durability, and stability. The best predictors of such high scandal are a unified group of hemophiliacs with a political identity, a compelling narrative appealing to the larger population, a paternalistic political culture, and a centralized decision-making regime.

Political Organization, Hemophiliacs, and Scandal

The Japanese story is a clear example of the role that interest groups played in the shaping of blood scandals. Japanese hemophiliacs, as Eric Feldman's chapter explains, had adopted a rights-based strategy by 1987 in response to proposed legislation (the AIDS Prevention Law) targeted at people with AIDS. Moreover, unlike what happened in other countries, Japanese hemophiliacs expanded their coalition to include students and others who were not hemophiliacs.[12] They sued the government and the pharmaceutical industry in 1989, stressing that litigation was not merely a plea for financial relief (which had already been offered in 1985),[13] but a demand for dignity. They sought an apology from a government that had failed to protect them.[14] The persistence of the Japanese hemophiliac community, coupled with further disclosures of both public and corporate wrongdoing, ultimately led to the long-sought apologies. Key figures in the formation of policy during the early 1980s subsequently faced criminal prosecution.

Unlike those in Japan, hemophiliacs in Canada did not organize themselves effectively until the 1990s. Canada, like many other countries, had established in 1989 a compensation scheme without admitting fault. But the details of the program angered many hemophiliacs. Families were compelled to forfeit rights to file separate legal actions, and to accept compensation by a certain date or forfeit it forever. Moreover, payments were limited to four years and excluded surviving spouses. But no organized political action resulted. Even the severe criticism of the Canadian Red Cross, deriving from its role as protector of the voluntary blood supply and from its control (along with the Canadian Blood Commission) of blood collection and fractionation, failed to motivate hemophiliacs to consolidate as a political force. What finally triggered organized national action was the persistence of a small, new provincial group that brought its cause to Ottawa after its lobbying success in Nova Scotia.

In 1990, many provinces jointly decided to provide no additional compensation to supplement what had already been provided in the national compensation program.[15] It was in this particular context—facing a 1993 expiration date for his benefits—that Randy Connors, an infected hemophiliac, and his wife, Janet, formed the group Infected Spouses. They convinced Nova Scotia to break with the other provinces, establish its own compensation scheme, and extend the scheme to spouses.[16] They then took their cause to the Canadian capital, where the House of Commons held hearings that led to the establishment of the Krever Commission. That commission's hearings, discussed by Norbert Gillmore and Margaret Somerville,[17] were to draw the nation's attention to the plight of hemophiliacs and their families. The Connors' lobbying tactics were subsequently adopted by other provincial groups, leading some provincial ministers to abandon the 1990 interprovincial pact and establish their own compensation schemes. The confidence of Canadians in their blood system has been indisputably shaken, and the Red Cross was compelled to withdraw from blood collection and distribution.

French hemophiliacs had the most limited political organization of those in the three high-scandal countries. In 1989, they, too, had accepted a lump-sum compensation plan offered by the national government. But Peter Garvanoff, the lawyer for the nation's hemophilia society, proved central to mobilizing French opinion. Garvanoff, an infected hemophiliac who had lost two brothers, rejected compensation and persisted with litigation. A journalist following the plight of hemophiliacs proceeded to publish a sensational series of disclosures, which kept the issues before the public, galvanized the hemophiliac community, and made further investigations inevitable.[18] Jean Marie Le Pen's right-wing National Front provided some hemophiliacs with counsel and used the legal cases and ongoing disclosures to excoriate the Socialist Party, which had been in control of the government since the initial outbreak of AIDS in the early 1980s. Monica Steffen notes that in addition to contributing to the Socialists' loss at the next election, the growing sentiment on behalf of hemophiliacs led to the revision of the French constitution itself, which now limits the immunities available to public officials for acts committed in office.[19]

Compelling Narrative

Consistent with the formation of a group identity, groups of hemophiliacs constructed narratives of betrayal, suffering, and stigmatization in every country. Those in the high-scandal group, however, broadened the agenda beyond their own claims for justice concerning a past injury. They engaged the public through champions and were persuasive in arguing that everyone's security was threatened.

In Canada, Randy and Janet Connors emerged as sympathetic symbols. They highlighted the debate about infection of the blood supply while engaging the media and broader community of Canadians. Anxious for the financial security of their son after Randy's impending death, they pressed the case for additional compensation.[20] Later that year *Maclean's* recognized their courage and achievements by naming them to its 1993 Honor Roll. Randy Connors's accusation before the Krever Commission was powerful: knowingly distributing unsafe products was "murder." This charge was supported by evidence that the Red Cross had kept a "Schindler's List" of hemophiliacs who were to receive safer, heat-treated products. Such charges led the press, in turn, to describe the Krever Commission hearings as "a damning portrait of the Canadian Red Cross . . . and of government officials."[21] After Randy's widely reported death, Janet Connors became the avenging angel of Canada's blood-supply victims,[22] a vocal and highly visible public presence, commenting on key testimony and arguments presented before the Commission, and conducting interviews on the yearly anniversaries of her husband's death.

An articulate, appealing woman, Janet Connors gave a human face to the tragedy and opened a window into the homes of infected families. Hemophiliacs' surviving spouses—almost always women and often infected with HIV themselves—had no life insurance. They owed medical bills beyond the limits of Canada's universal health insurance, and coped with their own infection and their anxiety about the children who would be orphaned after their deaths. A 1997 interview on Canadian television about the Red Cross' effort to limit the Krever inquiry highlighted Janet Connors's ability to go beyond appeals to pity for hemophiliacs and their families, and to address the concerns and values of the broader Canadian community: "This [limit] would set a precedent," Connors claimed. "If anyone in government is unhappy with the findings of any commission, they can just run off to the Supreme Court and have the truth hidden. If Justice Krever is not allowed to write his report, more Canadians will die."[23]

In Japan, as Eric Feldman's chapter illustrates, it was only after years of demonstrations, litigation, and settlement offers that the transmission of HIV through blood products came to be seen as involving broad social and political issues that concerned not just hemophiliacs, but the entire nation. Instead of being viewed as a devastating problem for a small fraction of the populace, the plight of hemophiliacs and their families was reframed in terms of an ongoing civic battle against secrecy, corruption, and betrayal of public trust by elected officials and career bureaucrats. The "Kan-Kan War"[24] was, indeed, instigated not by a hemophiliac, but by a new, ambitious minister of health and welfare, Kan Naoto, who took on the Japanese bureaucracy. In this context, the picture of the president of Green Cross, down on his knees with his forehead to the floor, was, to be sure, a symbol of the humiliation of Japan's political and industrial elites.[25] But for hemophiliacs and their families, it also signaled a new era in which their concerns were not isolated and separate from those of the Japanese mainstream.

In France, the compelling narrative with broad public appeal was constructed by neither a hemophiliac nor an ambitious government minister. Instead, the narrator was a tenacious medical reporter, Anne-Marie Casteret, whose story, as in Japan, involved secrecy, betrayal, and money.[26] Among other things, she obtained the minutes of the May 1985 meeting at which Dr. Michel Garretta, director of the national transfusion center, decided to keep his contaminated factor VIII on the market.[27] She published the minutes and also covered subsequent court proceedings at which the hemophiliac association's lawyer (Peter Garvanoff) called out "Assassins!" during the defendants' testimony. The stark contrast between the legal immunity of public officials and the deterioration and death of hemophiliacs undermined the French public's trust both in their blood-supply system and in their government.

Paternalism and Scandal Intensity

The media tactics of hemophiliacs in high-scandal countries exploited the shock value of public disclosures, especially in political cultures like those of Japan and France, which are marked by the tight control of information and presumptions of governmental paternalism. This tactic, revealing the seeming wrongdoing of elites who were supposed to "govern," in itself heightened the drama associated with the disclosures. The prospect of disclosure engendered, in turn, efforts to prevent disclosure — efforts that when known only further heightened the drama associated with the blood scandal.

The hierarchical structure of French and Japanese[28] government is highly visible, and the prevailing view of their governing elites is that they should attend to the public's business without too much interference from ordinary citizens. French and Japanese citizens have no legal right, for example, to see government documents; in France, even documents introduced in court proceedings can be obtained only by consent of the Justice Ministry.[29] It is no surprise, then, that after Casteret published the minutes of the Garretta meeting, the media, especially TV stations, took up the story with abandon. The credibility of France's medical establishment was severely shaken by the accusation that a respected physician and researcher, Dr. Jean-Pierre Allain, had knowingly given contaminated blood products to hemophiliacs.[30] The Japanese medical establishment was shaken in much the same way when Dr. Takeshi Abe was accused of accepting money from manufacturers, and of delaying clinical trials of heat-treated products so that Green Cross could catch up with US and European manufacturers.[31] More revelations followed, ones that undermined the credibility of both nations' revered "political class"[32]; the opening segment of the nightly news often featured a new disclosure, complete with a visual of a document stamped "Confidential." Most damaging of all were the accusations that government officials in France and Japan had, in order to promote domestic industry, refused to import heat-treated products.

The connections among paternalism, governmental hierarchy, and the intensity of scandal require further elaboration. The major claim is that both French and Japanese bureaucrats have traditionally been expected to do their public jobs with confidence, competence, and little interference. Entrance into the elite ranks of these bureaucracies is reserved for those who have demonstrated high intelligence, gone through established channels of socialization, and successfully competed with other talented contenders. They are expected to take care of the public policy issues in their separate domains and are, in that sense, paternalistic. Moreover, they are expected to do so with high levels of skill and reliability. It is because high-ranking bureaucrats had earned, and been entrusted with, such paternalistic authority that citizens came to feel betrayed by their failure to protect the public. Added to this mix was the rage that came from knowing that the policy of governmental secrecy, which was taken for granted, both protected the bureaucrats from disclosure and prevented citizens from knowing the truth. Put another way, expectations determine evaluations of behavior; in the case of Japan and France, those expectations of protective security were high, and, once disappointed, all the more angering.

The Canadian case does not fit easily into this portrait of the public's disappointed expectations for paternalistic elites. In Canada, citizens have easier access to government information than in France and Japan. Moreover, while governmental officials in Canada have traditionally had higher status than in, for example, the United States, Canadian political culture is not strongly hierarchical and paternalistic. So why did the level of scandal there come to rival that of France and Japan?

As the blood scandal evolved in Canada, the Canadian Red Cross—a nongovernmental organization—received increasingly prominent attention because of its central, paternalistic involvement in the world of Canadian blood donation, distribution, and regulation. The Red Cross was also presumed by most Canadians to be utterly reliable. In these respects, there is a limited parallel between the Red Cross in Canada and the governmental elites of France and Japan. An additional factor is that the Red Cross, as a private, nonprofit organization, enjoyed more protection for its internal documents than did Canadian governmental organizations, and that it attempted to block blood investigations by public officials. Indeed, many questions about the role of the Red Cross are still unanswered; for example, whether, as alleged, the Red Cross maintained secret lists of donors for heat-treated blood.[33] In this respect, too, there is a parallel with France and Japan; the sustained scandal of Canada hinged, in part, on the rage that elites provoke when they have disappointed public expectations and have shown themselves to be protecting themselves from scrutiny when challenged.

The cases we have characterized as instances of high-intensity scandal are a mix of features, some present in those countries alone, some present in other countries where similar features produced less conflict. For instance, the physician who violated his or her trust was a source of anger in many countries, and discredited physicians played a prominent role in moderate- and low-intensity countries as well. It is important to distinguish, however, between the generalized anger many hemophiliacs felt toward formerly trusted physicians, and the scandal created when physicians in high office are charged with misconduct. Rather than being individual physicians who disappointed their professional clients, actors in France and Japan, and the Canadian Red Cross, had official capacities—and positions of special trust—within the blood-regulation context.

The argument, then, is that configurations of culture and institutions distinguish the cases of high scandal, not distinctive levels of real or alleged misdeeds. To see that more clearly, we turn to national instances of iatrogenic tragedy that did not produce the same level of scandal experienced by France, Japan, and Canada.

Moderate-intensity Conflict

The countries with scandals of moderate intensity included, among the cases discussed in this volume, the United States, Denmark, Germany, Australia, and Italy.
In each, the discovery of infection led to episodes of panic or spasms of intense
anger, but there was a limited quality to the conflicts. To be sure, disputes over compensation and broader policy options persisted from the late 1980s until the late 1990s.
But, for present purposes, the important point is that in these cases the public's
attention to scandal was either brief or intermittent, in large part because of the role
hemophiliacs played politically. In Germany and Australia, hemophiliacs scored early
political victories that helped to defuse the momentum for later collective action. In
Denmark initial victories on compensation were also important, as Erik Albaek's
chapter makes plain.[34] Hemophiliacs in Italy and the United States were more divided than they were in Germany and Australia, making sustained collective action
of any kind difficult. The roads to intermittent conflict described in the earlier chapters are therefore understandable, but not identical.

Germany, like the other countries under study, experienced a panic. It was not
sustained over time, however, and it neither broadly eroded confidence in the government nor resulted in major reform. German hemophiliacs were treated early with
the Bonn cure, a treatment envied and sought after by their counterparts in other
countries. They did not develop a strong political identity as victims unjustly treated
or make powerful demands beyond that of compensation. The German Hemophilia
Society, physician dominated as in most countries,[35] appears to have taken little initiative to shape the response to the aftermath of infection.[36] No splinter group of
hemophiliacs emerged.[37] Nor did infected victims or any champion from the press
step forward to engage and sustain public attention.

There were, however, raw materials for a sustained German scandal involving
the fear of AIDS, the safety of the public, and malfeasance by a corporation. This
story involved an ambitious—and impetuous—federal health minister who caused
an international panic by issuing an alert that German transfusion recipients might
have AIDS.[38] The short-run political result in Germany was to blame the government for disclosure, not for secrecy. This relatively benign framing of the incident
all but guaranteed that it would not expand into broader areas of civic trust (which it
did not). Individuals were arrested at the companies involved, and there was minimal change in German blood regulation.

Hemophiliacs in Australia were better organized politically than they were in
Germany. They had been included in policy making for some time, a status and
position of influence that had eluded even their politically alert and aggressive
counterparts in Denmark. In view of the hemophiliac community's strong political
organization, Australia may well have turned into a high-scandal country had the
government responded ineffectively to their concerns, or had there been disclosures

of serious malfeasance, either governmental or corporate. The issue of wrongdoing, however, was moot; the country has responded very early on with blood safety measures. Though the government was initially resistant to compensating hemophiliacs infected with HIV, pressure from the hemophiliac community, parliament, and the courts led, in halting stages, to a generous compensation scheme for all citizens with medically acquired HIV. As in Germany, the issues remained narrowly defined throughout the process, and no major crisis resulted.

The United States, as Ronald Bayer notes, was marked by litigation, high emotions, and occasionally heated conflict, but also by deep divisions within the hemophiliac community about how to understand and address their situation. The National Hemophilia Foundation (NHF) itself became a political target of militants who had broken from that organization to form the Committee of Ten Thousand (COTT) and the Hemophilia/HIV Peer Association. These splinter groups charged that, beginning with its failure to heat-treat for hepatitis B and continuing through the early years of the HIV epidemic, the fractionation industry had placed profit over safety. They picketed NHF meetings, accusing the NHF and medical elites of "genocide"[39] (a charge that echoed the claims of gay-rights groups). They lobbied for public compensation and for congressional hearings, and initiated a class-action suit against the pharmaceutical industry. The results were emotional public hearings, a stinging 1995 report of institutional failures within the blood industry and public-health sector,[40] increased FDA surveillance of the blood industry (including the Red Cross), and settlement of their class action suit. Other compensation was left to the courts, although legislation to establish a compensation fund, called the Ricky Ray Hemophilia Relief Fund Act,[41] was as of mid-1998 still pending in Congress. There was no crisis, either governmental or nongovernmental, however, perhaps because of the dispersion of authority and therefore of blame in the United States, and because divisions within the hemophiliac community prevented the development of a more powerful and unified public movement. The results in the United States were relatively modest institutional reforms.

In Italy, as in the United States, differences within the hemophiliac community diffused efforts for redress. The national organization, the Italian Hemophilia Foundation (IHF), was closely tied to the medical profession and formally represented the interests of hemophiliacs. Cultural differences between the northern and southern regions of the country[42] had always meant that organizational unity was a great challenge. But whatever unity there was dissolved after the first data on HIV infection in Italy became available in 1988. With IHF's ties to the medical community, the organization preferred a course of accommodation (a "dialogue line") with authorities,[43] and the legislative redress they sought followed a social-insurance model. In contrast, Turin's regional association, more highly developed organizationally,[44] was considerably more aggressive, adopting a media-based strategy, and ultimately forming a new organization of transfusion recipients, the Italian Multi-Transfused Association (API). The legislation this group sponsored in 1990 called for recoverable damages—a radical divergence from the approach of IHF. The executive, not the legislative, branch ultimately took action, in part to avoid potential embarrassment during the soon to be held international conference on AIDS in Florence, and in part to close the door on new claims arising from a recent supreme court decision that approved just compensation for mandatory vaccination.[45]

Reflecting both the failure of the Italian hemophiliac community to present a unified position and the associated failure to galvanize public support, not only was the compensation fund modest, but there were administrative barriers to filing a claim. The victory was, as Umberto Izzo suggests, more symbolic than real.

The Danish case sits at the borderline between high- and moderate-intensity scandal politics. It involved the most protracted judicial sequel in Danish political/administrative history. Danish hemophiliacs were, in a number of respects, successful in having their demands met. They organized in the early 1980s to obtain the "Bonn protocol" and resisted the political fragmentation that had undercut hemophiliacs' efforts in Italy and the United States. They forced the resignation of a health minister ("Blood Britta"), helped ensure that heat-treated blood products were introduced and that all donated blood was screened for HIV antibody, gained institutional representation on the governmental body responsible for blood products, and received the highest compensation award ever granted by the nation's health system.[46] Within a broader social and political perspective, Danish hemophiliacs were also successful in publicizing the existence of danger to the entire Danish blood supply, and in highlighting gaps between government pronouncements and practice. All of these achievements, coming in bursts of public attention, were notable. But it was the very success of Danish hemophiliacs, coupled with the intermittent rather than continual attention they received, that defused the sustained resentment underlying the high-intensity scandals we have seen elsewhere.

In the countries that experienced moderate-intensity conflict, the road from angry criticism to sustained, high-intensity scandal was blocked for one reason or another. The explanation for the difference cannot be found, however, in the relative number of infected hemophiliacs or in the relative degree of neglect or wrongdoing by organizations and individual actors in the world of blood. The fact that the United States, for example, had a greater proportion of infected hemophiliacs than any other nation was not expressed in a substantial and sustained public debate over who was responsible and what should be done. The fragmentation of American political institutions meant that many channels of criticism were open and that it was difficult to focus on the specific failures of particular individuals or governmental organizations. Attention to the safety and stability of the blood supply was dispersed among many actors—from the FDA to blood banks, from the fractionators to the hematologists. And the review of their behavior was split among Congress, bodies like the

Institute of Medicine, and the courts. That disputes continue to this day surprises no one familiar with the litigiousness of American society.

The American experience is but one illustration of how culture, politics, and science come together to produce outcomes, in this case an example of what we have called moderate-intensity scandal politics. To put that level of scandal in better perspective, it is helpful to consider very briefly nations where the distribution of contaminated blood led to compensation for hemophiliacs, but little scandal or political impact.

Contaminated Blood Products and Low-intensity Politics

Though the Netherlands is not included in this volume, is represents an example of a country that escaped divisive social and political scandal. Some brief observations are in order.

The aftermath of infection in Holland was not one of confrontation. As was true with other areas of AIDS policy, there emerged a consensual effort both to provide a remedy for the victims of contaminated blood and blood products, and to work out acceptable ways of securing the blood supply. Consensus building had begun early. For example, in discussions that included the various interest groups involved, Holland had instituted a system of voluntary, but not mandatory, measures (such as self-exclusion) to protect the blood supply. But beyond that direct preventive goal, the process of consensus building also had the effect of reducing the likelihood of later rage. In 1992, for example, the Dutch Society of Hemophiliacs (NVHP) requested an investigation into cases of HIV contamination and then filed a formal complaint against the Dutch authorities. While these developments may have reflected a breakdown of the consensus model (or even just an instance of cross-national learning in the politics of hemophilia activism), the governmental response demonstrated its continuing commitment to pursue consensus in lieu of open political and legal conflict. The complaint was handled not by the courts—an inherently adversarial and confrontational forum—but through the National Ombudsman. The result was an official admission of liability from the government, accompanied by an increase in the compensation to victims to approximately the average level in other countries.

Conclusion

The tragic stories presented in this book continue to be troubling. Across the world, nations still struggle with the impact and meaning of the experience with contaminated blood and blood products. That experience bears not only on questions of political accountability, legal liability, and compensation, but also on issues of prudent prevention in the future. Contemporary discussions about risk, decision making under conditions of uncertainty, and the application of science to policy making all involve lessons drawn (and overdrawn) from the experiences this book has reviewed. Heightened awareness of the exposure of vulnerable groups, indeed of the whole community, to new pathways of infection has led to various policy changes — some that may threaten the pace of innovation, others that rank safety over cost in ways that will no doubt prove problematic. The excitement associated with earlier advances that improved the lives of hemophiliacs has in many contexts been replaced by grief, anger, and ambivalence about science and government.

The scandal politics analyzed in this chapter raise a broad issue concerning the media. Contemporary media has the ability to accelerate cross-national learning in ways that would have been hard to imagine in a world without the fax, e-mail, and institutions like CNN and Sky Television. It can transmit information (and myths) beyond traditional elites to ordinary citizens and in so doing fuel the possibility of scandal. To be sure, scandal politics may help to balance systems where power is distributed unequally. In the countries under study, the level of scandal, remedies, and punishments depended significantly on the level of organization of the hemophiliacs themselves, the institutional channeling of protest, and the tenacity of the press. The actual levels of infection or timing of responses explained far less than one might have expected.

As the case studies in this volume demonstrate, there is a highly uncertain relation between the realities of risk and the reactions of nations to them. The complex mix of factors that produce reactions are unlikely to yield simple prediction or lessons. There is the danger that, given the tragic experience of HIV-tainted blood, governmental regulators will be excessively cautious and restrictive in reacting to future threats — real or imagined — to the safety of medical products. There is also the likelihood that excessive caution will in turn yield to more relaxed regulation. Either way, the uncertainty that characterized battles over HIV and blood will reappear in an everchanging array of disguises. As in the recent conflict over hepititis C, once again the legal, policial, and social systems of the industrialized democracies will respond to common threats, and to the burdens that result from unforeseen dangers, in the most uncommon of ways.

NOTES

1. Although it has been argued that there was wide variation in initial responses (see, for example, M. J. Trebilcock, R. Howse, and R. Daniels, "Do Institutions Matter? A Comparative Pathology of the HIV-infected Blood Tragedy," *Virginia Law Review* 82(8) [1996] 1407–1492) and that differences in institutional arrangements account for this variation, what is most striking about the countries under study is the similarity of institutional responses during this period, especially in view of the obvious differences in their institutional arrangements — legal, political, and medical.

2. Centers for Disease Control and Prevention, *Morbidity and Mortality Weekly Report* (MMWR), 30 (June 5, 1981), pp. 250–52.

3. *MMWR*, 31 (December 10, 1982), pp. 644–52.

4. L. B. Leveton, H. C. Sox, Jr., and M. Stoto, eds., *HIV and the Blood Supply: An Analysis of Crisis Decisionmaking* (Washington, D.C.: National Academy Press, 1995), p. 212.

5. U. Izzo, this volume, quoting Rizzo et al., "Emofilia e lavoro," in *Difesa Sociale*, 6 (1992), p. 151 to the effect that 90% of Italian hemophiliacs died before entering their twenties.

6. *HIV and the Blood Supply*, p. 171

7. S. A. Larsson, "Life Expectancy of Swedish Haemophiliacs, 1831–1980," *British Journal of Haemotology*, 59(4) 1985, pp. 593–602.

8. M. Triemstra et al., "Mortality in Patients with Hemophilia: Changes in a Dutch population from 1986 to 1992 and 1973 to 1986." *Annals of Internal Medicine*, 123(11) (1995), pp. 823–827.

9. M. J. Trebilcock, R. Howse, and R. Daniels, *op. cit.*

10. This section reflects not only the case studies presented in this volume but further research and analysis by Patricia Dillon. For a full account of her treatment of this subject, see Patricia A. Dillon, "Hemophilia, AIDS, and Scandal: Worldwide Responses to Contamination" (Masters Thesis, Yale University, Epidemiology and Public Health), 1988.

11. D. Kirp, "The Politics of Blood: Hemophilia Activism in the AIDS Crisis," Eric Feldman and Ronald Bayer, eds., Blood Feuds: AIDS, Blood, and the Politics of Medical Disaster (New York: Oxford University Press, 1999).

12. E. Feldman, "HIV and Blood in Japan: Transforming Private Conflict into Public Scandal," Feldman and Bayer, *op. cit.*

13. *Ibid.*

14. Importantly, they chose not to sue the Japanese Red Cross; because the family of its honorary chair had been included in the Japanese royal family since the Meiji period, such an act would not only have been culturally unthinkable, but would also have alienated public support for their position. Feldman, *op. cit.*

15. R. Blassing, "Nova Scotia to Compensate People Who Contracted AIDS Virus from Tainted Blood," *Buffalo News*, April 18, 1993.

16. *Ibid.*

17. N. Gilmore and M. Somerville, "From Trust to Trajedy: HIV/AIDS and the Canadian Blood System," Feldman and Bayer, *op. cit.*

18. J. Kramer, "Bad Blood," *The New Yorker*, October 11, 1993, p. 80.

19. M. Steffen, "The Nation's Blood: Medicine, Justice, and the State in France," Feldman and Bayer, *op. cit.*

20. Blassing, *op. cit.*

21. T. Fennell, "Voices of the Victims: An Inquiry Reveals How the Blood System Failed," *Maclean's*, September 19, 1994, p. 28.

22. CBC-TV *National Magazine*, "Janet Connors: Private Pain, Public Battle: Why She Turned Personal Tragedy into Political Action," June 5, 1997 (follow-up on September 26, 1997, with related stories on October 10, 1996, and on January 17 and June 25, 1997).

23. Evening news, *CBC-TV*, September 26, 1997.

24. Feldman, *op. cit.*

25. *Ibid.*

26. Kramer, *op. cit.*, p. 94, and Steffen, *op. cit.*

27. *Ibid.* p. 82.

28. Feldman, *op. cit.* p. 11.

29. Kramer, *op. cit.*, and Steffen, *op. cit.* p. 94.

30. *Ibid.* p. 75.

31. "AIDS Advisors Disagree over Events in HIV Blood Scandal," *Nature*, April 25, 1996.

32. Kramer, *op. cit.*, and Steffen, *op. cit.* p. 93.

33. Nor has it been possible to determine whether, as alleged, the Canadian Blood Commission shredded public documents in order to frustrate investigations into individual liability. M. Kennedy, "Files Destroyed to Hide Facts: Information Czar Targets Federal Official," *Ottawa Citizen*, January 23, 1997. Though not directly involving the Red Cross, this continuing uncertainty concerning the Canadian Blood Commission added to public frustrations about the lack of access to information central to the investigation of the Canadian blood scandal.

34. E. Albaek, "The Never-Ending Story? The Political and Legal Controversies over HIV and the Blood Supply in Denmark," Feldman and Bayer, *op. cit.*

35. Dressler, "Blood 'Scandal' and AIDS in Germany," Feldman and Bayer, *op. cit.*

36. Dressler, *op. cit.* The dominance of physicians is important because they continued to support the use of extremely high doses of factor VIII, known as the Bonn protocol.

37. *Ibid.*

38. B. Groom, "A Case of Bloody Madness," *Scotland on Sunday*, November 7, 1993.

39. R. Bayer, "Blood and AIDS in America: Science, Politics, and the Making of an Iatrogenic Disaster," Feldman and Bayer, *op. cit.*

40. L. B. Leveton, H. C. Sox Jr., and M. Stoto, *op. cit.*

41. The Ray fund is targeted to hemophiliacs alone and excludes transfusion recipients.

42. U. Izzo, "Blood, Bureaucracy and Law: Responding to HIV-Tainted Blood in Italy," Feldman and Bayer, *op. cit.* Although Italy officially promotes the "gift" culture of donation, regions vary in their acceptance. Turin has a high collection rate, but the south is more tribal and less collective; loyalty is tied to family. The sale of "red gold" and charges of usury are not unusual.

43. *Ibid.*

44. *Ibid.*

45. *Ibid.*

46. E. Albaek, *op. cit.*

Index